D0488147

CENGAGE

Milady Standard Foundations
Milady

Vice President and General Manager, Milady:
Sandra Bruce

Product Director: Kara Melillo

Product Manager: David Santillan

Learning Design Manager: Jessica Mahoney

Senior Content Manager: Nina Tucciarelli

Learning Designer: Beth Williams

In-House Subject Matter Expert: Harry Garrott

Marketing Manager: Kim Berube

Marketing Director: Slavik Volinsky

Design Director, Creative Studio: Jack Pendleton

Cover Designer: Joe Devine

© 2020 Milady, a part of Cengage Learning, Inc.

Unless otherwise noted, all content is © Cengage.

ALL RIGHTS RESERVED. No part of this work covered by the copyright herein may be reproduced or distributed in any form or by any means, except as permitted by U.S. copyright law, without the prior written permission of the copyright owner.

For product information and technology assistance, contact us at
**Cengage Customer & Sales Support, 1-800-354-9706
or support.cengage.com.**

For permission to use material from this text or product, submit all requests online at **www.cengage.com/permissions.**

Library of Congress Control Number: 2019931164

ISBN: 978-1-337-09525-9

Cengage
20 Channel Center Street
Boston, MA 02210
USA

Cengage is a leading provider of customized learning solutions, with employees residing in nearly 40 different countries and sales in more than 125 countries around the world. Find your local representative at **www.cengage.com.**

Cengage products are represented in Canada by Nelson Education, Ltd.

To learn more about Cengage platforms and services, register or access your online learning solution, or purchase materials for your course, visit **www.cengage.com.**

Notice to the Reader

Publisher does not warrant or guarantee any of the products described herein or perform any independent analysis in connection with any of the product information contained herein. Publisher does not assume, and expressly disclaims, any obligation to obtain and include information other than that provided to it by the manufacturer. The reader is expressly warned to consider and adopt all safety precautions that might be indicated by the activities described herein and to avoid all potential hazards. By following the instructions contained herein, the reader willingly assumes all risks in connection with such instructions. The publisher makes no representations or warranties of any kind, including but not limited to, the warranties of fitness for particular purpose or merchantability, nor are any such representations implied with respect to the material set forth herein, and the publisher takes no responsibility with respect to such material. The publisher shall not be liable for any special, consequential, or exemplary damages resulting, in whole or part, from the readers' use of, or reliance upon, this material.

Printed in the United States of America
Print Number: 08   Print Year: 2021

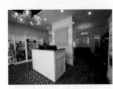

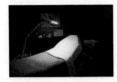

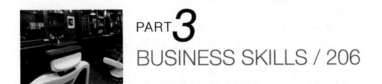

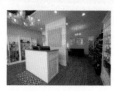

PART *1*
SOFT SKILLS TOOLBOX / 2

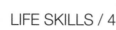

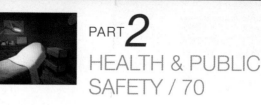
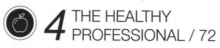

PART *2*
HEALTH & PUBLIC SAFETY / 70

6 CHEMISTRY & CHEMICAL SAFETY / 152

7 ELECTRICITY & ELECTRICAL SAFETY / 182

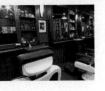

PART 3
BUSINESS SKILLS / 206

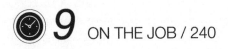

8 CAREER PLANNING / 208

9 ON THE JOB / 240

10 THE BEAUTY BUSINESS / 268

MILADY STANDARD FOUNDATIONS

Congratulations! You are about to begin a journey that can take you in many directions and that holds the potential to make you a confident, successful professional. At Milady, we believe that those who always pursue knowledge, step out of their comfort zone, and challenge themselves have the greatest chance to succeed.

You and your school have chosen the perfect course of study to accomplish your goals, starting with creating a strong foundation. *Milady Standard Foundations* was created to help you master the fundamental principles that you will use throughout your education and career, wherever it takes you. This resource includes the building blocks of your beauty and wellness education, including science basics, theory topics, soft skills, and business fundamentals. Combined with your discipline-specific Milady text, you have at your fingertips the most relevant, comprehensive education in your field.

As your school experience begins, consider how you will approach your course of study; even when the going gets tough, the right attitude, study skills, habits, and perseverance will see you through. Stay focused on your goal, reach out to your instructors when you need help, and don't be afraid to start thinking beyond getting licensed. A beauty career in this amazing industry can take you anywhere, but it all begins with a winning mindset and a good foundation!

THE INDUSTRY STANDARD

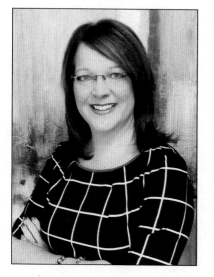

Since 1927, Milady has been committed to quality education for beauty professionals. Over the years, tens of millions of licensed professionals have begun their careers studying from Milady's industry-leading textbooks.

We at Milady are dedicated to providing the most comprehensive learning solutions in the widest variety of formats to serve you, today's learner. This first edition of *Milady Standard Foundations* is available to you in multiple formats including the traditional print version, an eBook version, and MindTap, which provides an interactive learning experience complete with activities, learning tools, and brand-new video content.

Milady would like to thank the educators and professionals who participated in surveys and reviews to best determine the content that needed to be included in this edition. We would also like to thank learners, past and present, for being vocal about your needs and giving Milady the opportunity to provide you with the very best in beauty and wellness education.

Thank you for trusting Milady to provide the valuable information you need to build the foundation for your career. Our content combined with your passion, creativity, and devotion to your craft and your customers will set you on the path to a lifetime of success. Congratulations for taking the first step toward your future as a beauty professional!

Sandra Bruce
Vice President and General Manager, Milady

NEW TO THIS EDITION

As part of the development of *Milady Standard Foundations*, this text includes many features and learning tools that may be new to learners familiar with previous Milady core books.

ORGANIZATION OF CHAPTERS

The information in this text, along with your teachers' instruction, will enable you to develop the abilities you need to build a loyal and satisfied clientele. To help you locate information more easily, the chapters are grouped into three main parts.

PART 1: SOFT SKILLS TOOLBOX

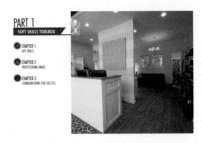

Soft Skills Toolbox consists of three chapters that focus on the personal and interpersonal skills you will need to become successful. Chapter 1, "Life Skills," emphasizes the ability to set goals and maintain a good attitude, along with examining the psychology of success. Chapter 2, "Professional Image," stresses the importance of cultivating your outward appearance, from proper hygiene and dressing for success to focusing on your soft skills, your portfolio, and your social media etiquette. Chapter 3, "Communicating for Success," describes the important process of building relationships based on trust and effective communication and is centered around the client consultation.

PART 2: HEALTH & PUBLIC SAFETY

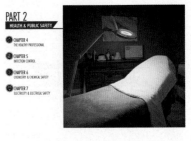

Health & Public Safety includes important information you need to know in order to keep yourself and your clients safe and healthy. Chapter 4, "The Healthy Professional," combines nutrition and ergonomics information with guidance on staying healthy, taking a sick day, and pregnant professionals and clients. Chapter 5, "Infection Control," offers the most current vital facts about identifying and preventing the transmission of pathogens in the salon, spa, and barbershop, in addition to specific safety precautions, such as the special needs of high-risk clients. Chapter 6, "Chemistry & Chemical Safety," covers basic concepts in chemistry as they relate to beauty and wellness, with a focus on the safe handling, storage, and disposal of chemicals. Chapter 7, "Electricity & Electrical Safety," similarly presents electrical theory with an eye toward understanding the possibilities and precautions of electrical devices in the salon, spa, and barbershop.

PART 3: BUSINESS SKILLS

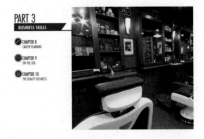

Business Skills opens with Chapter 8, "Career Planning." This chapter prepares students for licensure exams and job interviews and explains how to create a resume and a portfolio. What you will be expected to know and do as a newly licensed beauty professional is described in Chapter 9, "On the Job." It offers tips on how to make the most of your first job—including the importance of managing your money and learning all you can. The final chapter, "The Beauty Business," exposes students to the numerous types of business ownership options available to them, with a glimpse of the requirements and responsibilities involved.

ELEVATING LEARNING

In response to advances in learning science and the growing importance of competency-based education, *Standard Foundations* includes several changes that set it apart from the discipline texts you may be familiar with. Features have been added or tweaked with the hope of making your learning experience more intuitive, more effective, and, above all, more relevant.

TABLE OF CONTENTS

Whether you are getting started, reviewing for your exams, or just feeling lost, the table of contents at the beginning of this text will be your learning roadmap through these foundations. The **Contents** section not only shows you the structure of the text as a whole, making it easier to find the section you are looking for, but because the section headers double as learning objectives, this table of contents also shows you at a glance all the objectives you will need to complete in order to master each chapter.

CHAPTER ICONS

Each chapter of *Standard Foundations* has its own icon, which connects it across all of its supplements. Think of these icons as badges—once you have completed all of a chapter's learning objectives, you have successfully earned a chapter icon! And so much more.

LEARNING OBJECTIVES

LEARNING OBJECTIVES

AFTER COMPLETING THIS CHAPTER, YOU WILL BE ABLE TO:

1. EXPLAIN LIFE SKILLS.
2. LIST THE PRINCIPLES THAT CONTRIBUTE TO SUCCESS.
3. DESIGN A MISSION STATEMENT.
4. SET LONG-TERM AND SHORT-TERM GOALS.
5. DEMONSTRATE EFFECTIVE TIME MANAGEMENT.
6. EMPLOY SUCCESSFUL LEARNING TOOLS.
7. DEFINE *ETHICS*.
8. DEVELOP A POSITIVE PERSONALITY AND ATTITUDE.

At the beginning of each chapter is a list of learning objectives that tell you what important information you will be expected to know after studying the chapter. Throughout the chapter, these learning objectives are also used as the titles of the major sections themselves. This is done for ease of reference and to reinforce the main competencies that are critical to learn in each chapter to prepare for licensure. In addition, learning objectives have been written to focus on measurable results, helping you know what it is you should be able to do after mastering each section.

CHECK IN QUESTIONS

CHECK IN
What are the characteristics of a healthy, positive attitude?

Instead of placing review questions at the end of each chapter, check in questions have been added to the end of the section that they cover. This allows you to check your understanding as you progress through a chapter as opposed to waiting until you have finished the chapter to simply check your memory. **Check In** questions also make it easier to find any answers you need help with.

COMPETENCY PROGRESS

The list of learning objectives is repeated at the end of each chapter, with added checkboxes. At this point, you will be invited to review your progress through the content you have just covered, including checking off the learning objectives you feel you have mastered. Anything not checked off will stand out as a clear reminder of work you still need to do to complete that chapter.

COMPETENCY PROGRESS

How are you doing with Professional Image? Check off the Chapter 2 Learning Objectives below that you feel you have mastered; leave unchecked those objectives you will need to return to:

☐ EXPLAIN PROFESSIONAL IMAGE.
☐ EMPLOY IMAGE-BUILDING BASICS.
☐ DEMONSTRATE A PROFESSIONAL ATTITUDE.
☐ CREATE YOUR PERSONAL PORTFOLIO.
☐ IMPLEMENT SOCIAL MEDIA BEST PRACTICES.

EXPLAIN AND APPLY SECTIONS

The first and last sections of each chapter work a little differently from the standard content sections that make up the bulk of the text. A chapter begins with an **Explain** section, which serves as a brief introduction to the chapter and occasionally contains additional content. You will notice that this section has a learning objective, while **Apply** does not. This is because the **Explain** section is considered a higher-level objective of the chapter—in order to master the content of a chapter as a whole, you should be able to explain the importance of the chapter itself to your discipline.

Related to this, the **Apply** section that closes each chapter is an invitation to you, your study group, or your class to discuss how the general beauty and wellness topics of the chapter apply specifically to your discipline. This section provides a few suggestions, but the real discussion is up to you. This is why there is no learning objective for **Apply**, since you or your instructor will be doing the real work of connecting the chapter to your own career.

EXPLAIN LIFE SKILLS

While it is extremely important to master good technical skills, it is equally important to learn and apply sound life skills. Beauty and wellness is at heart a creative industry, where you are expected to exercise your artistic talent. To be successful in a salon, spa, or barbershop environment, you need to have well-developed communication, decision-making, image-building, customer service, self-actualization, goal-setting, and time-management skills. These life skills are the foundation of success for students and professionals. In addition, developing effective study skills will help you achieve your educational and professional goals.

APPLY LIFE SKILLS

Congratulations on completing this chapter! Before you move on, take a moment to think about how these Life Skills topics apply to your particular discipline. Discuss with a classmate or study group how success may be defined differently for your discipline; what unique demands your schedule may have; how you can address specific ethical dilemmas; and so on.

ADDITIONAL FEATURES

Many features are available in this text to help you master key concepts and techniques.

FOCUS ON

Throughout the text, short boxed sections draw attention to various skills and concepts that will help you reach your goal. The **Focus On** pieces target sharpening technical and personal skills, ticket upgrading, client consultation, and building your client base. These topics are key to your success as a student and as a professional.

FOCUS ON

The Whole Person
An individual's personality is the sum of their characteristics, attitudes, and behavioral traits. Attitude improvement is a process that continues throughout life. In both your professional and personal life, a pleasing attitude gains more associates, clients, and friends. You will know you have a pleasing attitude when you are able to see the good in difficult situations. People enjoy the company of individuals who can put a positive spin on things.

DID YOU KNOW?

This feature provides interesting information that will enhance your understanding of the material in the text and call attention to a special point.

DID YOU KNOW?

Seven percent of communication is verbal (involves actual words), 55 percent is visual (body language, eye contact), and 38 percent is tonal (pitch, speed, volume, tone of voice)[i]. To communicate effectively as a professional, project strong body language imbued with confidence, competence, and charisma.

HERE'S A TIP

There are many portfolio websites available; some require you to pay for their services after a trial period, and others are free (such as pathbrite.com). Alternatively, you can present your online portfolio through image-hosting sites, blogs, personal websites, or a Facebook gallery. All of these options have pros and cons that should be weighed before you begin to build a portfolio.

CAUTION

Use caution when using social media while still in school! Some states penalize students for posting service-related content, including photos. Check with your instructor and your state board to see what you are allowed to post and when. If you do post material, your portfolios and social media should make it clear that you are still a student and cannot accept clients.

ACTIVITY

Nutrition Tracking

Choose a food tracking program, such as the supertracker at USDA.gov or an app on your phone, and track what you eat in one week. After a week, discuss everyone's results as a class: What are some good habits? Some bad habits? What nutrients are especially lacking? What are some ways you could address this need?

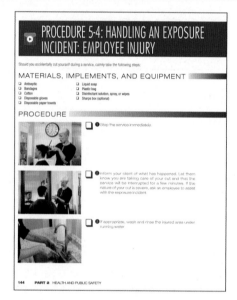

GLOSSARY

ethics ETH-iks	p. 19	the moral principles by which we live and work
game plan GAYM plan	p. 9	the conscious act of planning your life, instead of just letting things happen
goal setting GOHL SET-ing	p. 10	the identification of long-term and short-term goals that helps you decide what you want out of life
mind mapping MYND MAP-ing	p. 17	a graphic representation of an idea or problem that helps organize one's thoughts

A

Acid–alkali neutralization reactions, when acids are mixed with alkalis in equal proportions, balancing the total pH and forming water (H₂0) and a salt, 168

Acidic solution, a solution that has a pH below 7.0 (neutral), 166

Acquired immune deficiency syndrome, abbreviated AIDS: a disease that

Anode, positive electrode of an electrotherapy device; the anode is usually red and is marked with a *P* or plus (+) sign, 192

Antibacterial soaps, 117

Antibiotics, substances that kill or slow the growth of bacteria and other microorganisms, 80–81

Antiseptics, chemical germicides formulated for use on skin;

HERE'S A TIP

These helpful tips draw attention to situations that might arise and provide quick ways of doing things. Look for these tips throughout the text.

CAUTION

Some information is so critical for your safety and the safety of your clients that it deserves special attention. The text directs you to this information in the **Caution** boxes.

ACTIVITY

The **Activity** boxes describe hands-on classroom or personal exercises that will help you understand the concepts explained in the text.

PROCEDURES

All step-by-step procedures offer clear, easy-to-understand directions and multiple photographs for learning the techniques. At the beginning of each procedure, you will find a list of the needed implements and materials, along with any preparation that must be completed before the procedure begins.

In previous editions and texts, the procedures interrupted the flow of the main content, often making it necessary for readers to flip through many pages before continuing their study. In order to avoid this interruption, procedures have been moved to a special **Procedures** section at the end of each chapter. As you move through the main content of the chapter, you will be directed to the page number where any relevant procedure appears.

COMBINATION OF KEY TERMS AND GLOSSARY LIST

A complete list of key terms appears as part of the glossary at the end of each chapter. In addition to the key terms, you will find the *page reference* for where the key terms are defined and discussed in the chapter material. *Phonetic spellings* for all terms are included along with the glossary definitions. The combined key term and chapter glossary is a way to learn important terms used in the beauty and wellness industry and to prepare for licensure. This list is a one-stop resource to create flash cards or study for quizzes on a particular chapter.

All key terms are included in the **Chapter Glossary**, as well as in the **Glossary/Index** at the end of the text.

PHOTOGRAPHY AND ART

Standard Foundations provided a challenge, requiring photography that showed not only a diversity of professionals and clients, but also represented the range of disciplines that build on this text's foundations. The intent was to remain discipline agnostic by including imagery from across the beauty and wellness spectrum: barbers and stylists, estheticians and nail techs, even the occasional massage therapist and makeup artist. Our hope is that every student can find themselves and their future career somewhere in this text.

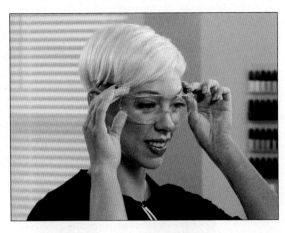

CONTRIBUTORS

LESLIE ROSTE

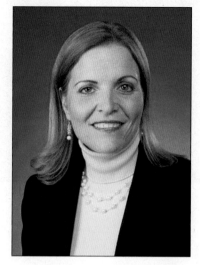

Chapter 4 The Healthy Professional
Chapter 5 Infection Control
Chapter 6 Chemistry & Chemical Safety
Chapter 7 Electricity & Electrical Safety

Leslie Roste, RN, BSN, graduated from the University of Kansas, where she studied nursing and microbiology. She worked in various nursing positions in such fields as obstetrical nursing and infection control in the Kansas City area prior to joining the cosmetology industry. Her main focus in the industry has been on health and safety in the professional beauty environment and general education about the sciences involved. Leslie has written many articles for publications and spoken to audiences large and small on infection control in the work environment, minimum health and safety standards, and safety-based licensure. She is very involved with the industry at all levels, from students to legislators, in making sure that professional beauty industry services are performed safely.

Leslie currently serves on several state and federal commissions connected to health and public safety and occupational licensing. She also spends a large portion of her time working with individual states to revise rules and/or legislation regarding infection control in the professional beauty industry. She is currently the national director of education for King Research.

PAST CONTRIBUTORS

- C. Jeanine Fulton, Persona Market Enterprises, Atlanta, GA
- Dr. Roychen Joseph, Farouk Systems, Inc, Houston, TX
- Mary Ann Kilgore, OC Minx Cosmetics, LLC, Laguna Niguel, CA
- Suzanne Mulroy, Beauty Changes Lives, Los Angeles, CA

ACKNOWLEDGMENTS

Milady recognizes, with gratitude and respect, the many professionals who have offered their time to contribute to *Milady Standard Foundations* and wishes to extend enormous thanks to the following people who have played an invaluable role in the creation of this edition:

- Daesha Devon Harris, Michael Gallitelli, Tom Stock, and Julie Moscheo for lending us their photography powers and bringing their cameras to bear in the name of upping Milady's imagery game.
- Paul Mitchell The School (Schenectady, NY), Capri Cosmetology Learning Center (Newburgh, NY), 560 Salon and Spa (Cobleskill, NY), Make Me Fabulous (Saratoga Springs, NY), and Henry Street Barbershop (Saratoga Springs, NY) for graciously hosting our photo and video shoots. Heartfelt thanks go out to all these establishments for their generosity and assistance in the pursuit of photographic excellence.
- Special thanks to Devin, Rasi, and Josh at Henry Street Barbershop. Their barbershop is a business that emphasizes community as evidenced by their donation of free haircuts for the homeless and veterans the first Sunday of each month.
- Danielle Valachovic for her makeup skills at multiple photo and video shoots as well as modeling on demand.
- Michelle Whitehead for working tirelessly to stock, orchestrate, and execute many of Milady's shoots during her tenure, including those for this book. We could not have done this without her help.
- The army of Beauty Operatives for providing their feedback throughout this project's development. We are grateful for your assistance in making this happen!

REVIEWERS OF *MILADY STANDARD FOUNDATIONS*

- Yota Batsaras, QueenB Parlor, Cypress, CA
- Jenny Berglund, Independent Stylist, Duluth, MN
- Adrienne Bishop, Nail Crazed, LLC, Spanish Fork, UT
- Bonita Branch, Bennett Career Institute, Washington, DC
- Dina Costello, Benes Career Academy, New Port Richey, FL
- Kimberly Cutter-Williams, Savannah Technical College, Savannah, GA
- Cheryl Duarte, Greater Lowell Technical High School, Tyngsborough, MA
- John Halal, Chemistry Simplified, McCordsville, IN
- Donna Haynes, Jackson Barber College, Houston, TX
- Cindy Heidemann, ABC School of Cosmetology, Esthetics & Nail Technology Inc., Lake in the Hills, IL
- Sarah Herb, Evergreen Beauty College, Everett, WA
- Tammy Hingten, TONI&GUY Hairdressing Academy, Albuquerque, NM
- Mike Kennamer, Northeast Alabama Community College, Rainsville, AL
- Joanne Myers, Pulse Beauty Academy, Downingtown, PA
- Barbara Padget, Kenneth Shuler School of Cosmetology, Columbia, SC
- Juanita Darlene Ray, CND, Chattanooga, TN
- Kathy Davis Rees, National Institute of Medical Aesthetics, South Jordan, UT
- Jean Schlaiss, Kenneth Shuler School of Cosmetology, Rock Hill, SC
- Sharicka Washington, Institute of Skin Science, Stratham, NH
- Madison Weinrich, Continental School of Beauty, Rochester, NY
- Patrice Wilson, Bennett Career Institute, Washington, DC
- Debbie Yandow, Gaston Community College, Dallas, NC

PART 1

SOFT SKILLS TOOLBOX

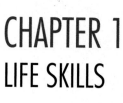

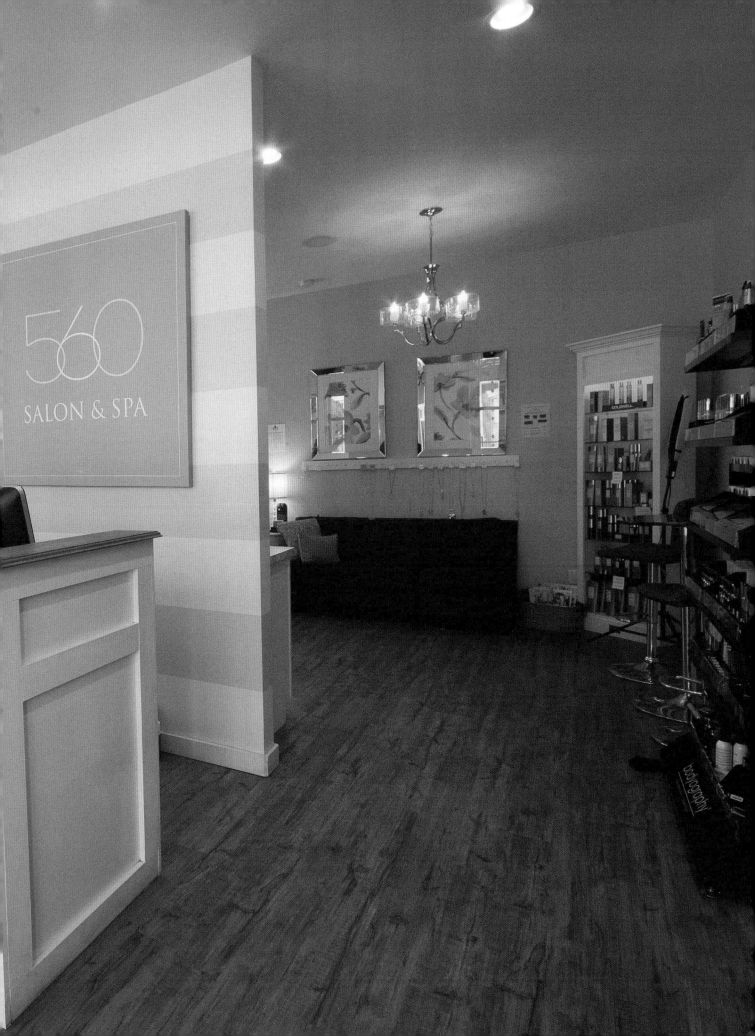

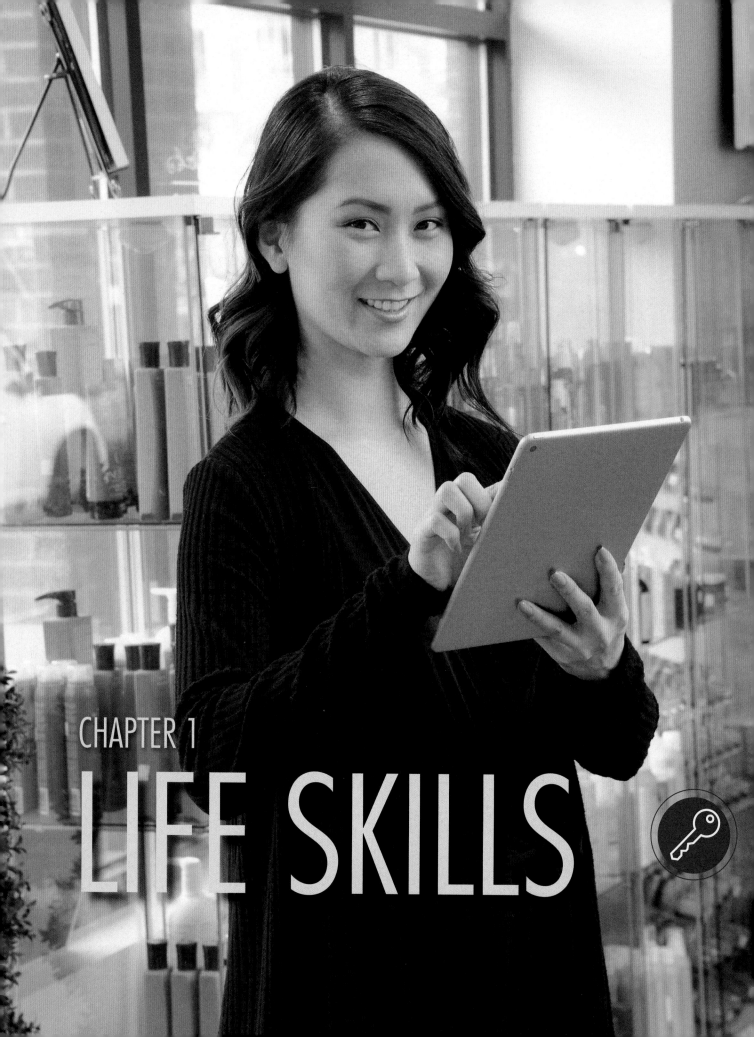

CHAPTER 1
LIFE SKILLS

"Everything you've ever wanted is on the other side of fear."
-George Addair

LEARNING OBJECTIVES

AFTER COMPLETING THIS CHAPTER, YOU WILL BE ABLE TO:

1. EXPLAIN LIFE SKILLS.
2. LIST THE PRINCIPLES THAT CONTRIBUTE TO SUCCESS.
3. DESIGN A MISSION STATEMENT.
4. SET LONG-TERM AND SHORT-TERM GOALS.
5. DEMONSTRATE EFFECTIVE TIME MANAGEMENT.
6. EMPLOY SUCCESSFUL LEARNING TOOLS.
7. DEFINE *ETHICS*.
8. DEVELOP A POSITIVE PERSONALITY AND ATTITUDE.

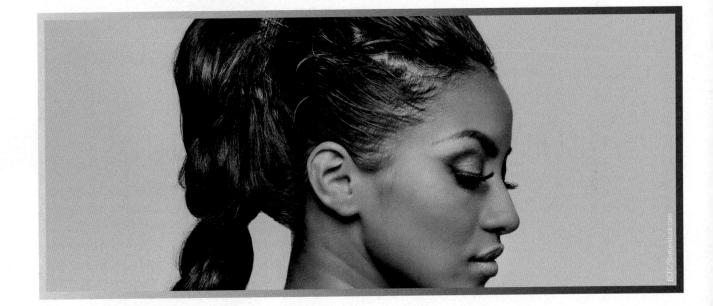

EXPLAIN LIFE SKILLS

While it is extremely important to master good technical skills, it is equally important to learn and apply sound life skills. Beauty and wellness is at heart a creative industry, where you are expected to exercise your artistic talent. To be successful in a salon, spa, or barbershop environment, you need to have well-developed communication, decision-making, image-building, customer service, self-actualization, goal-setting, and time-management skills. These life skills are the foundation of success for students and professionals. In addition, developing effective study skills will help you achieve your educational and professional goals.

Beauty professionals should study and have a thorough understanding of life skills because:

- Practicing good life skills will lead to a more satisfying and productive beauty and wellness career.
- Beauty professionals work with many different types of clients, and life skills can help keep interactions positive in any situation.
- The ability to deal with difficult circumstances comes from having well-developed skills.
- Having life skills builds self-esteem, which helps individuals achieve their goals.

LIFE SKILLS IN ACTION

Life skills are day-to-day actions and capabilities that help you to be a productive and well-rounded person. Some of the most important life skills for you to remember and practice include:

- Being helpful and caring for others.
- Making good friends.
- Feeling good about yourself.
- Having a sense of humor.
- Maintaining a cooperative attitude.
- Approaching work with a strong sense of responsibility.
- Being consistent in your work.
- Adapting successfully to different situations.
- Sticking to a goal and seeing a job through to completion.
- Mastering techniques to become more organized.
- Developing sound decision-making skills.

LIST THE PRINCIPLES THAT CONTRIBUTE TO SUCCESS

Success has been defined in many ways over the years, varying from person to person. What is your definition of success? Take a few minutes to think and then write down your answer. The process of self-actualization (self ack-chew-uh-lih-ZAYE-shun), fulfilling one's full potential, requires a lifelong commitment. Stay the course and fuel your passion by following proven success-building steps (**Figure 1-1**).

ACTION STEPS FOR SUCCESS

Being successful in life requires hard work and effort. Continually focusing on the following action steps will create a solid foundation for achieving your goals.

- **Build self-esteem.** Self-esteem is based on inner strength and begins with trusting your ability to achieve set goals. It is essential that you begin developing high self-esteem while you are in school. Reading positive affirmations is a great way to start.
- **Visualize success.** Imagine working in your dream shop. You are competently handling clients, loving the job and the environment.

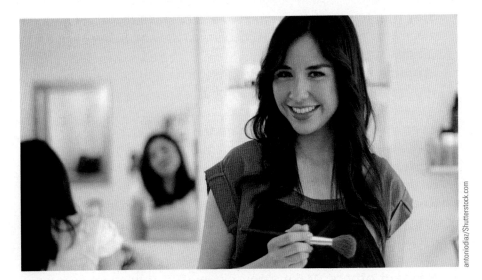

▲ FIGURE 1-1 Loving your work is critical to your success.

The more you practice visualization, the more easily you will turn your vision into reality.

- **Build on your strengths.** Practice doing whatever helps you maintain a positive self-image. If you are good at something (e.g., playing the guitar, running, cooking, gardening, singing), the time you invest in that activity will allow you to feel good about yourself (**Figure 1-2**). Remember that there may be things you are good at that you do not realize. You may be a good listener, for instance, or a caring and considerate friend.

- **Be kind to yourself.** This action step may be the hardest, but it is the most important one for success. Eliminate counterproductive self-critical or negative thoughts. If you make a mistake, view it as a learning opportunity to improve yourself and get it right the next time.

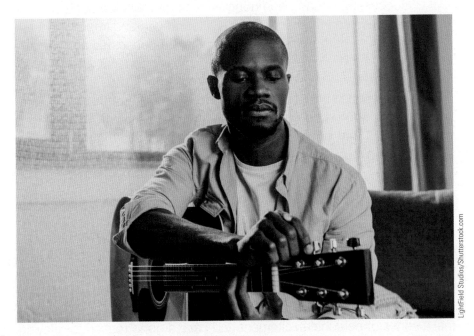

▲ FIGURE 1-2 Spend time on things you do well.

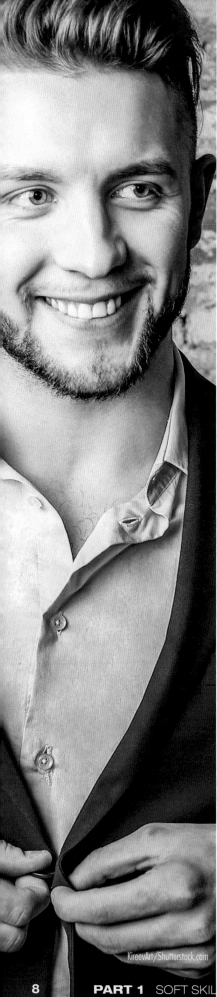

KireevArt/Shutterstock.com

- **Stay true to yourself.** Be yourself and be professional! It takes too much time and effort to be someone you are not. Being unique is a valuable asset.
- **Practice new behaviors.** Because achieving success is a skill, you can develop it by practicing positive new behaviors, such as speaking with confidence, standing tall, and using proper grammar.
- **Keep your personal life separate from your work.** Talking about your personal life at work is counterproductive and can cause the whole shop to suffer. Try to separate your work life from your home life and develop a healthy work–life balance.
- **Keep your energy up.** Successful beauty professionals take care of themselves. Get the proper amount of sleep, eat healthy foods, and manage your time wisely. Also, create balance by spending time with family and friends, having hobbies, and enjoying recreational activities.
- **Respect others.** Make a conscious effort to respect everyone. Exercise good manners by using words such as please, thank you, and excuse me. Practice being a good listener and remember not to interrupt others when they are speaking.
- **Stay productive.** Three bad habits can keep you from maintaining peak performance: (1) procrastination, (2) perfectionism, and (3) lacking a game plan. You will see an almost instant improvement in your productivity when you eliminate these troublesome tendencies.

    1. Procrastination (pro-CRASS-tin-aye-shun) is putting off until tomorrow what you can do today. For example, "I will study tomorrow instead of today." This thought process may be attributed to scheduling too many tasks at one time, which is a symptom of faulty organization.
    2. Perfectionism (pur-FEK-shun-izm) is an unhealthy compulsion to do things perfectly. Success is not defined as doing everything perfectly. As long as you learn from your mistakes, you will be successful. In fact, someone who never makes a mistake may not be taking the necessary risks for growth and improvement.
    3. Having a game plan (GAYM plan) is the conscious act of planning your life, instead of just letting things happen. While an overall game plan is usually organized into large blocks of time (five or ten years), it is just as important to set daily, monthly, and yearly goals. Where do you want to be in your career five years from now? What do you have to do this week, this month, and this year to move closer to that goal?

MOTIVATION AND SELF-MANAGEMENT

Starting something new can be both exciting and intimidating. For example, many new students feel nervous about starting beauty and wellness school. Whatever emotions you may feel, motivation and self-management skills will help you move to the next level in your career. To achieve success, you need more than an external push: You must feel a sense of personal excitement and have a good reason for staying the course. You are in charge of managing your own life and learning. Embracing your creativity will help you to achieve this goal successfully.

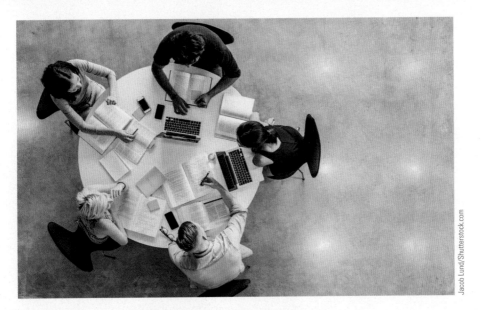

▲ FIGURE 1-3 Build strong relationships for support.

YOUR CREATIVE CAPABILITY

Being creative means having a talent, such as painting, acting, playing an instrument, writing, cutting hair, applying makeup, or creating nail art. Creativity is also an unlimited inner resource of ideas and solutions. To enhance your creativity, keep these guidelines in mind:

- **Be positive.** Criticism blocks the creative mind from exploring ideas and discovering solutions to challenges.
- **Look around for creative inspiration.** Tap into the creative energy of art museums, music, fashion shows, and magazines.
- **Improve your vocabulary.** Build a positive vocabulary by using active problem-solving words like *explore, analyze, and determine*.
- **Surround yourself with others who share your passion.** In today's hectic and pressured world, many talented people find that they are more creative in an environment where people work together and share ideas. This is where the value of a strong team comes into play **(Figure 1-3)**.

CHECK IN
What principles contribute to personal and professional success?

DESIGN A MISSION STATEMENT

An essential part of business is the **mission statement** (MISH-uhn STATE-ment), which establishes the purpose and values by which an individual or institution lives and works. It provides a sense of direction by defining guiding principles and clarifying goals as well as indicating how an organization operates. Often you will find the mission statement of

Mission Statement

Building a TEAM that values the importance
of each of its MEMBERS
where our GUESTS, by our positive attitudes,
will enjoy the excellent CUSTOMER SERVICE
they all come to expect.

Thanks to our team's continuing education,
our CLIENT will receive the best
quality of work possible.

▲ FIGURE 1-4 Mission statements should be displayed with pride. Statement courtesy of Jean Paul Salon & Spa.

a company posted for customers to read. Look for one the next time you are in a hotel, fast-food restaurant, or other service-related business. The mission may be more than just a statement; it often becomes the cultural pulse of an organization (**Figure 1-4**). A well-thought-out sense of purpose in the form of a mission statement will also help individuals on their journey to success.

Try to prepare a one- or two-sentence mission statement that communicates who you are and what you want from your life. One example of a simple yet thoughtful mission statement is: "I am dedicated to pursuing a successful career with dignity, honesty, and integrity." Your mission statement can lead you in the right direction and help you feel secure when things temporarily go off course. For reinforcement, keep a copy of your mission statement where you can see it, and read it frequently.

CHECK IN
How is having a mission statement useful, both now and in the future?

SET LONG-TERM AND SHORT-TERM GOALS

Do you have direction, drive, desire, and a dream? If so, do you have a reasonable idea of how to go about meeting your goal(s)?

Goal setting (GOHL SET-ing) is the identification of long-term and short-term goals. When you know what you want, you can draw a circle around your destination and chart the best course to get there. By mapping out your goals, you will see where to focus your attention in order to fulfill your dreams.

The Goal
Determine whether your goal-setting plan is effective by asking yourself these key questions:

- Are there specific skills I will need to learn in order to meet my goals?
- Is the information I need to reach my goals readily available?
- Am I willing to seek out a mentor or a coach to enhance my learning?
- What is the best method or approach to accomplish my goals?
- Am I open to finding better ways of putting my plan into practice?

HOW GOAL SETTING WORKS

When setting goals, categorize them based on the amount of time it takes to accomplish them. An example of a short-term goal is to get through an exam successfully. Another short-term goal is to graduate from beauty and wellness school. Short-term goals can usually be accomplished in a year or less.

Long-term goals are measured in larger increments of time, such as two, five, or ten years—or even longer. An example of a long-term goal is becoming a spa owner in five years.

Once you have organized your thoughts, create two columns labeled "Short Term" and "Long Term." List your goals in the corresponding column. Then, break up your goals into smaller pieces so they don't seem out of sight or overwhelming. For example, if you are a part-time beauty and wellness student, one of your long-term goals should be to become a licensed beauty professional. At first, getting this license might seem to require an overwhelming amount of time and effort. However, when larger aspirations are divided into short-term goals (such as going to class on time, completing homework assignments, and mastering techniques), you will find that accomplishing each short-term goal progressively leads to the accomplishment of the larger goal.

Remember to set feasible goals, create a plan of action, and revisit the plan often. While adjusting goals and action plans may be necessary from time to time, successful people know that focusing on their goals will move them toward additional successes (**Figures 1-5** and **Figure 1-6**).

ACTIVITY

Screen Time
On average, a person spends about four hours checking e-mail, looking at websites, and watching videos. The average teenager sends nearly 80 text messages a day! To find out if you are managing your time well, try this exercise:

- Write down the time in the morning when you first go online, check e-mail, or send a text message.
- Do what you normally do online. Note the time you finish these activities.
- Throughout the day, try to estimate (and add to your list) how much additional time you spend on these activities.
- At the end of the day, total up the time you spent online.

Are you surprised? Time-management experts recommend that people work for the first 45 minutes or hour of the day, avoiding e-mailing, web browsing, and texting. You too can use this time to plan the day, review reading materials for school, or do other work. The first hour of the day—quiet and often free of interruptions—is often the best time to accomplish something concrete.

HOW TO SET AND TRACK SHORT-TERM GOALS

Number	Goal Setting Checklist	Completion Date	Done
1.	Read Chapter 1. Action Steps: Read first part at lunch; finish it after dinner.	6/09	✓
2.	Practice speaking to clients in a pleasing voice. Action Steps: Do with family tonight.	6/10	✓
3.	Create my own mission statement. Action Steps: Review sample in Chapter 1; write my own.	6/15	✓
4.	Start learning trends. Action Steps: Search online, read trade and beauty magazines. Make a five-word "trend list."	6/20	✓
5.	Prepare to pass the Chapter 1 exam. Action Steps: Review what I read, ask instructor any questions, have study session with two friends.	7/10	✓
6.	Practice being on time! Action Steps: Set alarm for 15 minutes earlier. Give self $1 every time I get to class 10 minutes early.	Start 6/20 5 days in a row by 7/20	
7.	Build my vocabulary. Action Steps: Buy book or find website. Learn one new word a day.	Daily	

▲ FIGURE 1-5   Break down goals, as in this example of short-term goal tracking.

MY GOALS

Number	Goal Setting Checklist	Completion Date	Done
1.			
2.			
3.			
4.			
5.			
6.			
7.			

▲ FIGURE 1-6   Photocopy this template and fill in your own goals!

DEMONSTRATE EFFECTIVE TIME MANAGEMENT

Effectively managing your time will help you reach your goals more quickly. Here are some ways you can be more effective at time management:

- Learn to **prioritize** (pry-OR-uh-tize) by ordering tasks on your to-do list from most important to least important.
- When designing your time management system, make sure it will work for you. For example, if you are a person who needs a fair amount of flexibility, schedule some blocks of unstructured time.
- Never take on more than you can handle. Learn to say *no* firmly but kindly, and mean it. It will be easier to complete tasks if activities are limited.
- Learn problem-solving techniques that will save you time and needless frustration.
- Give yourself some downtime whenever you are frustrated, overwhelmed, worried, or feeling guilty. You lose valuable time and energy when you are in a negative state of mind. Unfortunately, there may be situations where you cannot get up and walk away. To handle these difficult times, try practicing the technique of deep breathing. Fill your lungs as much as you can and exhale slowly. After about 5 to 10 breaths, you will usually find that you have calmed down and your inner balance has been restored.
- Have a notepad, organizer, tablet, or other digital application accessible at all times.
- Make daily, weekly, and monthly schedules that show exam times, study sessions, and any other regular commitments. Plan leisure time around these commitments rather than the other way around (**Figure 1-7**).
- Identify times during the day when you are energetic and times when you want or need to relax. Plan your schedule accordingly.
- Reward yourself with a special treat or activity for work done well and efficient time management.

DID YOU KNOW?

In a salon, spa, or barbershop environment, it takes a team effort to efficiently manage time. Shops book appointments based on the types of services being provided, the clientele, and the shop type. Some businesses operate without setting appointments, and instead work on a walk-in or first-come, first-served basis. Both methods require beauty professionals to practice effective communication with fellow professionals and peers.

Making sure that you arrive on time, start your first client as soon as they arrive, and stay on schedule will take you a long way toward success as a beauty professional. The front desk and manager can be a tremendous help if you find yourself falling behind or if you have the opportunity to add-on a service and need help fitting it into your day. With experience, you'll learn to accommodate late clients and add-on services like a pro.

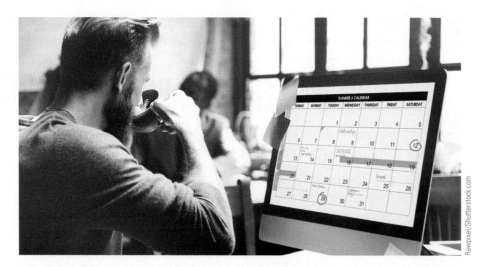

▲ **FIGURE 1-7** Schedules help keep track of your commitments, including your downtime.

- Do not neglect physical activity. Remember that exercise and recreation stimulate clear thinking (**Figure 1-8**).
- Schedule at least one block of free time each day. This will be your hedge against events that happen unexpectedly, such as car trouble, childcare problems, helping a friend in need, or other unforeseen circumstances.
- Understand the value of to-do lists for the day and the week. These lists help prioritize tasks and activities, a key element to organizing time efficiently.
- Make effective time management a habit.

CHECK IN
What are some of the most effective ways to manage time?

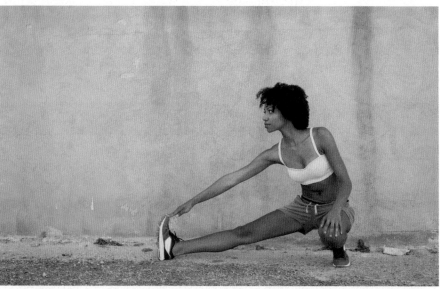

▲ **FIGURE 1-8** Make time for exercise and recreation.

EMPLOY SUCCESSFUL LEARNING TOOLS

Having a successful career as a beauty professional begins by employing key learning tools while you are in school. To realize the greatest benefits education can provide, commit yourself to do the following:

- Attend all classes.
- Arrive for class early.
- Have all necessary materials ready.
- Listen attentively to your instructor.
- Take notes.
- Highlight important points.
- Pay close attention during summary and review sessions.
- When something is not clear, ask for clarification. If you are still unsure, ask again for assistance.

HERE'S A TIP

After becoming a licensed professional, seek continuing education opportunities. Never stop learning! The beauty and wellness industry is constantly changing; there are always new trends, techniques, products, and information. Reading magazines, joining industry associations, attending trade shows, and enrolling in advanced educational classes are all ways to continue learning.

Everyone learns in their own personal and unique ways. Your study skills should use those methods or tools that will help you absorb and retain new information. Learning about all of the study skills available will help you find what works best for you and make valuable use of your time.

REPETITION

Whether you repeat information in your head, say it out loud, write it down, or practice it hands-on, repetition (reh-peh-TIH-shun) helps your short-term memory secure a firmer grasp on the information, making it easier to retrieve when you need it.

ORGANIZATION

Organization (or-gan-ih-ZAY-shun) can be used to process new information for both short-term and long-term memory use. If a new topic seems particularly overwhelming, categorize the information into smaller segments. For example, rather than trying to learn about all the layers of skin at once, study one skin division at a time.

MNEMONICS

A mnemonic (new-MON-ick) is a device that helps you remember or recall information; it can be a word association, acronym, song or rhyme, or any other form of memory trigger that helps you to recall information.

WORD ASSOCIATIONS

To promote better long-term memory, try to associate new information with prior knowledge by using word association techniques. For example, the outermost layer of the epidermis is the *stratum corneum*. It is also known as the *horny layer* because it consists of tightly packed cells that are similar to an animal's horn or hoof. The outer cells are continually shed and replaced with new cells from the underlying layers of the epidermis. In this example, *corn* in *corneum* rhymes with *horn*, providing an easy way to remember both technical and alternate terminology.

Using word associations can be helpful for remembering most information; however, be sure to create associations that mean something to you. Meaningful associations will assist you in actually learning the material and make it easier for you to retrieve it from your long-term memory when you need it.

ACRONYMS

You can create an acronym by using the first letters in a series of words. For example, the bones of the skull can be remembered using the phrase PEST OF—Parietal, Ethmoid, Sphenoid, Temporal, Occipital, and Frontal (**Figure 1-9**). Another acronym covers the functions of the skin with the word SHAPES—Sensation, Heat regulation, Absorption, Protection, Excretion, and Secretion. SHAPES is a particularly good acronym because the skin also gives shape to the body.

SONGS OR RHYMES

Songs or rhymes do not have to be complicated. Something as simple as "keep the air and the hair moving when blowdrying" to prevent burning the client's scalp or "rock 'n' roll rodding creates a spiral perm" to illustrate a rodding technique can be an effective reminder during application procedures.

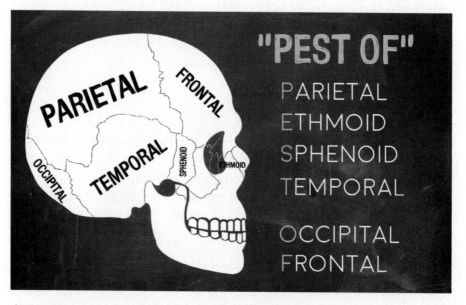

▲ FIGURE 1-9 Acronyms connect related ideas and make them more memorable.

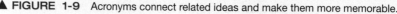

VISUAL STUDY SKILLS

For some, the need to visually lay out thoughts, plans, and ideas is key to retaining information. For these learners, the more visual study skills of mind mapping and note taking can be effective learning tools.

MIND MAPPING

Mind mapping (MYND MAP-ing) is a method you can use to create a visual representation of your thoughts, ideas, or class notes (**Figure 1-10**). Here are some basic guidelines for mind mapping a topic:

- Write the main topic or problem in the center of a piece of paper.
- Think about the topic and allow your ideas to flow.
- Write down key words or ideas that come to mind.
- Use lines to connect the key words to the main topic.
- Expand on the key words by creating new connections to additional thoughts or information.
- Use colors and/or symbols to highlight important information.

NOTE TAKING

Note taking is a valuable skill to develop for studying and for working in the business world. Effective note takers listen carefully and pay attention to verbal cues that alert them to important information. When taking notes, listen and watch for these cues:

- The speaker emphasizes words or phrases.
- You hear a directive, such as "You need to know" or "You might want to remember."

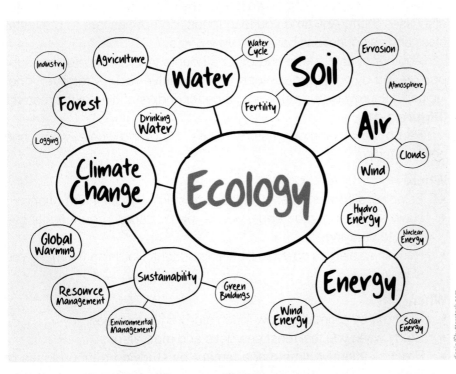

dizain/Shutterstock.com

▲ FIGURE 1-10   Mind mapping the topic "ecology."

"THE Expert AT ANYTHING WAS ONCE A Beginner"

—HELEN HAYES

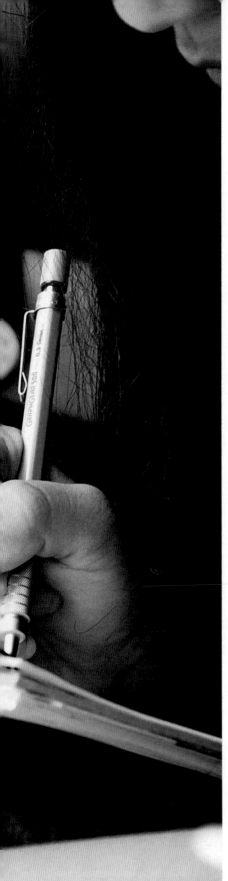

- The speaker uses definitive words, such as *main* or *first,* that provide the importance or the order of something.
- If it gets written on the board, it is usually important.

Although most of us develop our own way of taking notes, here are some general tips to get you started. Remember, you need to take notes in a way that makes sense to you and that will help you make the most of the process.

- Develop or select a note-taking template that works best for the way you like to organize new information.
- Date and number the note pages for easier organization when you need to review them.
- Listen carefully to lesson introductions and summaries.
- Use key words or phrases to identify main points.
- Use complete and accurate sentences when the instructor says, "You need to know …" or "This is important …" or when technical definitions are used.
- Use marks or symbols to emphasize important words, definitions, and so on.
- Use symbols, pictures, and diagrams to create visual reminders or to illustrate a concept.
- Use colored pens or highlighters to emphasize important points.

ESTABLISHING GOOD STUDY HABITS

If you find studying overwhelming, focus on small tasks, one at a time. For example, instead of trying to study for three hours at a time, set the bar lower by studying in smaller chunks of time. If your mind tends to wander in class, try writing down key words or phrases as your instructor discusses them. Any time you lose focus, do not hesitate to stay after class and ask questions based on your notes.

Another study tip is to find other students who are helpful and supportive. Studying in groups can bring positive results for everyone, including improved study skills and a better understanding of the material (**Figure 1-11**).

Part of developing good study habits is knowing where, when, and how to study.

Where
- Establish a comfortable, quiet place to study without interruptions.
- Have everything you need—books, pens, paper, proper lighting—prior to studying.
- Remain as alert as possible by sitting upright. Reclining will make you sleepy!

When
- Start out by estimating how much study time you need.
- Study when you feel most energetic and motivated.
- Practice effective time management by studying during blocks of time that would otherwise be wasted—such as while you are waiting in the doctor's office or taking a bus across town.

Chanlawut/Shutterstock.com

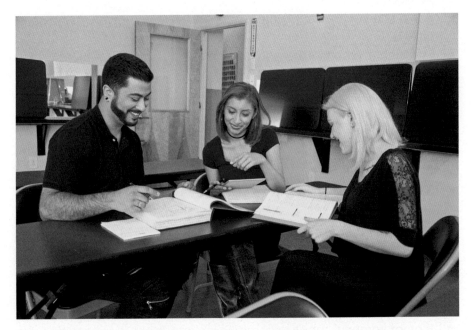

▲ FIGURE 1-11 Studying with friends can be effective and fun.

How

- Study just one section of a chapter at a time and review key points. This method is more effective than reading the entire chapter at once.
- Highlight key words and phrases as you go along.
- Test yourself on each section to ensure that you understand the information.

Remember that every effort you make to follow through on your education is an investment in your future. The progress you make with your learning will increase your confidence. In fact, when you have mastered a range of information and techniques, your self-esteem will soar right along with your grades.

CHECK IN
How do you describe good study habits?

DEFINE ETHICS

Ethics (ETH-iks) are the moral principles by which we live and work. In a shop setting, ethical standards should guide your conduct with clients and fellow employees. When your actions are respectful, courteous, and helpful, you are behaving in an ethical manner.

Practice ethical behavior in the shop by employing these five professional actions:

- Provide skilled and competent services.
- Be honest, courteous, and sincere.

- Avoid sharing clients' private matters with others—even your closest friends.
- Participate in continuing education and stay on track with new information, techniques, and skills.
- Give clients accurate information about treatments and products.

PROFESSIONAL ETHICS

To be an ethical person, you should embody the following qualities:

- **Self-care.** To be helpful to others, it is essential to take care of yourself. Try the Self-Care Test to assess how you are doing (**Figure 1-12**).

- **Integrity.** Maintain your integrity by aligning your behavior and actions to your values. For example, recommending products that clients do not really need is unethical behavior. On the other hand, if you feel that a client would benefit from certain products and additional services, it would be unethical not to give the client that information.

- **Discretion.** Do not share your personal issues with clients. Likewise, never breach confidentiality by repeating personal information that clients have shared with you.

The Self-Care Test

Some people know intuitively when they need to stop, take a break, or even take a day off. Other people forget when to eat. You can judge how well you take care of yourself by noting how you feel physically, emotionally, and mentally. Here are some questions to ask yourself to see how you rate on the self-care scale.

1. Do you wait until you are exhausted before you stop working?
2. Do you forget to eat nutritious food and substitute junk food on the fly?
3. Do you say you will exercise and then put off starting a program?
4. Do you have poor sleep habits?
5. Are you constantly nagging yourself about not being good enough?
6. Are your relationships with people filled with conflict?
7. When you think about the future are you unclear about the direction you will take?
8. Do you spend most of your spare time watching TV?
9. Have you been told you are too stressed and yet you ignore these concerns?
10. Do you waste time and then get angry with yourself?

Score 5 points for each yes. A score of 0-15 says that you take pretty good care of yourself, but you would be wise to examine those questions you answered yes to. A score of 15-30 indicates that you need to rethink your priorities. A score of 30-50 is a strong statement that you are neglecting yourself and may be heading for high stress and burnout. Reviewing the suggestions in Chapter 1 will help you get back on track.

▲ FIGURE 1-12 Take the Self-Care Test.

- **Communication.** Your responsibility to behave ethically extends to your communications with customers and coworkers. Be aware of what you say and how you say it. Also, be conscious of your nonverbal communication, such as facial expressions and body language, which is just as important as verbal communication.

CHECK IN
What are some examples of unethical conduct in the beauty industry?

DEVELOP A POSITIVE PERSONALITY AND ATTITUDE

Beauty professionals interact with people from all walks of life—every day, all day. It is useful, therefore, to have a sense of how different personality traits work together. Refer regularly to the following characteristics of a healthy, positive attitude:

- **Diplomacy.** Being assertive may help people to understand your position. However, it is a short step from assertive to being aggressive or even bullying. Take your attitude temperature to see how well you practice the art of diplomacy. Diplomacy—also known as *tact*—is the ability to deliver truthful, even sometimes critical or difficult, messages in a kind way.
- **Pleasing tone of voice.** The tone of your voice is a personality trait; however, if your natural voice is harsh or if you tend to mumble, you can consciously improve it by speaking more softly or more clearly. Another technique is to smile when speaking (if it is appropriate). Smiling will help lift the tone of your voice, so practice it when speaking in person and when talking on the phone.

FOCUS ON

The Whole Person
An individual's personality is the sum of their characteristics, attitudes, and behavioral traits. Attitude improvement is a process that continues throughout life. In both your professional and personal life, a pleasing attitude gains more associates, clients, and friends. You will know you have a pleasing attitude when you are able to see the good in difficult situations. People enjoy the company of individuals who can put a positive spin on things.

- **Emotional stability.** Learning how to handle a confrontation and how to share your feelings in a professional manner is important to building emotional stability and control.
- **Sensitivity.** Being sensitive means being compassionate and responsive to other people.
- **Values and goals.** Values and goals guide our behavior and give us direction.

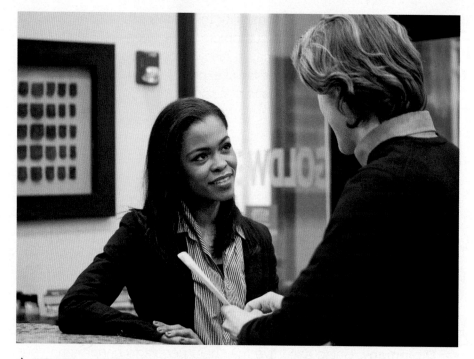

▲ FIGURE 1-13 Exercise good listening skills when discussing client requests.

- **Receptivity.** Be interested in other people and responsive to their opinions, feelings, and ideas. Receptivity involves taking the time to really listen to others. Also, be open-minded and willing to work with all personality types.
- **Effective communication skills.** Commit to practicing effective communication through active listening and both verbal and nonverbal skills (**Figure 1-13**).

CHECK IN
What are the characteristics of a healthy, positive attitude?

APPLY LIFE SKILLS

Congratulations on completing this chapter! Before you move on, take a moment to think about how these Life Skills topics apply to your particular discipline. Discuss with a classmate or study group how success may be defined differently for your discipline; what unique demands your schedule may have; how you can address specific ethical dilemmas; and so on.

COMPETENCY PROGRESS

LIFE SKILLS

How are you doing with Life Skills? **Check off the Chapter 1 Learning Objectives below that you feel you have mastered; leave unchecked those objectives you will need to return to:**

- ☐ EXPLAIN LIFE SKILLS.
- ☐ LIST THE PRINCIPLES THAT CONTRIBUTE TO SUCCESS.
- ☐ DESIGN A MISSION STATEMENT.
- ☐ SET LONG-TERM AND SHORT-TERM GOALS.

- ☐ DEMONSTRATE EFFECTIVE TIME MANAGEMENT.
- ☐ EMPLOY SUCCESSFUL LEARNING TOOLS.
- ☐ DEFINE *ETHICS*.
- ☐ DEVELOP A POSITIVE PERSONALITY AND ATTITUDE.

GLOSSARY

ethics ETH-iks	p. 19	the moral principles by which we live and work
game plan GAYM plan	p. 8	the conscious act of planning your life, instead of just letting things happen
goal setting GOHL SET-ing	p. 10	the identification of long-term and short-term goals that helps you decide what you want out of life
mind mapping MYND MAP-ing	p. 17	a graphic representation of an idea or problem that helps organize one's thoughts
mission statement MISH-uhn STATE-ment	p. 9	a statement that establishes the purpose and values by which an individual or institution lives and works; it provides a sense of direction by defining guiding principles and clarifying goals as well as how an organization operates
mnemonic new-MON-ick	p. 15	any memorization device that helps a person recall information
organization or-gan-ih-ZAY-shun	p. 15	a method used to store new information for short-term and long-term memory
perfectionism pur-FEK-shun-izm	p. 8	an unhealthy compulsion to do things perfectly
prioritize pry-OR-uh-tize	p. 13	to make a list of tasks that need to be done in the order of most-to-least important
procrastination pro-CRASS-tin-aye-shun	p. 8	putting off until tomorrow what you can do today
repetition reh-peh-TIH-shun	p. 15	repeatedly saying, writing, or otherwise reviewing new information until it is learned
self-actualization self ack-chew-uh lih-ZAYE-shun	p. 6	fulfilling one's full potential

CHAPTER 2
PROFESSIONAL IMAGE

"Be so good they can't ignore you."
-Steve Martin

LEARNING OBJECTIVES

AFTER COMPLETING THIS CHAPTER, YOU WILL BE ABLE TO:

1. EXPLAIN PROFESSIONAL IMAGE.

2. EMPLOY IMAGE-BUILDING BASICS.

3. DEMONSTRATE A PROFESSIONAL ATTITUDE.

4. CREATE YOUR PERSONAL PORTFOLIO.

5. IMPLEMENT SOCIAL MEDIA BEST PRACTICES.

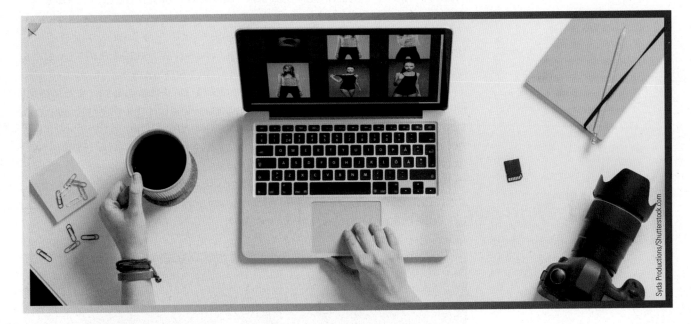

Syda Productions/Shutterstock.com

EXPLAIN PROFESSIONAL IMAGE

Whichever beauty discipline you are working toward, the path ahead will be a journey full of twists and turns filled with exciting opportunities. The important thing is to remain true to yourself while staying open to the many career options and opportunities available. Being flexible, open, willing, and ready to work will be the keys to unlocking future success. These are some of the qualities that will define your professional image, most of which are already a part of who you are. Successful beauty professionals are representations of themselves and their beliefs; trying to be someone you are not will hinder your creativity and detract from the uniqueness that defines you.

Beauty professionals should study and have a thorough understanding of professional image because:

- Your knowledge, talent, and professional reputation define you as a professional and are your most valuable assets.
- Clients rely on beauty professionals to look good and be well groomed. Having a professional image helps build trust with clients and leads to repeat business.
- Finding a salon, spa, or barbershop whose culture complements your image standards and goals is important for career growth and achievements.
- The most successful professionals stay informed, educated, and up-to-date, and are on the cutting edge of what is new and trending in their industry.

YOUR PROFESSIONAL IMAGE

Your professional image (pruh-FESH-un-al IM-aje) is the impression you project through your outward appearance and your conduct in the workplace. Skill and talent may get you to the top, but it is your professional image and reputation that will keep you there. Although we are not always able to control circumstances, we are always able to control how we respond to them. A constant awareness and fine-tuning of the qualities that represent a beauty professional will set you apart and present a complete package to clients, coworkers, and employers.

If you asked five different people to define *professionalism*, you would likely get five completely different answers. What frequently gets us into trouble is that professionalism oftentimes is quite literally in the eye of the beholder—your professional image is ultimately how clients, colleagues, and employers perceive you. Nevertheless, there are universal qualities that all professionals can aspire to, from surfers and musicians, to doctors and politicians, and plenty of work you can do to enhance and control your brand's message (**Figure 2–1**).

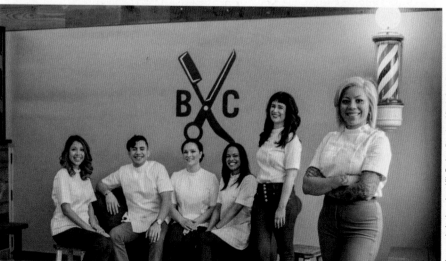

Photography by Jason Lott. Lilly Benitez, Founder of Blade Craft Barber Academy

▲ **FIGURE 2-1** Always present yourself professionally.

ACTIVITY

Get Professional

Select 10 qualities from the list below that you think demonstrate professionalism. These qualities will become the template through which you begin to shape your career and reputation. There are no right or wrong selections: Your choices will simply help guide you to become the outstanding professional you are meant to be.

Key Qualities

- Specialized knowledge
- Expert in chosen field
- Confident
- Communicates positively
- Responsible
- Accountable
- Integrity
- Respected
- High standards
- Ethical
- Professional appearance
- Prepared
- Organized
- Creative
- Team player
- Works well under pressure
- Looks for solutions, not blame
- Savvy business knowledge
- Time management skills
- Current and up-to-date on trends, techniques, and products

These are the qualities that you will bring to every job, every project, and every client you work with. Make a note of these qualities and review them often. Ask yourself whether you are living up to your professional image.

EMPLOY IMAGE-BUILDING BASICS

Fashion is, naturally, a creative outlet for the beauty professional. Being in the beauty industry gives us more creative freedom when it comes to our appearance; in many cases, the beauty professional is expected to present a professional appearance that is both fashionably put together and trendy. It is when we go a little beyond the boundaries in our quest for individual expression that we may get into trouble. When it comes to your professional image, keep the 7/11 rule in mind: Within 7 seconds, someone will establish 11 impressions of you. One of those first 11 impressions is a direct result of your appearance.

Being well groomed advertises a professional's commitment to the industry. Consider yourself a walking billboard and make following personal grooming and hygiene habits the first step in constructing your professional image.

CAUTION

Salons, spas, and barbershops often have a no-fragrance policy for staff members because a significant number of people are sensitive or allergic to a variety of chemicals, including perfume oils. Whether or not your place of business has a no-fragrance policy, you should not wear cologne and perfume at work.

PERSONAL GROOMING

Many owners and managers view appearance and personality as being just as important as technical knowledge and skills. Personal grooming (PURR-son-al GROOM-ing) is the process of caring for parts of the body and maintaining an overall polished look. How a person dresses and takes care of their hair, skin, and nails reflects one's personal grooming habits.

DRESS FOR SUCCESS

While working, your wardrobe selection should express a professional image that is consistent with the image of your salon, spa, or barbershop (**Figure 2–2**). Your clothes must be pressed and clean—not simply free of the dirt that you can see, but stain free. Be mindful about spills and drips when using chemicals and avoid leaning on counters in

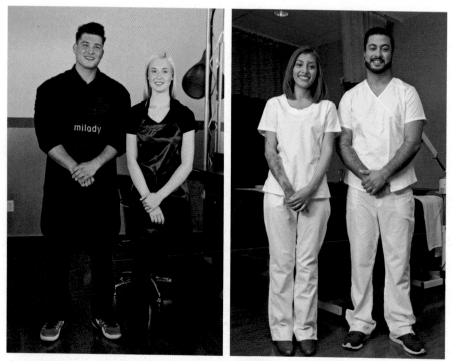

▲ FIGURE 2-2 Your work wardrobe should complement the image of your salon, spa, or barbershop.

the work area, particularly in the dispensary. Although some owners do not require their professionals to wear standard uniforms, they may have a specific dress code for the salon, spa, or barbershop. For example, some barbers may be required to wear a barber's jacket, some a smock, and others a tie. In the case of estheticians, scrubs may be mandatory, although some spas require only all white, and others something else entirely. These requirements are examples of a business's culture and dictate what successful dressing will mean there.

When shopping for work clothes, visualize how you would look in them while performing services. Is the image you will present one that

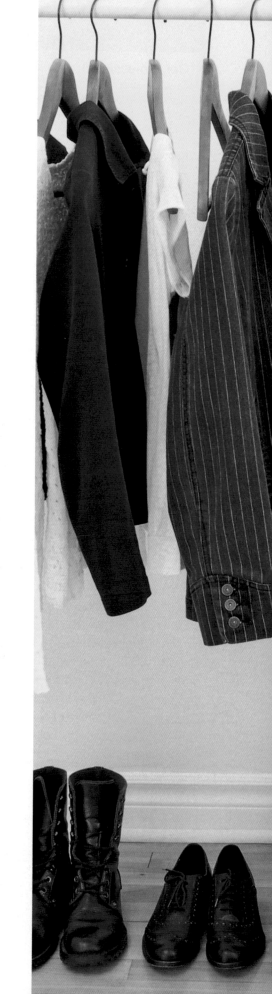

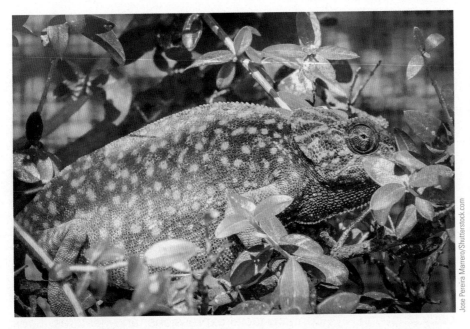

▲ FIGURE 2-7 Your ability to adapt to your environment is beneficial to your career.

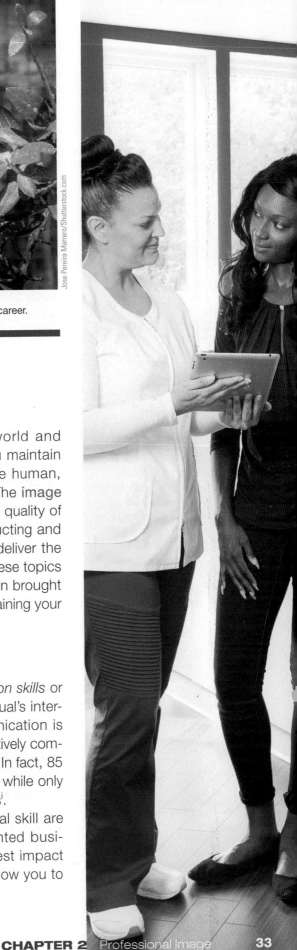

ADAPT YOUR ATTITUDE USING IMAGE ENHANCERS

Our attitude is the platform from which we view the world and through which the world views us. It is imperative that you maintain the professional image you are creating. However, we are human, and we all need an attitude adjustment from time to time. The **image enhancers** (IM-uj en-HAN-sers)—behaviors that improve the quality of your professional image through specific methods for conducting and representing yourself—detailed in this section will help you deliver the best professional image every day, in every way. Note that these topics are covered in greater depth in other chapters, but have been brought together here to illustrate the complexity of crafting and maintaining your professional image.

IMAGE ENHANCER #1: SOFT SKILLS

Soft skills (SAWFT SKILZ), often thought of as *communication skills* or *people skills*, are personal attributes that enhance an individual's inter-actions, job performance, and career prospects. Communication is absolutely a key component of soft skills—your ability to effectively communicate will dramatically contribute to your level of success. In fact, 85 percent of success comes from your ability to communicate, while only 15 percent of your success is attributed to your technical skills[i].

As a beauty professional, your artistic eye and technical skill are essential; that said, the beauty industry is a people-oriented business, and being able to communicate will have the greatest impact on your career. Good speaking—and listening!—skills will allow you to communicate your vision to your client effectively and ensure that their expectations and needs are met. Successful communication between professional and client can be the difference between a satisfied client and success, or an unhappy client and failure.

DID YOU KNOW?

Seven percent of communication is verbal (involves actual words), 55 percent is visual (body language, eye contact), and 38 percent is tonal (pitch, speed, volume, tone of voice)[ii]. To communicate effectively as a professional, project strong body language imbued with confidence, competence, and charisma.

While the importance of verbal communication skills cannot be downplayed, we have to acknowledge that an overwhelming amount of all communication is unconscious. Nonverbal communication (non-VERR-bul com-yoon-ih-KAY-shun) is the communication expressed by body language, eye contact, facial expressions, and gestures. Look around wherever you are and observe the unconscious communication of those around you. Take notice of anything you see—from rolling eyes to sighs, fidgets, quizzical looks, smiles, frowns, or nods. The more you work with people, the more adept you will become at reading body language: Actions often do speak louder than words. Tone of voice, facial expression, posture, and even eye movement and expression become invaluable tools in indicating whether you are on track with your clients and meeting their needs.

Be particularly aware of nonverbal actions that send a negative message and actively work to curb these actions in yourself:

- Avoiding eye contact
- Not smiling
- Tapping your foot
- Crossing your arms
- Standing with shoulders slouched
- Chewing your lip
- Furrowing your brows

As a professional, you will need to be acutely aware of your own body language and the message it is sending to your client. Your posture, tone of voice, facial expressions, and, most importantly, your confidence will indicate the level of your professionalism to clients and coworkers (**Figure 2–8**).

ACTIVITY

People Watching

Take 15 minutes outside of the classroom to sit and watch the people around you. Observe how they interact with others. See if you can identify five positive and five negative nonverbal behaviors. As a beauty professional, your awareness of your own actions will strengthen your awareness of your clients and everyone around you. These skills will enhance your ability to interact with different personalities and in different professional settings.

To pay Attention, this is our Endless — and — Proper Work.

-Mary Oliver

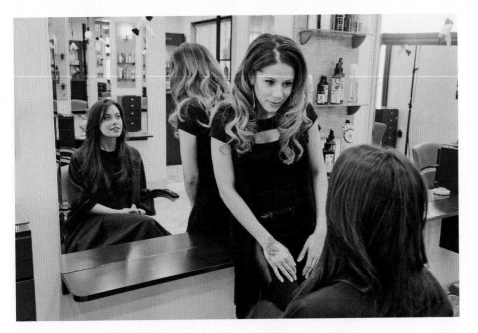

▲ FIGURE 2-8 Recognize and control your nonverbal communication.

IMAGE ENHANCER #2: CUSTOMER SERVICE

Due to the nature of your profession, you will inevitably be providing a service for clients to purchase. It is up to you to provide every potential customer with the best experience possible. Think of customer service as providing a memorable experience that the person receiving your services wants to experience over and over again. Good customer service meets the client's expectations; *great* customer service exceeds your client's expectations.

It is your job to deliver results that exceed the needs and expectations of your clients. When your clients walk away from their service satisfied, happy, and feeling beautiful/handsome/rejuvenated/stylish, you have a client for life. Every customer is a learning experience and an opportunity to not only fine-tune your technical skills, but to enhance your soft skills. To exceed your clients' expectations, you must combine your professional image, a positive attitude, and the information you obtain during the consultation process into one complete service package. Once you begin to make this process part of every service you perform, you will easily exceed client expectations every time and promote a professional image and reputation that fosters success (**Figure 2–9**).

IMAGE ENHANCER #3: WORK ETHIC

You may often hear someone described as an ethical person. What exactly does this mean? Remember that ethics are the moral principles by which we live and work. In the business of beauty, having a strong work ethic (WERK ETH-ik) means taking pride in your work and committing yourself to consistently doing a good job for your clients; employer;

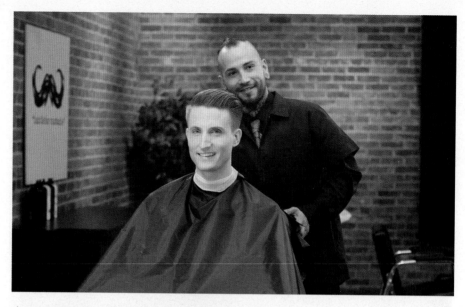

▲ FIGURE 2-9 Effective customer service is key.

and salon, spa, or barbershop team. A solid work ethic incorporates doing what is right and being honest by staying motivated, displaying integrity, practicing good communication skills, and being enthusiastic in all of your endeavors.

- **Motivation** is having the drive to take the necessary actions to achieve a short- or long-term goal. Although motivation can come from external sources—parental or peer pressure, for instance—the best motivation is internal, such as the desire to perfect your makeup artistry skills. Motivation and drive will place opportunity all around you.
- **Integrity** is staying committed to a strong code of moral and artistic values. Integrity is the compass that keeps you on course over the length of your career.
- **Good technical and communication skills.** While you may excel at either technical or communication skills, you must develop both to reach the level of success you desire. Being able to employ good communication skills will always ensure that expectations are clear and correct results are delivered.
- **Enthusiasm and passion** are the flame that lights the fire! Never lose your eagerness to learn, grow, and expand your skills and knowledge. The beauty and wellness industry evolves every day, with new products, styles, techniques, and trends constantly emerging in the market place. A successful beauty professional is not only aware of new technologies and trends, but is also immersed in the details and incorporates these dynamic elements into their professional practice.

DID YOU KNOW?

People tell one friend about good customer service and ten friends about bad customer service. With the popularity of social media, that number can easily quadruple.

IMAGE ENHANCER #4: TIME MANAGEMENT

Whether you are hired as an independent contractor or an employee, you are expected to show up on time at a given location to deliver a service. Being on time is a critical component of being a professional. We would not stay in practice or in demand very long if we were unable to be on time and balance the time with each client wisely. On the job, punctuality is a professional responsibility. Oftentimes your role will not be independent, even if you are an independent contractor. There will always be other professionals who rely on you and your ability to manage your schedule. If you run late, you will impact the entire team of individuals, who also have jobs to do (**Figure 2–10**). In the beauty business, time is money. Poor time-management skills will adversely affect your professional image and can have a catastrophic effect on your professional reputation and future success.

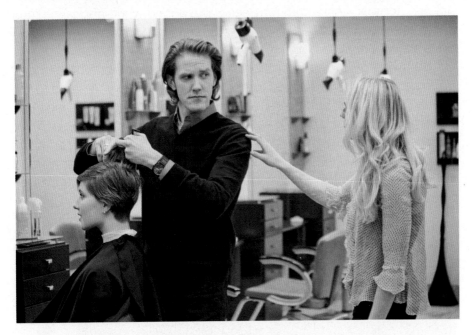

▲ FIGURE 2-10   Poor time management on your part can throw off the entire team.

Remember that you are responsible for your own time management. Sometimes, certain predicaments or instances arise that are unforeseen and unavoidable, and we do run late. If this happens, communicate with those it will affect immediately—both clients and coworkers—and be prepared to offer solutions to make up for the lost time.

IMAGE ENHANCER #5: CONTINUING EDUCATION

Regardless of your age, experience, or skill, there are always new products, cosmetic ingredients, and techniques emerging in the beauty industry. The most successful beauty professionals stay informed and up-to-date on the cutting edge of what is new and trending in their profession. There are many ways to stay informed and to gain the experience that will position you at the forefront of your contemporaries.

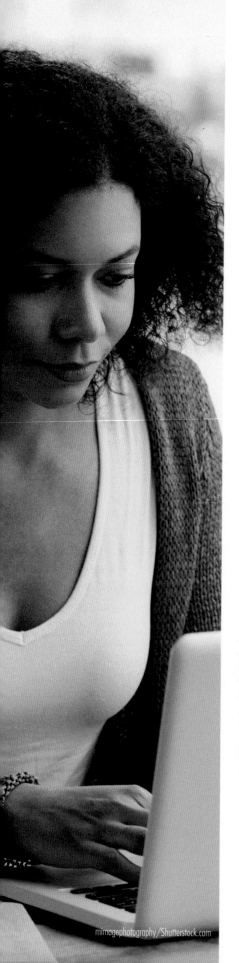

Consumer and professional magazines have been long-standing sources for what is new and exciting in the industry. Consumer magazines keep you informed of what your clients are being exposed to, so that you can answer their questions about new trends, techniques, products, and ingredients. Professional trade magazines, on the other hand, are published specifically for the industry professional, with topics on techniques, ingredients, jobs, education, products, trends, colors, FDA issues, supplies, tools, and styles, along with other aspects of the various beauty professions.

The Internet is obviously a powerful source of information, and one that you can be sure your clients are tapped into. As with consumer magazines, it will serve you well to be aware of current trends that your clients are likely to ask about. Thanks to the Internet, these days you may have to field even more unrealistic requests from clients inspired by images they have found somewhere! While keeping abreast of the Internet and apps like Instagram may seem like added work, appearing (and being) knowledgeable is a great boost to your professional image—and odds are, you're already doing this research in your downtime.

Speaking of knowledge, there are over a dozen conferences and trade shows across the United States that are specifically targeted to the beauty professional, both general and discipline specific. Dates and locations may vary, but are usually set one year in advance, making it easy for attendees to include at least one conference into their schedule annually. Conferences are great places to network with other professionals and industry representatives, learn about emerging trends, and take classes to expand your soft and hard skills (**Figure 2–11**).

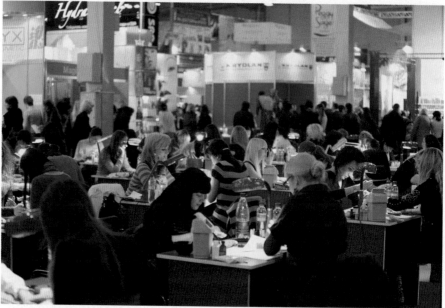

▲ **FIGURE 2-11** Conferences and trade shows are exciting events at which to network and learn.

Check with local beauty institutions, supply stores, or distributors for additional education opportunities, which increasingly include online classes. Many classes provide certification that you can use to pump up your professional image and testify to your expanding skill set. Naturally, before attending any class, be sure to ask for the references of graduates and instructors. You want to ensure that your time and money are well spent on a reputable class and institution.

CHECK IN
Why is a positive attitude important in shaping your professional image?

CREATE YOUR PERSONAL PORTFOLIO

The Internet is a world unto itself, whose population increases daily, thanks in particular to the mobile market. There is a saying in marketing: "If you're not on the Internet, then you don't exist." Your online portfolio (port-FOE-lee-oh) or website is a personal calling card where you display your talents and work for potential customers and employers to evaluate your professional skills. The Internet is also where potential employers and clients will look for you. In the beauty industry, your online portfolio and presence is just as important, and oftentimes more important, than your resume, client list, and physical portfolio. Your online portfolio is a visual representation of your talent and skill and contributes as much to your professional image as the physical display of professional qualities (**Figure 2–12**).

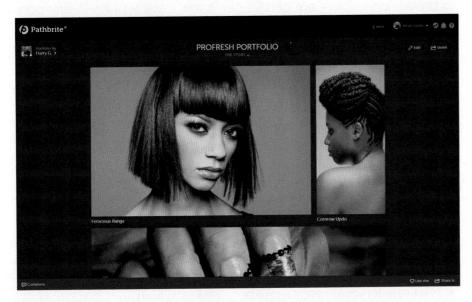

▲ FIGURE 2-12 There are distinct advantages to hosting your portfolio online.

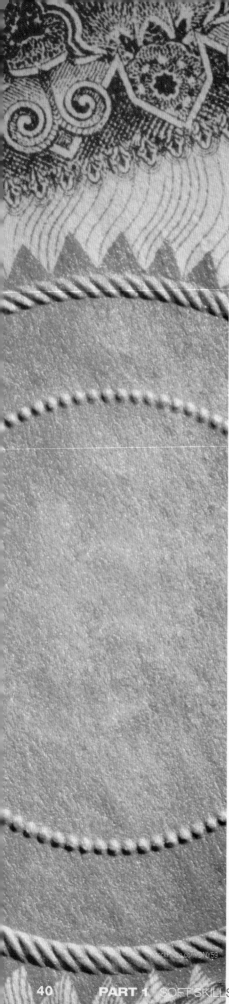

HERE'S A TIP

There are many portfolio websites available; some require you to pay for their services after a trial period, and others are free (such as pathbrite.com). Alternatively, you can present your online portfolio through image-hosting sites, blogs, personal websites, or a Facebook gallery. All of these options have pros and cons that should be weighed before you begin to build a portfolio.

Think of a portfolio as an exhibit of your work on display for potential clients and employers that allows them to evaluate your professional skills and technical artistry. Your portfolio should contain a wide range of photos and show a diversity of styles. Start an online portfolio while you are still in school in order to clearly show the progression of your skills and expertise. The important thing is to establish your presence in the industry as soon as you can.

Do your homework, research carefully, and think long-term—you want your presence, your portfolio, and your web address to be around for years to come. Investigate and discover what other beauty professionals are doing online by looking up and viewing their websites or professional pages.

If creating a website is currently not in your budget, use a portfolio website or create a fan page on Facebook to showcase your work. Remember: Your fan page is your business page and a representation of your professional image.

PORTFOLIO CONTENTS

While the actual contents of the portfolio will vary from professional to professional, there are certain items that have a place in any portfolio. The goal is to create a collection of photos and documents that reflect your skills, accomplishments, and abilities in your chosen career field.

A powerful online or printed portfolio includes the following elements:

- Diplomas, including high school and beauty school
- Student awards and achievements
- Current resume, focusing on accomplishments
- Letters of reference from former employers
- Summary of continuing education and/or copies of training certificates
- Statement of membership in industry and other professional organizations
- Statement of relevant civic affiliations and/or community activities
- Before-and-after photographs of services you have performed on clients or models
- Release forms for photographs
- Brief statement about why you have chosen a career in your discipline
- Any other information that you regard as relevant

When you write the statement about why you chose a career in your field, you might include the following elements:

- A statement that explains what you love about your new career
- A description about the importance of teamwork and how you see yourself as a contributing team member
- A description of methods and ideas you would use to increase service and retail revenue

As for including photos of your best work, your photo selection should be above all diverse—this will show that you are capable of adapting to different clients, needs, environments, techniques, products, styles, and designs. Include services performed on teens, brides, men, fashion or glamour models, camouflage or special needs subjects, fantasy makeup models, or any other unique application that you perform. Before-and-after photos will clearly depict the transformative power of your work (**Figure 2–13**).

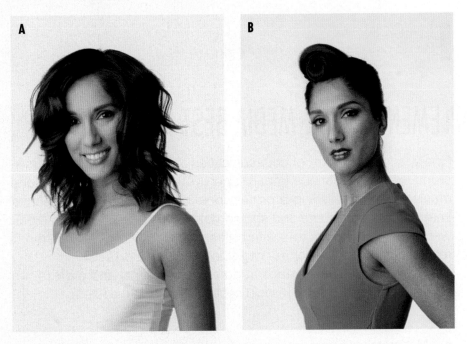

▲ FIGURE 2-13 Use before (A) and after (B) photos of services to showcase your skills.

PORTFOLIO BINDER

If you are not in a position to create an online portfolio or website, you can begin with a portfolio binder. These binders can be purchased at any photography or office supply store, in various sizes and colors. Choose a size that is easy to carry and show to potential employers and clients. Keep in mind that your portfolio and photos should be the same size. For example, if your portfolio is 8" × 10", all the photos inside should be 8" × 10". The presentation and layout of your portfolio will be critiqued along with the photos within. The organization of your portfolio is not only a representation of your personal organization skills and technical artistry, but also a demonstration of your professional image.

ONLINE AND BINDER PORTFOLIO GUIDELINES

Once you have assembled your portfolio, online or otherwise, ask yourself whether it accurately portrays you and your career skills. If it does not, identify what needs to be changed. If you aren't sure, run it by a neutral party and ask for feedback about how to make it more interesting and accurate. The portfolio should be prepared in a way that projects professionalism:

- For ease of use, you may want to separate sections of a printed portfolio with tabs.
- A bound portfolio should be easy to carry and show to potential employers and clients.
- The photos should all have the same dimensions.
- If you are showing your online portfolio, be sure your electronic device is fully charged and the web page is bookmarked for easy retrieval.
- Have a printed copy of your digital portfolio on hand, just in case.

CHECK IN
List the items that should be included in your portfolio.

IMPLEMENT SOCIAL MEDIA BEST PRACTICES

Finally, a frequent form of communication that can easily be misunderstood, yet has a serious impact upon your business, is online communication. Establishing a professional online image is an essential image-building attribute and should not be taken lightly. Social media websites, including photo-sharing sites, can quickly diminish a person's reputation if media etiquette is neglected (**Figure 2–14**).

Follow some simple steps in both your personal and professional social media venues to help avoid costly mistakes in the future:

DO

- Moderate your personal pages or walls.
- Use social media to communicate with peers and clients.
- Post helpful content.

DON'T

- Use foul language.
- Participate in or entertain arguments online.
- Post nude or embarrassing photographs.
- Forward spam.
- Bully or promote bullying.

You will need to build a little time into your schedule to maintain your social media presence; however, it needn't be much time and will likely happen naturally during breaks or meals. Maintaining your professional image online is a daily process—it is also an investment of time that can have huge returns for your business. Social media allows you to share your professional image—including proof of your skills, your creativity,

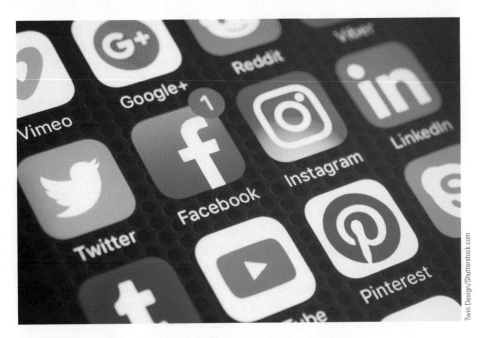

▲ FIGURE 2-14 Social media is a powerful tool when used correctly.

and your passion—with an enormous world of potential clients and fellow beauty professionals. It's up to you to make sure that this image is your best!

> **CAUTION**
>
> Use caution when using social media while still in school! Some states penalize students for posting service-related content, including photos. Check with your instructor and your state board to see what you are allowed to post and when. If you do post material, your portfolios and social media should make it clear that you are still a student and cannot accept clients.

SOCIAL MEDIA AS A BUSINESS TOOL

Getting likes and shares is a good self-esteem booster, but getting appointments from social media puts money in your pocket (and clients in your book). These three tips can turn your social media accounts into powerful business tools.

1. **Include a link to your appointment form.** When you see something on social media that you want (a delicious-looking dessert, a pair of shoes, etc.), you need to know how to get it, right? Potential clients will wonder the same thing if they see your work or promotions on social media. Update your social media profiles to include a link to your website form or appointment-management system so that interested customers can make an appointment. *Pro Tip:* Use a URL shortening tool to simplify a long URL. Some tools will also track how many people have clicked on the link so you know how many visitors your account is attracting.

2. **Take branded photos of your clients and tag them.** This involves some pre-appointment work. Choose an area in your salon, spa, or barbershop where you can set up a photo backdrop. This could be a decorative wall or a supply door (just cover it with luxe wrapping paper). Next, create or buy some props for your clients to pose with. The prop should include the name of your business and the name of the client (if you want to simplify it, just your business name works). Before you take photos of your clients, be sure to ask their permission. If they agree, take multiple photos and invite them to choose the images you post. Next, ask for their social media name or handle and tag them. Now when you take photos of clients, you'll be advertising your business to their friends and family.

3. **Tag your business.** It seems simple, but tag your business in your posts and add the location. When the posts get likes or comment or are included in messages, viewers will know exactly where the work was done and perhaps come by for a visit themselves. If you have one, add your company hashtag too!

FOCUS ON

Social Media Marketing

Each specific form of social media—Facebook, Twitter, Pinterest, Instagram—has its own tips and tricks. Here are 10 general guidelines to keep in mind:

1. Completely fill out your profile info.
2. Always respond.
3. Don't oversell.
4. Moderate spam and negative comments.
5. Focus on engagement, not likes.
6. Keep it short.
7. Don't post too much *and* don't post too little.
8. Always ask: Does this post help my fans?
9. Be personable.
10. *Be visual!*

CHECK IN

What are four things you should *not* do when it comes to social media?

APPLY PROFESSIONAL IMAGE

Congratulations on completing this chapter! Before you move on, take a moment to think about how these Professional Image topics apply to your particular discipline. Discuss with a classmate or study group how you expect to dress on the job; what conventions or trade shows currently exist for your discipline; what apps or websites you should follow to stay informed; and so on.

COMPETENCY PROGRESS

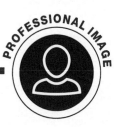

How are you doing with Professional Image? **Check off the Chapter 2 Learning Objectives below that you feel you have mastered; leave unchecked those objectives you will need to return to:**

☐ EXPLAIN PROFESSIONAL IMAGE.

☐ EMPLOY IMAGE-BUILDING BASICS.

☐ DEMONSTRATE A PROFESSIONAL ATTITUDE.

☐ CREATE YOUR PERSONAL PORTFOLIO.

☐ IMPLEMENT SOCIAL MEDIA BEST PRACTICES.

GLOSSARY

image enhancers IM-uj en-HAN-sers	p. 33	behaviors that improve the quality of your professional image through specific methods for conducting and representing yourself
nonverbal communication non-VERR-bul com-yoon-ih-KAY-shun	p. 34	communication expressed by body language, eye contact, facial expressions, and gestures
personal grooming PURR-son-al GROOM-ing	p. 28	the process of caring for parts of the body and maintaining an overall polished look
personal hygiene PURR-son-al HY-jene	p. 31	daily maintenance and cleanliness by practicing good healthful habits
portfolio port-FOE-lee-oh	p. 39	a display of your talents and work for potential clients and employers to evaluate your professional skills
professional image pruh-FESH-un-al IM-aje	p. 26	the impression projected by a person engaged in any profession, consisting of outward appearance and conduct exhibited in the workplace
soft skills SAWFT SKILZ	p. 33	personal attributes that enhance an individual's interactions, job performance, and career prospects
work ethic WERK ETH-ik	p. 35	taking pride in your work and committing yourself to consistently doing an excellent job for your clients; employer; and the salon, spa, or barbershop team

CHAPTER 3

COMMUNICATING FOR SUCCESS

"Communication works for those who work at it."

-John Powell

LEARNING OBJECTIVES

AFTER COMPLETING THIS CHAPTER, YOU WILL BE ABLE TO:

1. EXPLAIN COMMUNICATING FOR SUCCESS.

2. PRACTICE COMMUNICATION SKILLS.

3. CONDUCT THE CLIENT CONSULTATION.

4. HANDLE COMMUNICATION BARRIERS.

5. FOLLOW GUIDELINES FOR WORKPLACE COMMUNICATION.

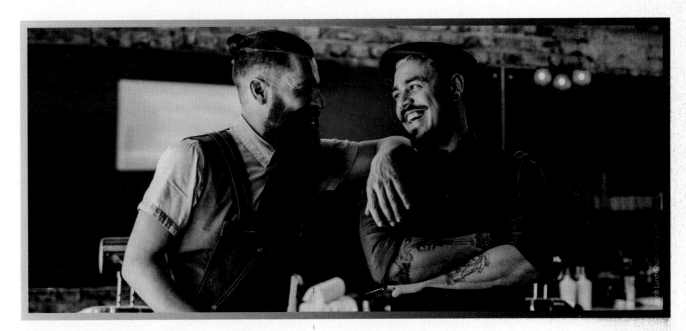

EXPLAIN COMMUNICATING FOR SUCCESS

In order to have a thriving clientele, commit to mastering the art of communication (**Figure 3-1**). Effective human relations and communication skills build lasting client relationships, accelerate professional growth, and promote a positive work environment.

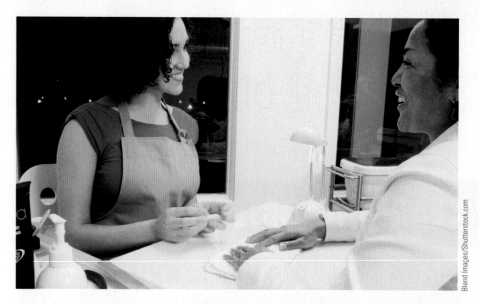

▲ **FIGURE 3-1** Communication is key in building lasting professional–client relationships.

Beauty professionals should study and have a thorough understanding of communicating for success because:

- Communicating effectively is the basis of all long-lasting relationships with clients and coworkers.
- The communication process will help beauty professionals perfect the consultation process with clients.
- Effective communication fosters a positive team environment.
- Good communication skills reduce potential workplace conflict.
- Learning how to communicate effectively can help beauty professionals improve retail and service sales.
- Practicing professional communication ensures that clients will enjoy their experience and encourages continued patronage.
- Effectively expressing ideas is a necessary skill for career advancement.

PRACTICE COMMUNICATION SKILLS

The ability to understand people is the key to operating effectively in many industries. It is especially important in beauty and wellness, where customer service is the cornerstone of success. Most of a beauty professional's achievements will depend on their ability to communicate successfully with a wide range of people: supervisors, coworkers, clients, and various vendors who come into the shop.

Here are practical steps for effectively communicating in the workplace:

- **Respond instead of reacting.** A man was asked why he did not get angry when a driver cut him off. "Why should I let someone else dictate my emotions?" he replied. A wise fellow, don't you think? He may have even saved his own life by not reacting with an "eye for an eye" mentality.

- **Believe in yourself.** When you do, you trust your judgment, uphold your values, and stick to what you believe is right. It is easy to believe in yourself when you have a strong sense of self-worth. Believing in yourself makes you feel strong enough to handle almost any situation in a calm, helpful manner.
- **Talk less, listen more.** There is an old saying that we were given two ears and one mouth for a reason. Listen more than you talk. When you are a good listener, you are fully focused on what other people are saying.
- **Be attentive.** Each client is different. Some clients are clear about what they want, some are demanding, and still others may be hesitant. If you have an aggressive client, ask your manager for advice. You will likely be advised that what usually calms difficult clients down is agreeing with them. Follow up by asking what you can do to make the service more satisfactory (**Figure 3-2**).
- **Take your temperature.** If you are tired or upset, your interactions with clients may be affected. An important part of succeeding in a service profession is taking care of your personal conflicts first so that you can take the best possible care of your clients.

THE GOLDEN RULES OF COMMUNICATION

Follow these golden rules of communication to build a successful beauty and wellness career:

- Project a professional demeanor at all times.
- A smile can be your best asset. Wear one every day.
- Be aware of your body language. For example, don't cross your arms when listening to clients or team members. Instead, nod your head to acknowledge or accept their points of view.
- Always remember that listening is the best relationship builder.
- Speak clearly and loudly enough for people to hear. Don't mumble.
- Avoid using slang.

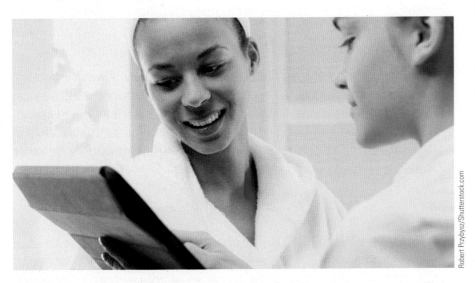

Robert Przybysz/Shutterstock.com

▲ FIGURE 3-2 Be attentive to your client's needs.

THE MOST *Important* THING IN *communication* IS TO HEAR WHAT ISN'T BEING *Said.*

— Peter Drucker

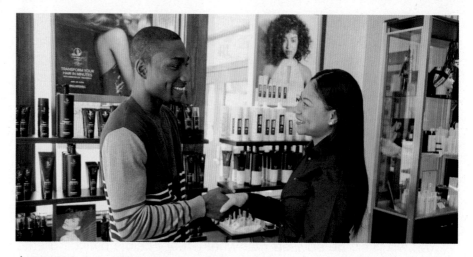

▲ FIGURE 3-3 Welcome your clients with a smile.

THE IMPORTANCE OF EFFECTIVE COMMUNICATION

Effective communication (uh-FEK-tiv com-yoon-ih-KAY-shun) is the act of successfully sharing information between two people (or groups of people) so that the information is understood. You can communicate through words, voice inflections, facial expressions, body language, or visual tools (e.g., a portfolio of your work). When you and your client are both communicating clearly about an upcoming service, your chances of pleasing that client soar.

MEETING AND GREETING NEW CLIENTS

One of the most important encounters you will have is meeting a client for the first time. Be polite, genuinely friendly, and inviting (**Figure 3-3**). Remember that your clients are coming to you for services and paying for your expertise. Communicate professionally by using the proper terminology and thoroughly explaining the features and benefits of the products and services.

To earn a client's trust and loyalty, you should:

- Be consistent by always having a positive attitude. Always introduce yourself and remember to use the client's name throughout the service. Set aside a few minutes to take new clients on a quick tour of the shop.
- Introduce clients to people they may have interactions with while in the salon, spa, or barbershop, including potential providers for other services, such as skin care or nail services.

THE CLIENT INTAKE FORM

Every new client should fill out a client intake form (KLY-ent IN-tayk FORM)—also called a *client questionnaire*, *consultation card*, or *health history form*. This form can prove to be an extremely useful communication and business tool (**Figure 3-4**). The client intake form is used in beauty and wellness services as a questionnaire that discloses the

Client Intake Form

Dear Client,

Our sincerest hope is to provide you with the best beauty and wellness services you've ever received! We want you to be happy with today's visit, and we sincerely hope to build a long-lasting relationship with you. In order for us to do so, we would like to learn more about you, your hair care needs, and your preferences. Please take a moment now to answer the questions below as completely and as accurately as possible.

Thank you, and we look forward to building a lasting relationship!

Name: _____

Address: _____

Phone Number: (day) _____ (evening) _____ (cell) _____

E-mail address: _____

Gender: _____   Age: _____

How did you hear about our salon? _____

If you were referred, who referred you? _____

Please answer the following questions in the space provided. Thanks!

1.   Approximately when was your last salon visit? _____

2.   In the past year have you had any of the following services either in or out of a salon?

   _____ Haircut   _____ Manicure

   _____ Haircolor   _____ Artificial Nail Services (please describe)

   _____ Permanent Wave or Texturizing Treatment   _____ Pedicure

   _____ Chemical Relaxing or Straightening Treatment _____ Facial/Skin Treatment

   _____ Highlighting or Lowlighting   _____ Other (please list any other services you've
                                                                       enjoyed at a salon that may not be listed here).
   _____ Full Head Lightening

3.   What are your expectations for your service(s) today? _____

4.   Are you now, or have you ever been, allergic to any of the products, treatments, or chemicals you've received during any salon service—hair, nails, or skin? (please explain)

   _____

5.   Are you currently taking any medications? (please list)

   _____

6.   Please list all of the products that you use on a regular basis.

   _____

   _____

7.   What styling tools do you use at home? _____

8.   What is the one thing that you want your stylist to know about you? _____

9.   Are you interested in receiving a skin care, nail care, or makeup consultation? _____

10. Would you like to be contacted via e-mail about upcoming promotions and special events?

   Yes _____ No _____

▲ FIGURE 3-4 This sample salon client intake form represents an early opportunity to build an excellent relationship with clients. Additional samples can be found in your specific discipline's text.

client's contact information, products used, hair/nail/skin care needs, preferences, and lifestyle. The form also includes all medications, both topical (applied to the skin) and oral (taken by mouth), along with any known medical issues, skin or scalp disorders, or allergies that might affect services.

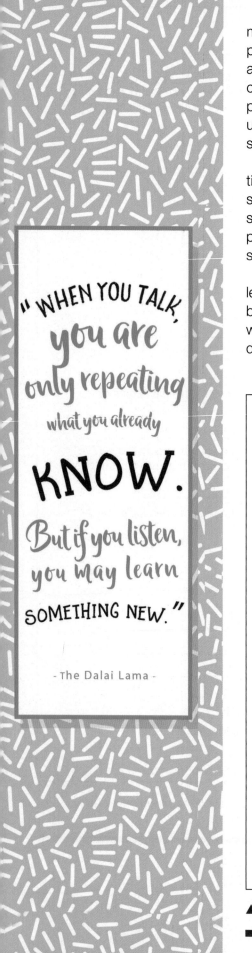

" WHEN YOU TALK,
you are
only repeating
what you already
KNOW.
But if you listen,
you may learn
SOMETHING NEW. "

- The Dalai Lama -

Allergies or sensitivities must also be noted, highlighted, and documented on the service record card (SIR-viss REK-urd KARD)—the client's permanent progress record of services received, results, formulations, and products used during the service or purchased. The service record card is not intended for the client's use and is completed by the beauty professional performing the service. It is the technician's responsibility to update or note changes on this document with each client visit. Some shops use a customer database to record this pertinent information.

The amount of information requested on the intake form or questionnaire varies depending on your workplace. In beauty and wellness school, the intake form may be accompanied by a release statement and service notes in which the client acknowledges that the service is being provided by a student who is under instruction. This helps protect the school and the student from legal action (**Figure 3-5**).

Whatever the specific content, remember that client intake forms are legal documents and should be kept confidential. Physical forms should be secured in lockable, fireproof cabinets and electronic forms protected with firewalls and adequate passwords. Failure to maintain client confidentiality can have legal ramifications.

RELEASE FORM

I, the undersigned,_____
(name)

residing at_____
(street, address)

_____
(city, state and zip)

about to receive services in the Clinical Department of
_____

and having been advised that the services shall be performed by either students, graduate students, and/or instructors of the school, in consideration of the nominal charge for such services, hereby release the school, its students, graduate students, instructors, agents, representatives, and/or employees, from any and all claims arising out of and in any way connected with the performance of these services.

The Proprietor is not Responsible for Personal Property

Signed_____

Date_____

Witnessed_____

THIS RELEASE FORM MUST BE SIGNED BY THE PARENT OR GUARDIAN IF THE CLIENT BEING SERVED IS UNDER 18 YEARS OF AGE.

▲ FIGURE 3-5 A school release form is used when performing services in a school setting.

HOW TO USE THE INTAKE FORM

The client intake form can be used from the moment a new client calls to make an appointment. When scheduling the appointment, let the client know that you and the shop will require some information before you can begin the service, and that it is important to arrive 15 minutes ahead of the appointment time. Also, allow time in your schedule to do a 5- to 15-minute client consultation.

FOCUS ON

Understanding the Total Look Concept

While the enhancement of your client's image should always be your primary concern, it is important to remember that nails, skin, and hair are reflective of an entire lifestyle. How can you help a client make choices that reflect a personal sense of style? Start by doing a little research. Look for books or articles that describe different fashion styles and become familiar with them. This exercise is useful for developing a profile of the broad fashion categories that you can refer to when consulting with clients (**Figure 3-6**).

Changes can occur between visits, so remember to have your returning clients refer to their notes on the intake form recorded at their last visit. Any significant changes should be recorded on the service record card as well.

CHECK IN

What are the golden rules of communication?

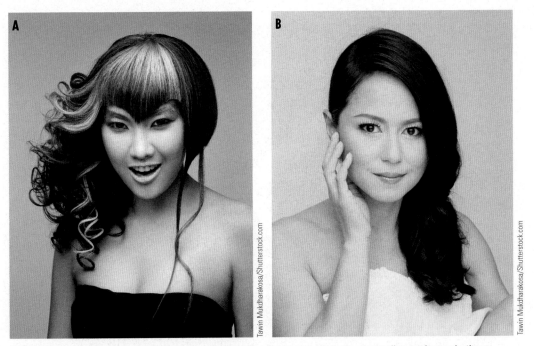

▲ **FIGURE 3-6** Your client's image matters. Cater services to fit their personality, such as whether a dramatic look (A) or a more classic style (B) is preferred.

CONDUCT THE CLIENT CONSULTATION

The **client consultation** (KLY-ent kon-sul-TAY-shun) is the discussion with a client that determines the client's needs and how to achieve the desired results. The consultation is one of the most important parts of any service and should always be done before starting the actual service. A consultation should be performed as part of every single service and shop visit. Effective client consultations keep your clientele looking current, feeling good, and above all satisfied with your services. A happy client means rebookings and referrals for both the business and you.

PREPARING FOR THE CLIENT CONSULTATION

Be prepared to make the most of this dialogue and have certain important items on hand:

- a pen and client intake form
- a selection of styling books, pamphlets, literature, and/or digital images that your clients can look through
- material showcasing a variety of available service options
- a portfolio of your work with before and after photos (**Figure 3-7**)
- additional material that can help the client visualize potential results, such as treatment brochures, nail rings, or hair swatches (**Figure 3-8**); these items are often provided by product manufacturers as selling tools

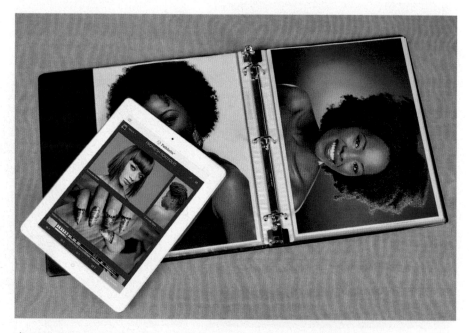

▲ FIGURE 3-7 Use a photo collection to help confirm your client's choice.

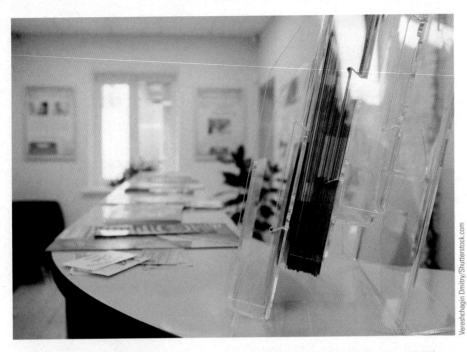

Vereshchagin Dmitry/Shutterstock.com

▲ FIGURE 3-8 Pamphlets and brochures can help present services and their possibilities to clients.

THE CONSULTATION AREA

It is the beauty professional's responsibility to find out the client's needs and to make recommendations accordingly. To do so effectively, you will need a freshly cleaned and uncluttered workspace. Make sure that the product bottles, cans, and jars are also clean (**Figure 3-9**). Clients should be able to look at themselves in the mirror without having to compete with sticky product bottles, implements, and tools on the station. While it may take time and effort to make your station aesthetically pleasing, the payoff of an effective consultation is worthwhile.

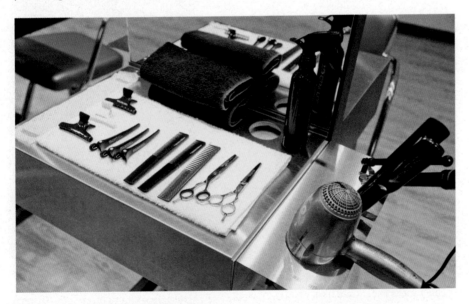

▲ FIGURE 3-9 Tidy up your workstation in preparation for every consultation.

10-STEP CONSULTATION METHOD

Every consultation should be structured so that you cover all the key points that lead to a successful conclusion. While this may seem like a lot of information to memorize, it will become second nature as you become more experienced. To ensure that you cover all the bases, keep a list of the following 10 key points at your station. Modify the list as needed for each actual service:

1. **Review** – Review the intake form. Feel free to make comments that break the ice and initiate conversation with the client. Read the intake form carefully, referring to it often during the consultation process. Also make notes on the service record card (some shops will have a joint intake form and service record card). After the service, record any formulations or products that were used and include any specific techniques or goals. This information will be needed for future visits.

2. **Assess** – Perform a needs assessment. Discover what the client wants and needs. Start off by assessing the client's current style. Is it classic? Avant-garde? For skin, are they looking to remedy a skin condition or relax and unwind? For nails, are the nails long, short, or somewhere in between?

3. **Preferences** – Discover and rate the client's preferences. This will help determine what services will best help the client. Here is a sample question: How would you rate the manageability of your hair on a scale of 1 to 10, where 1 is poor and 10 is excellent? These numerical values will serve as a measuring tool for total customer satisfaction. Other examples of probing questions include: When was the last time you loved your nails? What challenges are you having with maintaining your beard?

4. **Analyze** – Analyze the client's characteristics. Assess the state of the client's hair, fingernails, skin, or whatever you will be working on (**Figure 3-10**). Taking hair as an example, examine

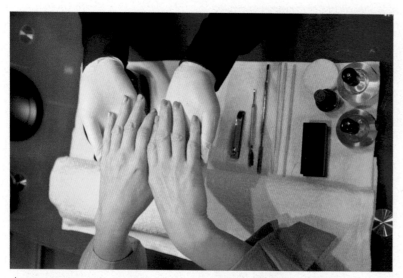

▲ FIGURE 3-10 Analyze the condition of your client's fingers and nails when performing a nail consultation.

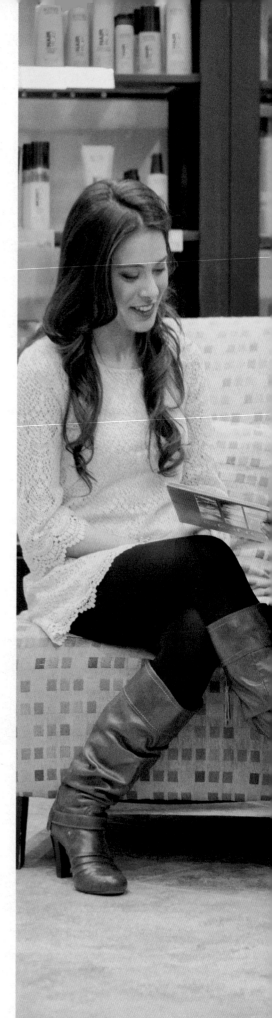

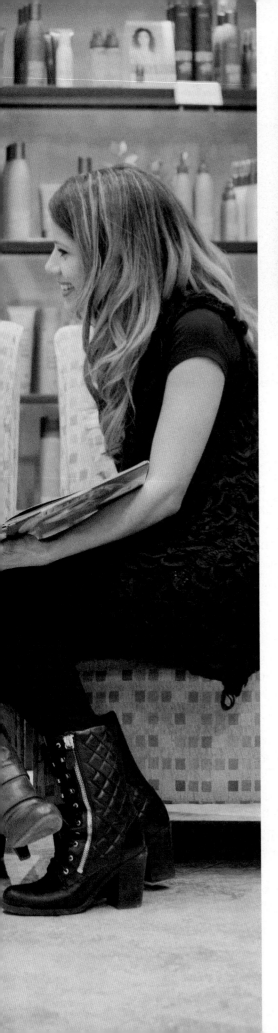

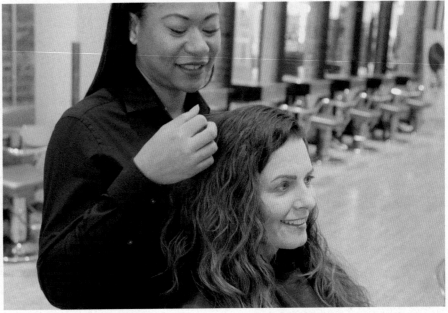

▲ **FIGURE 3-11** A hair analysis should check for thickness, texture, manageability, and condition.

its thickness, texture, manageability, and condition. Is the hair particularly thin on top or at the temples? Check for strong hair growth patterns, including unruly cowlicks. Ask your client what products they use at home and if the products are effective (**Figure 3-11**).

5. **Lifestyle** – Review the client's lifestyle. Ask the following questions about career and lifestyle:

- Do you spend a great deal of time outdoors? Do you swim frequently? Do you work with your hands?
- How much sun exposure do you get?
- What is your occupation? Describe your personal style.
- What are your skin, hair, or nail care habits? How much time do you want to invest in maintaining your nails, hair or skin?

6. **Show and Tell** – Encourage your client to describe styles or services that they like (**Figure 3-12**). Monitor the choices to ensure the services are feasible for the client's hair (skin, nail) type and personal style. Many times, clients desire a service that they may have seen on a friend or heard of a celebrity getting. If the desired result cannot be achieved, create a plan, offer alternative options, and set future goals.

In addition, listen to how the client describes their expectations. If the client says they want their hair short, for instance, does that mean shoulder length? Above the ears? One-inch long all over the head? When the client's bangs are dry, should they be long enough to touch their eyebrows? In order to make sure you understand what your client is saying, repeat what they tell you, using specific terms like *chin length* or *resting on the shoulders*—as opposed to vague terms like *short* or

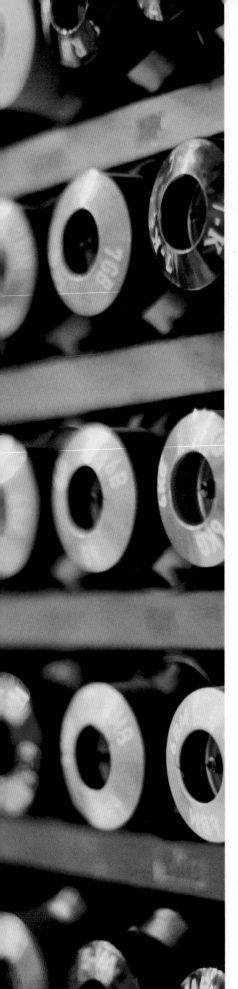

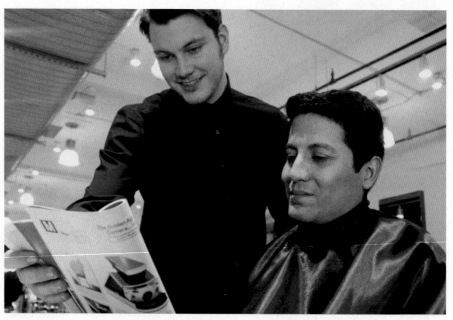

▲ FIGURE 3-12 Use style books, magazines, and other image sources to help discuss style specifics with your client.

long—and reinforce your words both with pictures and by pointing to where the hair would fall. Listening to the client and then repeating, in your own words, what you think the client is telling you is known as reflective listening (ree-FLEK-tiv LIS-en-ing). It is important to focus on the client and not interrupt while they are speaking. After the client is finished, restate and confirm what was said. Then ask for confirmation to make certain you understand what the client wants or needs.

7. **Recommend** – Make recommendations as part of the needs assessment. Once you have enough information, ask the client if you may make some recommendations. Before giving any suggestions, wait for them to give you permission to do so, then base your recommendations on the client's needs and desires. Narrow your selections in keeping with the following criteria:

- **Lifestyle.** The services you choose must fit the client's maintenance ability, meet the client's needs, and provide options as required.
- **Hair (nail, skin) type.** Base your recommendations on the client's characteristics. In the case of skin, do they have dry, normal, oily, or combination skin? For nails, make suggestions based on the client's preferred nail lengths and shapes.
- **Face shape.** For hair, point out hairstyles that would look good with the client's face shape. Is the face narrow across the temple area? If so, you should suggest styles that add

a little fullness in this area. The same applies for makeup options.

When you make suggestions, qualify them by referencing the above parameters. For example: "I think this hairstyle would work well with the texture of your hair." Tactfully discuss any unreasonable expectations that the client expresses, based on their characteristics or personal needs. If their hair (nail, skin) is damaged, address intensive treatments, better home-care products, and lifestyle changes.

8. **Upsell** – Upsell services. Unless a client absolutely does not want to talk about adding on other services, these recommendations should be part of every consultation service. For example, almost everyone can use a paraffin treatment to soften the skin of the hands; or makeup services after a facial, hair, or nail service to complement a new look and feel (**Figure 3-13**).

Never hesitate to suggest additional services (be sure to offer two or more) that will complete the look or improve it in some way. In addition to color, this could be a texture service for added hair movement or body, a straightening service to tame curls, a makeup lesson to complement your client's new style, a manicure with matching nails, a massage or facial service, and so on.

When talking about any beauty service, be very careful to make sure you and the client are speaking the same language. Beauty professionals are accustomed to the technical side of services and tend to use terms like *multidimensional highlighting*, or *monomer liquid and polymer powder*. This can be very confusing and misleading to clients. Use pictures as much as possible. The term *blond* to a beauty professional might be platinum blond; to

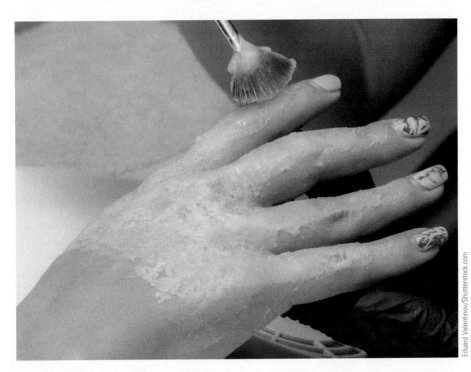

Eduard Valentinov/Shutterstock.com

▲ FIGURE 3-13 Paraffin wax treatments are an upsell service with broad appeal.

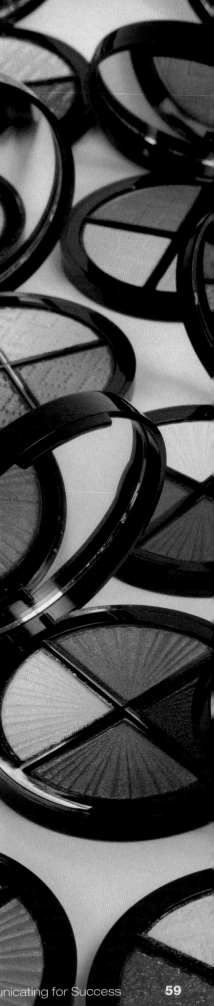

a client, it may mean a few fine streaks of medium-blond around the hairline. Let photos be your guide.

ACTIVITY

Service Experience

When was the last time you went to a salon, spa, or barbershop for a service yourself? Putting yourself in the client's shoes will help you improve your communication skills in every way. First, recall your most recent shop visit. Now, write down the following information:

- Your first impression of your beauty professional
- Your beauty professional's best verbal and nonverbal communication
- Any questions you asked your beauty professional, and their reply
- Questions you wanted to ask but did not, and why not
- What you would change, knowing what you know now about how to communicate with clients. Would you have asked more questions to make certain you got what you wanted? Would you have avoided a certain subject?
- Do you think you communicated exactly what you wanted? What questions did you ask that your clients may not know to ask, since they are not beauty professionals?

9. **Maintenance** – Discuss upkeep and maintenance. Counsel every client on maintenance services, lifestyle limitations (clients receiving exfoliation, for example, should avoid sun exposure), and at-home maintenance needed in order to look their best. Let the client know that throughout the service, you will be educating them on various products that you would recommend for home use, and that at the end of the service, there will be an opportunity to choose the products they need.

10. **Repeat** – Review the consultation. Reiterate everything that you have agreed upon by using a phrase like, "What I heard you say is…." Make sure to speak in measured, precise terms. Use visual tools to demonstrate the intended end result. This is the most critical step of the consultation process because it determines the ultimate service(s). Always take your time and be thorough. Pause for your client's confirmation and ask the client for feedback on the consultation process (**Figure 3-14**). After a successful consultation, it is time to conduct the service.

FOCUS ON

Retailing

The best way to make retailing recommendations is to use this three-step plan to discuss the What, Why, and How of the recommendation:

- Once you have chosen a product for the client, explain, "This is WHAT I recommend…."
- Next, explain WHY you recommend the product. This is the perfect time to refer back to the concerns that the client expressed during the consultation.
- Finally, describe HOW the client should use the product at home.

Educating clients using these three steps helps them better understand your recommendations and makes selling the home care products much easier.

dean bertoncelj/Shutterstock.com

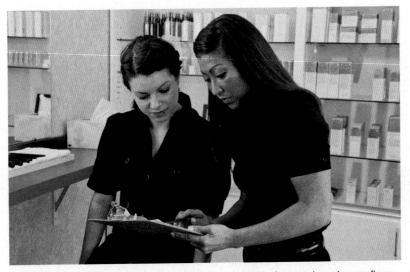

▲ FIGURE 3-14 Review the completed consultation form and receive confirmation before performing any services.

CONCLUDING THE SERVICE

Once the service is finished and the client is satisfied, take a few minutes to record the results on a service record card (**Figure 3-15**). Note anything you did that you want to do again, and things you would do differently next time. Also, make note of the final results and any retail products that the client purchased. Be sure to date your notes and file them in the proper place. Depending on your place of work, some shops may enter the information on each client into a client record database.

CHECK IN
What are the 10 steps of the consultation method?

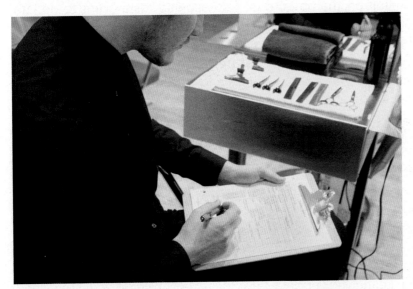

▲ FIGURE 3-15 Take time to record your results on a service record card after each and every service.

HANDLE COMMUNICATION BARRIERS

Although you may do everything in your power to communicate effectively, you will sometimes encounter situations that are beyond your control. Your reactions to situations and your ability to communicate effectively in the face of challenges are critical to being successful in a people profession.

DID YOU KNOW?

When referring to patrons, some salons and barbershops use the word *client*, while others use *guest*. Spas are more likely to use *guest* because of the amount of time the client spends on the premises and the fact that spa patrons often have lunch during visits. Some salons and barber shops have adopted this practice; others feel it personalizes the relationship too much. Medical spas have returned to using *client* because many spas are bound by medical privacy laws when it comes to record keeping. Additionally, *guest* is never used in the professional medical field. Go with the culture of the business in which you're working and you won't go wrong.

MANAGING TARDINESS

Tardy clients can greatly affect work flow. Because beauty professionals depend on appointments and scheduling to maximize working hours, a client who is overly late for an appointment or habitually late causes problems. One tardy client can set back an appointment calendar and make beauty professionals late for other services. The pressure involved in making up for lost time can be stressful. Beyond being rushed and feeling harried, you risk inconveniencing clients who are prompt for appointments. Here are a few guidelines on managing late appointments:

- Know and abide by your shop's appointment policy. Many shops set a limit on the amount of time allowed for a client to be late before requiring a reschedule. Generally, if clients are more than 15 minutes late, they should be asked to reschedule. Most clients will accept responsibility and be understanding about the rule; however, you may come across a few clients who insist on being serviced immediately. Explain to them that you have other appointments and are responsible to those clients as well. Also explain that rushing through the service would be unacceptable to both of you.
- If a client arrives late and you have the time to take the appointment without jeopardizing other appointments, politely advise the client of the late policy. You can deliver this information diplomatically and still remain pleasant and upbeat.
- As you get to know your clients, you will learn who is habitually late. You may want to schedule such clients for the last appointment of the day or ask them to arrive earlier than their actual appointment time.
- If you are running very late, have the receptionist call your clients and let them know. The receptionist can give them the opportunity to reschedule or to come in a little later than their scheduled times.

MANAGING SCHEDULING MIX-UPS

We are all human, and we all make mistakes. Chances are you have gone to an appointment only to discover that you are in the wrong place at the wrong time. The way you are treated at that moment determines whether you patronize that business again. When you, as a professional, are involved with a scheduling mix-up, always remember to be polite. Never argue about who is correct.

Once you have the chance to consult your appointment book, you can say, "Oh, Mrs. Montez, I have you in my appointment book for 10 o'clock, and unfortunately I already have clients scheduled for 11 and 12 o'clock. I'm so sorry about the mix-up. Can I reschedule you for tomorrow at 10 o'clock?" Even though the client may be fuming, you need to stay detached. Move the conversation away from who is at fault and squarely into resolving the confusion. Make another appointment for the client and be sure the shop has their telephone number so that the appointment can be confirmed (**Figure 3-16**).

RESOLVING UNHAPPY CLIENT PROBLEMS

Once in a while, you will inevitably encounter a dissatisfied client. Remember the ultimate goal: Make the client happy. Happy clients build trust with their beauty professionals and will return for future services.

Here are some guidelines:

* Try to find out why the client is unhappy. Ask for specifics.
* If it is possible to change what the client dislikes, do so immediately. If not, look at your schedule book to see how soon you can fit them in to make the adjustment. You may need to enlist the help of the receptionist if you have to reschedule other appointments.

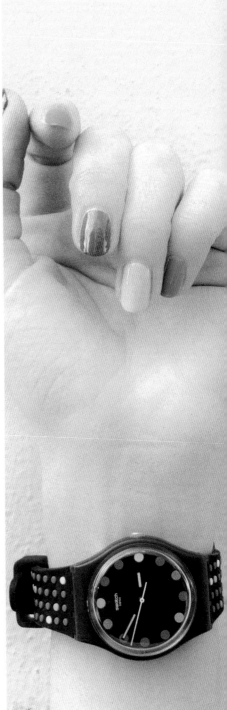

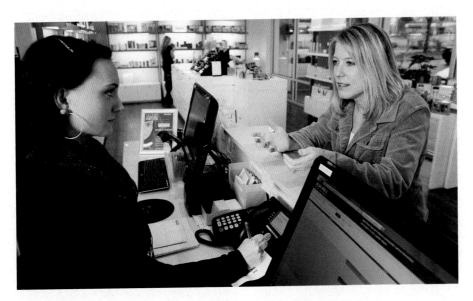

▲ **FIGURE 3-16** Accommodate an unhappy client promptly and calmly.

Photo by Analia Baggiano on Unsplash

- If the problem cannot be fixed, honestly and tactfully explain why. The client may not be happy but will usually appreciate your honesty. Sometimes you can offer other options that minimize the client's disappointment.
- Never argue with the client or try to force your opinion.

ACTIVITY

Unhappy Clients

At some point in your career you will have a client who is unhappy about something, either related to service or scheduling. The best way to prepare for this scenario is to practice. Role-play with a classmate, taking turns being the client and the beauty professional.

As you play the role of client:

- Act out different personalities: first shy, then aggressive.
- Act out a problem that was your (the client's) fault. Then evaluate your classmate's (the beauty professional's) reaction.
- Continue the conversation until you are satisfied.

As you play the role of beauty professional:

- Pay attention to the tone and level of your voice.
- Make certain you understand the problem.
- Avoid being defensive.
- Offer more than one solution.
- Determine when you should involve a manager (played by your instructor).
- Do not hesitate to ask for help from a more experienced beauty professional or your manager. If, after you have tried everything, you are unable to satisfy the client, defer to your manager's advice on how to proceed.
- Confer with your manager after the experience. A good manager will not hold the event against you, but will view it instead as an inevitable fact of life from which you can learn. Follow your manager's advice and move on to your next client.

MANAGING DIFFERENCES

As a beauty professional, you'll find the clients you are most likely to attract are similar to yourself in age, style, and taste. On the other hand, you will also service clients who are very different from you; this is a positive element of your career as a beauty professional. Without both older and younger clients, and ones from different social groups, you won't be able to build a solid client base for future business.

When working with clients who come from a different generation, the basic rules of professionalism should guide you. Older clients, in particular, may not like gum chewing, slang, or the use of *yeah* instead of *yes*. They like to hear *please* and *thank you*. They prefer to keep the topics of conversation professional. Some like to be addressed by the honorific, such as "Mr. Smith," rather than by their first names. When you meet an older client for the first time, ask how they would like to be addressed. Some clients are sensitive to verbiage about aging. When delivering skin care services, do not refer to aging skin; instead, talk about dryness and solutions to remedy the condition.

If these clients are your peers, relate to their image needs but don't act too much like a peer; it is always better to maintain a professional demeanor. When it comes to slang, the same word can have a different meaning across cultures, which is why it is always best to avoid using slang. If the word is fashion-related and your client uses it, you can too, indicating that you understand and are aware of current trends. Never use cultural slang or regionalisms you do not fully understand. When in doubt say, "I have never heard that expression before. What, exactly, do you mean?"

FOCUS ON

Talking Points

Let's imagine a long-time client reveals to you that she and her husband are going through a messy divorce. You care for her and want to be understanding as she reveals increasingly personal details. Other practitioners and their clients are soon listening to every word of this conversation. You want to be helpful and supportive, but this is not the right time or place. What can you do? Decide which of these solutions you might use:

- Tell her you understand that the situation is very difficult, but that while she is in the shop you want to do everything in your power to give her a break from it. Let her know gently that while she is in your care, you should both concentrate on her enjoyment of the services and not on the things that are causing her stress.
- Change the subject. What topic could you shift to that seems the most natural?
- Find a reason to excuse yourself. When you return, change the subject.
- Acknowledge her by saying, "I'm sorry to hear that." Suggest a mini relaxation service the shop is promoting.

GETTING TOO PERSONAL

Sometimes when a client forms a bond of trust with a beauty professional, the client can have a hard time differentiating between a professional and a personal relationship. Manage client relationships tactfully and sensitively, with professionalism and respect. Do not engage in an attempt to fulfill the role of counselor, career guide, parental sounding board, or motivational coach for any of your clients.

If your client gets too far off topic, use neutral subjects to bring the conversation back to beauty needs. If the client tells you about a personal problem, simply listen and tell the client you are sorry. Then ask, "What can we do to make your visit better today?"

If your client is gossiping, change the subject as soon as you can. Try something like, "I just noticed your ends are drier than I thought. We'll do a deep-conditioning treatment after your color." Then describe the treatment and home care.

Books, movies, and celebrities can all be used to move into conversations about a particular look or style. As a rule, avoid discussing religion and politics. When you cannot find a way to move the conversation back to something beauty-related, simply listen and then change the subject.

CHECK IN

How should you handle an unhappy client? List at least four points to keep in mind.

FOLLOW GUIDELINES FOR WORKPLACE COMMUNICATION

Behaving in a professional manner is the first step in making meaningful in-shop communication a reality. The salon, spa, or barbershop is a close-knit community in which people spend long hours working side by side. For this reason, it is important to maintain boundaries. Remember, this is your place of business and, as such, communication within it should occur with respect and mindfulness.

COMMUNICATING WITH COWORKERS

In a work environment, you will not have the opportunity to handpick your colleagues. There will always be people you like or relate to better than others. Keep these points in mind as you interact and communicate with coworkers:

- **Treat everyone with respect.** Regardless of whether you like someone, your colleagues are professionals who deserve respect.
- **Remain objective.** Different types of personalities working together over long and intense hours can breed some degree of dissension and disagreement. Make every effort to remain objective. Resist being pulled into spats and cliques.
- **Be honest and sensitive.** Many people use the excuse of being honest as a license to say anything to anyone. While honesty is always the best policy, using unkind words or actions at work is never a good idea. Be sensitive and think before you speak.
- **Remain neutral.** There may be times where you are persuaded to choose sides. Avoid taking sides in a dispute.
- **Avoid gossip.** Gossiping never resolves a problem, it only makes it worse. Participating in gossip can be just as damaging to you as it is to the object of the gossip.
- **Seek help from someone you respect.** If you find yourself at odds with a coworker, seek out someone who is not involved and can be objective, such as the manager. Ask for advice about how to proceed and then really listen.
- **Do not take things personally.** How many times have you had a bad day, or been thinking about something totally unrelated to work, when a colleague asks you what is wrong or if you are mad at her? Just because someone is behaving in a certain manner, and you happen to be there, does not mean the behavior involves you. If you are confused or concerned by someone's actions, find a private place and an appropriate time to get clarification.
- **Keep your private life private.** The work environment is never the place to discuss your personal life and relationships.

FOCUS ON

Communicating with Managers

Another important relationship is the one a person builds with their manager. The salon, spa, or barbershop manager is usually the person with the most responsibility regarding overall operations. The manager's job is a demanding one. Often, in addition to running a hectic shop, managers also have personal clientele of their own.

The manager is the person who hires staff and is responsible for training. Managers have a vested interest in the success of staff members. Employees might perceive managers as powerful figures of authority, but it is important to remember that managers are human beings. Staff members should support management by following the rules and guidelines that are set.

Here are some guidelines for interacting and communicating with your manager:

- **Be a problem solver.** When seeking advice about an issue or problem, think of possible solutions beforehand. This will indicate that you are working in the business' best interest.
- **Get your facts straight.** Make sure that information is accurate before you speak to management. This proactive approach to problem solving will save time.
- **Be open and honest.** Advise the manager immediately when uncertainty compromises your decision-making skills.
- **Do not gossip or complain about colleagues.** If you are having a legitimate problem with someone, and have tried everything you can to handle the problem with your own resources, only then is it appropriate to go to your manager.
- **Be open to constructive criticism.** It is never easy to hear that you need improvement in any area, but keep in mind that part of your manager's job is to help you achieve professional goals and ensure the shop's success. It is the manager's job to evaluate your skills and offer suggestions on how to improve and expand those skills. Keep an open mind and do not take the criticism personally.

COMMUNICATING DURING AN EMPLOYEE EVALUATION

Well-run salons, spas, and barbershops make it a priority to conduct frequent and thorough employee evaluations. Sometime during the course of your first few days of work, your manager will tell you when to expect your first employee evaluation. If the manager does not mention it, you might request a copy of the form or list of the criteria on which you will be evaluated. The following are some points to keep in mind as you begin your tenure in the shop:

- Take some time to look over the employee evaluation document. Be mindful that the behaviors and activities most important to the shop are likely to be the ones on which you will be evaluated. You can begin to review and rate yourself in the weeks and months ahead, so you can assess your progress and performance.

- Remember, the criteria are created for the purpose of helping you become a better beauty professional and to ensure the shop's success. Make the decision to approach the evaluation positively.

- As the time for the evaluation draws near, try filling out the form yourself. In other words, perform a self-evaluation, even if the shop has not asked you to do so. Be objective, and carefully think out your comments.

Darren Baker/Shutterstock.com

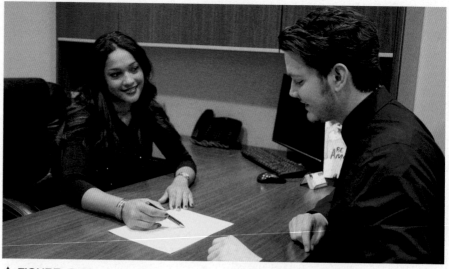

▲ FIGURE 3-17 Your employee evaluation is a good time to discuss your progress with your manager.

- Before your evaluation meeting, write down any thoughts or questions so you can share them with your manager. Do not be shy. If you want to know when you can take on more services, when your pay scale might be increased, or when you might be considered for promotion, this meeting is the appropriate time and place to ask. Many beauty professionals never take advantage of this crucial communication opportunity to discuss future advancement because they are too nervous, intimidated, or unprepared to discuss these issues. Participate proactively in your career and in your success by communicating your desires and interests.
- When you meet with your manager, share your self-evaluation and express that you are serious about your improvement and growth. Your manager will appreciate your input and your initiative. If you are being honest with yourself, there should be no surprises.
- At the end of the meeting, thank your manager for taking the time to do the evaluation and for the feedback and guidance offered (**Figure 3-17**).

CHECK IN
List at least five things to remember when communicating with your coworkers.

APPLY COMMUNICATING FOR SUCCESS

Congratulations on completing this chapter! Before you move on, take a moment to think about how these Communicating for Success topics apply to your particular discipline. Discuss with a classmate or study group how the 10-step consultation method should be adapted for your discipline; what some service-related complaints you may receive could be, and how to tackle them; how to accommodate clients with special or medical needs; and so on.

COMPETENCY PROGRESS

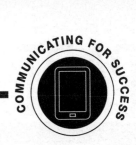

COMMUNICATING FOR SUCCESS

How are you doing with Communicating for Success? **Check off the Chapter 3 Learning Objectives below that you feel you have mastered; leave unchecked those objectives you will need to return to:**

☐ EXPLAIN COMMUNICATING FOR SUCCESS.

☐ PRACTICE COMMUNICATION SKILLS.

☐ CONDUCT THE CLIENT CONSULTATION.

☐ HANDLE COMMUNICATION BARRIERS.

☐ FOLLOW GUIDELINES FOR WORKPLACE COMMUNICATION.

GLOSSARY

client consultation KLY-ent kon-sul-TAY-shun	p. 54	communication with a client that determines what the client's needs are and how to achieve the desired results
client intake form KLY-ent IN-tayk FORM	p. 50	also known as a *client questionnaire*, *consultation card*, or *health history form*; used in beauty and wellness services as a questionnaire that discloses the client's contact information, products used, hair/nail/skin care needs, preferences, and lifestyle; the form also includes all medications, both topical (applied to the skin) and oral (taken by mouth), along with any known medical issues, skin or scalp disorders, or allergies that might affect services
effective communication uh-FEK-tiv com-yoon-ih-KAY-shun	p. 50	the act of sharing information between two people (or groups of people) so that the information is successfully understood
reflective listening ree-FLEK-tiv LIS-en-ing	p. 58	listening to the client and then repeating, in your own words, what you think the client is telling you
service record card SIR-viss REK-urd KARD	p. 52	the client's permanent progress record of services received, results, formulations, and products purchased or used

PART 2
HEALTH & PUBLIC SAFETY

 CHAPTER 4
THE HEALTHY PROFESSIONAL

 CHAPTER 5
INFECTION CONTROL

 CHAPTER 6
CHEMISTRY & CHEMICAL SAFETY

 CHAPTER 7
ELECTRICITY & ELECTRICAL SAFETY

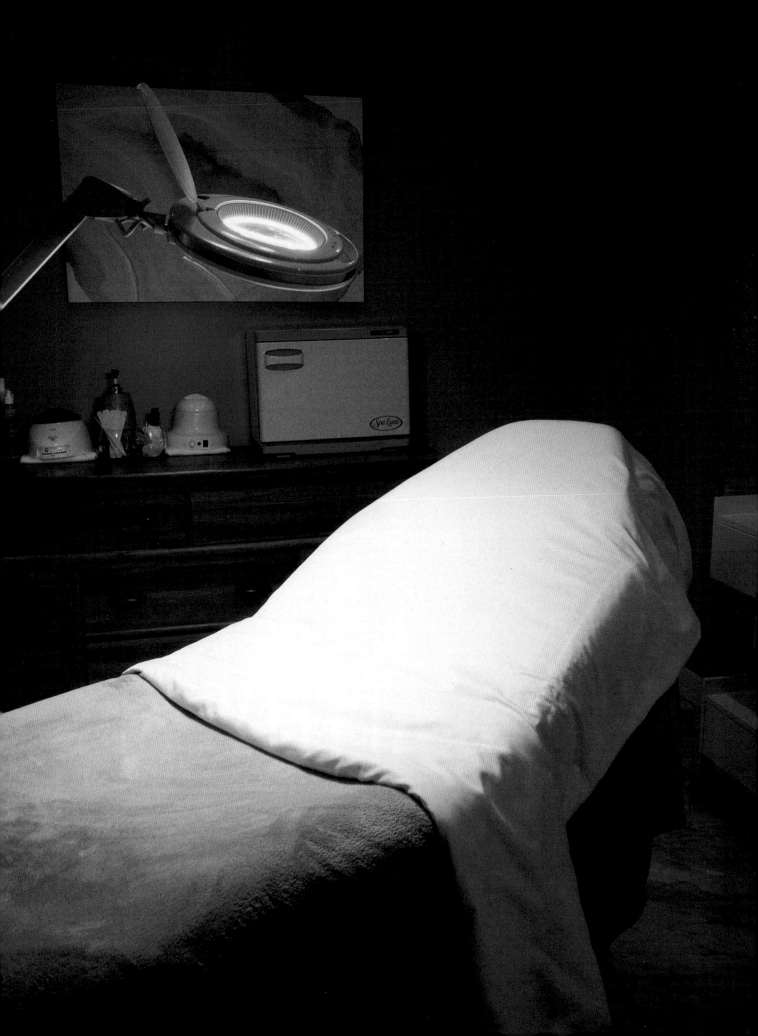

THE HEALTHY PROFESSIONAL

"Stay hungry. Stay foolish."
-Steve Jobs

LEARNING OBJECTIVES

AFTER COMPLETING THIS CHAPTER, YOU WILL BE ABLE TO:

1. EXPLAIN THE HEALTHY PROFESSIONAL.

2. DISCUSS NUTRITIONAL NEEDS IN A BEAUTY CONTEXT.

3. PRACTICE PROPER HYDRATION.

4. DESCRIBE HOW IMMUNITY KEEPS THE BODY SAFE.

5. EXPLAIN WHEN TO TAKE A SICK DAY.

6. IDENTIFY COMMON BEAUTY PROFESSIONAL HEALTH ISSUES.

7. PROTECT YOURSELF WITH PROPER BODY MECHANICS.

8. RECOGNIZE THE CHALLENGES POSED BY PREGNANCY.

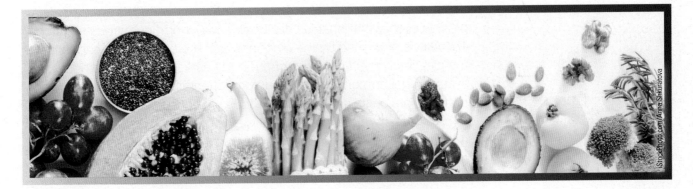

iStockPhoto.com/Anna Shkuratova

EXPLAIN THE HEALTHY PROFESSIONAL

For your own benefit, as well as for the benefit of your clients and the longevity of your career, you should have a basic understanding of how to maintain your health and well-being on the job. Making the right nutritional choices and drinking plenty of water is a good place to start. You've heard people say, "You are what you eat," so strive to be well balanced, vitamin-rich, and hydrated! On the flipside, skin disorders, fatigue, stress, depression, poor focus, and some diseases can be caused by an unhealthy diet or improper hydration.

Beyond eating and drinking properly, healthy professionals are also aware of their body movements at work, moving safely and efficiently to avoid putting unneeded stress on their body in what are physically demanding service jobs. You've got a long career ahead of you; an understanding of ergonomics will help you make it through a little less painfully.

Beauty professionals should study and have a thorough understanding of the healthy professional because:

- Maintaining a strong, healthy body directly impacts the health of your practice, and your practice itself is related to nutrition and wellness in many ways.
- Understanding proper nutrients for the body to maintain optimum energy levels throughout the day is beneficial for all practitioners and their clients.
- Knowing when to take a sick day when you feel ill is an important responsibility regarding your coworkers and clients.
- Avoiding work-related injuries through care and ergonomics leads to longer careers with less overall pain.
- You should be aware of the unique challenges presented by pregnancy in the salon, spa, or barbershop to ensure your or your clients' safety.

DISCUSS NUTRITIONAL NEEDS IN A BEAUTY CONTEXT

All bodily functions, including the building of tissues, are directly related to nutrition (noo-TRISH-un), the processes involved in taking in nutrients and assimilating and utilizing them. The foods we eat and the water we drink are the basic building blocks of life. Foods are broken down into basic molecules that are then delivered to every cell in the human body. These molecules are used by the cells to repair damage, form new cells, and conduct all biochemical reactions that run the body's systems. They provide energy that enables our bodies to perform numerous functions. The skin is nourished by the blood through the arteries and capillaries in the circulatory system. Think of the body as a factory. All the necessary systems, departments, units, and components for the factory to function optimally are contained within the foods we consume.

As we know, beauty professionals are not licensed dietitians, nor are we adequately trained in nutrition to legally recommend dietary changes to our clients. Clients may be taking medications for health conditions (such as diabetes or high blood pressure) that can be negatively affected by misleading advice, including supplement recommendations; however, it is beneficial for anyone practicing personal care services, such as esthetics, to have a good working knowledge of nutrition and how the body is affected by the foods we consume. Good nutrition is necessary for healthy skin, hair, and nails.

ESSENTIAL NUTRIENTS

There are six classes of nutrients that the body needs:

1. Carbohydrates (kahr-boh-HY-draytz) – needed for energy to run every function within the body.
2. Vitamins (VY-tuh-minz) – required for many body functions to occur, including normal metabolism.
3. Fats (FATS) – needed for many body functions, including hormones, sebum production, and absorption of fat-soluble vitamins A, D, E, and K.

4. Minerals (MIN-ur-ulz) – used by cells to produce important biochemicals that have many body functions.
5. Proteins (PRO-teens) – important for building muscle and blood tissues and for cell repair and replacement.
6. Water (WAW-tur) – necessary for virtually every function of the cells and body; makes up 50 to 70 percent of the body's weight.

These essential nutrients are obtained through eating and drinking. The body cannot make nutrients in sufficient amounts to sustain itself properly.

DID YOU KNOW?

If you want more information about nutrition, visit the USDA's special website at http://www.choosemyplate.gov. There are many information sources on this easy-to-use page that offer daily nutrition advice, healthy recipes and meal planning, and weight loss information.

The United States Department of Agriculture (USDA) developed a program called MyPlate to help people determine the amounts of food they need to eat from the five basic food groups. The food groups are:

- Grains
- Dairy
- Vegetables
- Protein foods (such as meat, poultry, seafood, beans, and eggs)
- Fruits

Eating the recommended amounts of foods from the five basic groups is the best way to support and maintain the health of the body, skin, and nails. See the recommended daily food amounts in **Figure 4-1**.

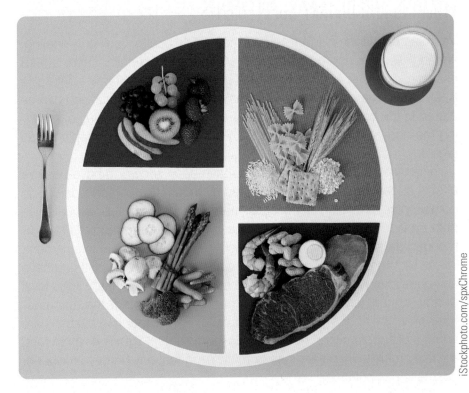

iStockphoto.com/spxChrome

▲ **FIGURE 4-1** MyPlate shows the five food groups and their appropriate proportions.

iStockPhoto.com/Petar Chernaev

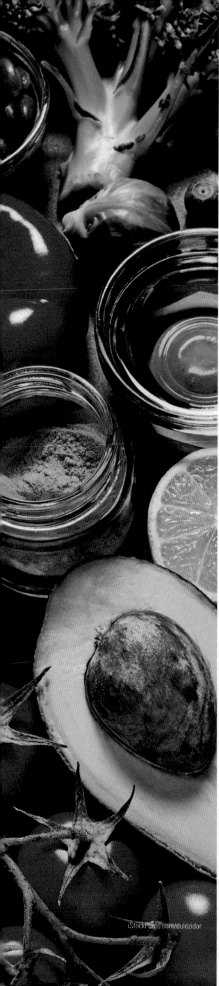

iStockPhoto.com/dulezidar

In addition to creating the recommendations included in the MyPlate program, the USDA and the United States Department of Health and Human Services have established dietary guidelines to assist people with achieving a balanced diet:

- Eat a variety of foods.
- Select a diet that is high in fresh fruits, vegetables, and grain products, and low in fats, saturated fat, and cholesterol.
- Consume moderate amounts of salt and sugar, including the sodium and modified sugars that are in prepared food products.
- Drink an appropriate amount of water.
- Keep consumption of alcoholic beverages to a minimum.
- Balance your diet with the right amount of physical activity.
- Maintain or improve your weight.

For much more information on necessary vitamins and minerals in the diet, visit the National Institutes of Health (NIH) at https://medlineplus.gov/ and search for *vitamins*.

ACTIVITY

Nutrition Tracking

Choose a food tracking program, such as the supertracker at USDA.gov or an app on your phone, and track what you eat in one week. After a week, discuss everyone's results as a class: What are some good habits? Some bad habits? What nutrients are especially lacking? What are some ways you could address this need?

VITAMINS AND DIETARY SUPPLEMENTS

Vitamins play an important role in the body's health, aiding in healing; fighting disease; and maintaining the skin, hair, and nails. There are 13 essential vitamins: A, C, D, E, K, and eight B-complex vitamins. Vitamins A, D, E, and K are fat-soluble vitamins, found in fats in foods, and can be stored in the body. Vitamins C and B-complex are water-soluble, meaning the body uses and loses them quickly, so they must be replenished regularly.

Vitamins such as A, C, D, and E have been shown to have positive effects on the skin's health when taken by mouth. If a person's daily food consumption is lacking in nutrients, vitamin and mineral supplements can help provide some of the nutrients needed. Be sure to read the recommended daily allowance (RDA) for each vitamin and mineral supplement. These recommendations are listed on all supplement labels. If you have any questions or concerns about the supplements, especially if the level of any nutrient is over 100 percent of the RDA, contact the manufacturer either by phone or through a website. Remember that vitamins are nutritional supplements, not cosmetic ingredients (**Figure 4-2**). In fact, the law prohibits manufacturers from claiming that any beauty product or cosmetic has nutritional value.

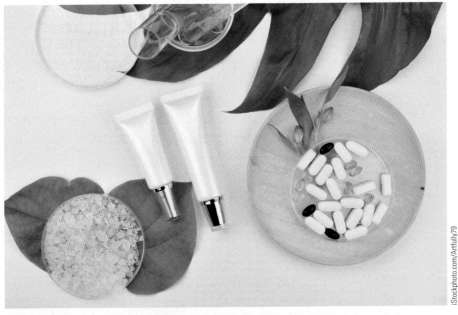

▲ **FIGURE 4-2** Vitamin and mineral supplements are not cosmetic ingredients, but they can still have positive effects on the hair, skin, and nails.

iStockphoto.com/Artfully79

The following vitamins have particularly significant effects on the skin:

- Vitamin A (VY-tuh-min AYE) supports the overall health of the skin and aids in the health, function, and repair of skin cells. It has been shown to improve the skin's elasticity and thickness.

- Vitamin C (VY-tuh-min SEE) is an important substance needed for the proper repair of the skin and tissues. This vitamin aids in and accelerates the skin's healing processes as well as boosting the immune system. Vitamin C also is vitally important in fighting the aging process and promotes the production of collagen in the skin's dermal tissues, keeping the skin healthy and firm.

- Vitamin D (VY-tuh-min DEE) enables the body to properly absorb and use calcium, the element needed for proper bone development and maintenance. Vitamin D also promotes rapid healing of the skin.

- Vitamin E (VY-tuh-min EE) helps protect the skin from the harmful effects of the sun's UV light. Some people claim that vitamin E helps to heal damage to the skin's tissues when taken by mouth.

Because the nutrients the body needs for proper functioning and survival must come primarily from what we eat and drink, you should not depend on supplements to make up for poor nutrition. If your daily food consumption is lacking in nutrients, you should strive to improve your diet rather than relying on vitamins and mineral supplements to provide nourishment.

Clients may occasionally ask you about nutrition and their skin. You can refer them to some of the informational websites listed within this chapter. If clients ask you detailed questions about nutrition, you should tell them to seek the advice of a physician or a registered dietician or nutritionist.

CHECK IN

What are the six classes of nutrients that the body needs?

PRACTICE PROPER HYDRATION

There is one essential nutrient no person can live without, and that is water (**Figure 4-3**). Drinking pure water is indispensable to keeping the body healthy: It sustains cell health, aids in elimination of toxins and waste, helps regulate body temperature, and aids in proper digestion. When all of these functions perform properly, they help the skin, hair, and nails stay healthy, vital, and attractive.

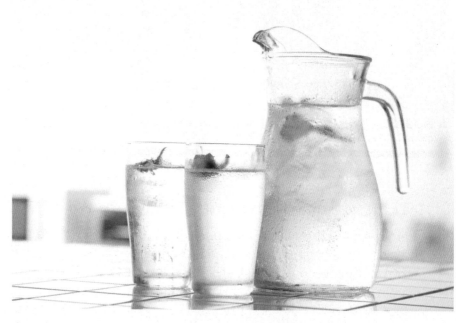

▲ FIGURE 4-3   Water is essential for life and for maintaining healthy hair, skin, and nails.

WATER FACTS

- An estimated 75 percent of Americans are chronically dehydrated. Research suggests that the benefits of water on human health and functioning are many.
- Even mild dehydration will slow metabolism by as much as 3 percent.
- Drinking lots of water can help stop hunger pangs for many dieters.
- Lack of water is the number one cause of daytime fatigue.
- A 2 percent drop in body water can trigger fuzzy short-term memory, trouble with basic math, and difficulty in focusing on a computer screen or printed page.

HERE'S A TIP

Keep a large bottle of water on hand daily to keep the body hydrated. Offer clients water during their services (**Figure 4-4**).

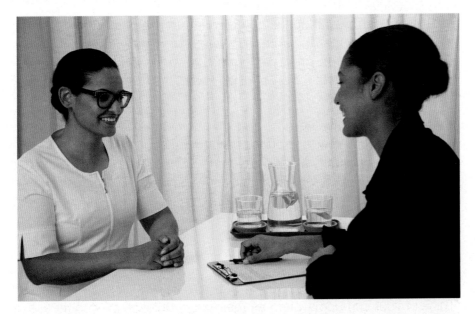

▲ FIGURE 4-4 Make water available to your clients, starting with your initial consultation.

WATER INTAKE REQUIREMENTS

The amount of water needed by an individual varies, depending on body weight and level of daily physical activity. The human body requires approximately 2 liters of fluid a day just to replace the fluid lost from simply existing: walking, standing, breathing. That's eight 8-ounce glasses of water per day at a bare minimum! Drinking nine to twelve glasses (2 to 3 liters) of water a day is an average recommendation.

Here is an easy formula to help you determine how much water is needed every day for *maximum* physical health: Take your body weight and divide by 2, then divide this number by 8. The resulting number approximates how many 8-ounce glasses of water you should drink every day. For instance, if you weigh 160 pounds, you should drink ten glasses of water a day. If you engage in intense physical activity each day, add two extra glasses of water to the final number. This will help replace extra fluids lost while exercising. Drinking excessive amounts of water is not recommended, so increase the amount further only if you are thirsty or dehydrated. As with all healthy habits, moderation is usually the best choice for nutritional balance.

CHECK IN
How many glasses of water should you drink every day?

DESCRIBE HOW IMMUNITY KEEPS THE BODY SAFE

Given all of the pathogens we encounter every day, it seems amazing that most of us are generally healthy. We owe that to our immune system. Immunity (im-YOO-net-ee) refers to the ability of the body to resist and destroy pathogens and respond to infection. A key element of this is the ability of the immune system to identify potential threats and protect the body, often without us knowing we are at risk. Immunity against disease is a sign of good health and can be either natural or acquired.

- Natural immunity (NATCH-uh-rul im-YOO-net-ee) is partly inherited and partly developed through healthy living.
- Acquired immunity (uh-KWY-erd im-YOO-net-ee) is developed after overcoming a disease, through inoculation (such as flu vaccinations), or through exposure to natural allergens (such as pollen, cat dander, and ragweed).

IMPROVE YOUR IMMUNE SYSTEM

Think of your immune system as the military defense of a country: It is constantly aware of potential threats and works behind the scenes to reduce risks and fight against intruders. Much like the military, its success is dependent on having functioning components. For your immune system to work well and protect and heal your body, it must be healthy. For some people, illness or medication may impair their immune systems; however, for most of us, a healthy immune system is the result of lifestyle choices. The most important of these choices, as far as the immune system is concerned, are:

- Proper nutrition – Choose foods that provide a variety of nutrients.
- Sleep – Most adults require eight to nine hours a night.
- Not smoking – The use of tobacco products significantly damages all systems of the body, including the immune system.

While other factors, such as exercise, alcohol use, and stress, certainly play a part in the health of the immune system, nutrition, sleep and not smoking are key.

BE CAREFUL WITH ANTIBIOTICS

We get sick when prevention and immunity fail us. While some illnesses have to run their course, such as those caused by viruses, those caused by bacteria can generally be treated with antibiotics (**Figure 4-5**). Antibiotics (ant-ih-by-AHT-iks) are substances that kill or slow the growth of bacteria and other microorganisms. While antibiotics seem commonplace today, they are relatively new, becoming widely prescribed only in the late 1950s. Indeed, the discovery of antibiotics changed healthcare and allowed many to live who might have otherwise died.

Unfortunately, today antibiotics are widely overused, leading to the development of new, stronger strains of bacteria that are often resistant to these miracle drugs. For antibiotics to continue to save lives, we must be good stewards of their use today. This means that you should take them only when you have a bacterial illness, take only those that have

iStockPhoto.com/Gang Zhou

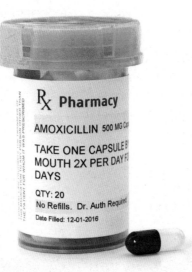

Sherry Yates Young/Shutterstock.com

▲ **FIGURE 4-5** Antibiotics are miraculous drugs that run the risk of being overused.

been prescribed for you, and complete the full course of a treatment. As a beauty professional, remember that some antibiotics can create skin sensitivity and reactions that you may see in your clients. If a client tells you that they are on antibiotics or are experiencing skin sensitivity, it is extremely important to patch test any chemicals prior to a service. A patch test (PACH TEST), also known as a *predisposition test*, is a test for identifying a possible allergy in a client.

CHECK IN
What can you do to improve your immune system?

EXPLAIN WHEN TO TAKE A SICK DAY

When you are employed by a salon, spa, or barbershop, you will be made aware of various company policies, including the official sick policy. From time to time you may find yourself feeling under the weather, forced to balance the expectations of this policy with your busy schedule. In these cases you will have to make a choice: go to work sick or stay home.

STAYING HOME

For beauty professionals, time is money, and the decision to stay home is a big one both for your clients and your bank account. However, some illnesses are highly contagious and put not only your clients but also the health of your salon, spa, or barbershop at risk. If you are running a fever or experiencing vomiting or diarrhea, you should stay home until you have been cleared by a physician or your symptoms have disappeared. Even a simple cold, while not generally dangerous, can be easily spread to your clients (and their families) as well as to your coworkers, which hurts the business as a whole.

If you do decide to go into work, it is important to remember that you are possibly contagious and practice the following:

- Avoid shaking hands. Nothing spreads illness faster than this simple act intended to be welcoming and polite.
- Wash hands prior to every client. While this is the rule in most states, very few professionals have the time to actually do this in practice, even if hand washing can reduce the risk of spreading illness by up to 70 percent.
- Sneeze into your elbow. When you know you are going to sneeze, bring the crook of your elbow to your face, forcing respiratory droplets to the ground (**Figure 4-6**). Avoid sneezing into your hands!

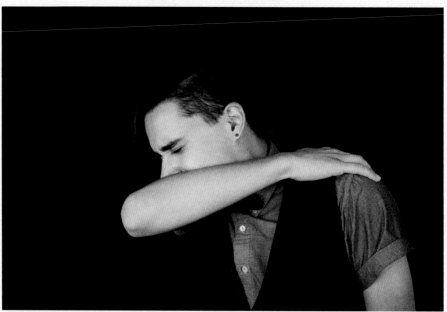

Brenda Carson/Shutterstock.com

▲ FIGURE 4-6 Sneeze into your elbow to avoid spreading potential illnesses.

- Consider covering up. Protective equipment (like gloves and masks) is highly effective at reducing the spread of illness-causing bacteria. While wearing a mask or gloves may seem awkward to you, your clients will understand and appreciate the precaution.
- Increase fluids. Give your body the resources it needs to allow your immune system to do its job. Water is always essential.
- See a doctor if symptoms persist.

Everybody gets sick! Your manager, coworkers, and clients all know this and will be ready to help you reschedule appointments and make sure you're covered. In the meantime, just focus on feeling better.

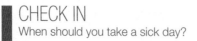

CHECK IN
When should you take a sick day?

IDENTIFY COMMON BEAUTY PROFESSIONAL HEALTH ISSUES

All professions run the risk of certain health problems; however, some are much more common for beauty professionals. These are also mostly preventable or easily treated, and ignoring them could lead to more complex issues.

ALLERGIES (OVEREXPOSURE)

Allergies (AL-ur-jees) are hypersensitivity disorders of the immune system. Allergic reactions occur when a person's immune system reacts negatively to normally harmless substances in the environment; such reactions are often manifested by itchy eyes, a runny nose, wheezing, a skin rash, or diarrhea. Many of the allergies that develop in beauty professionals are related to a few common sources:

- Fragrances in products
- Preservatives in products
- Chemicals used in services
- Excessive exposure to moisture

You may work for many years with a product without any issues and suddenly notice signs of a developing allergy. This may begin as an irritation only and then develop into something that can make it painful to do your job.

While it may be difficult to determine the source of the allergic reaction, the symptoms will continue to get worse with repeated exposure. If you cannot remove the allergen, a visit to your physician may offer some solutions. While the use of gloves can limit your exposure to chemicals, it is important to wash and thoroughly dry your hands after you take them off. In fact, the importance of thoroughly drying your hands after every exposure to moisture cannot be overstated. Once you have dried your hands, use a lotion or cream to restore moisture to the skin and enhance skin integrity. Always be conscious of ongoing irritation or symptoms and be vigilant about limiting exposure.

BACK, HIP, AND FOOT PAIN

Proper ergonomics is the best prevention for many of the bone and joint pains associated with being a beauty professional. However, there are several other things you can do to avoid and reduce the pain associated with your profession:

- While style is important, one of the most important decisions you will make is what footwear you choose to wear at work every day. Particularly for those who stand for 8 to 10 hours a day, improper footwear creates a tremendous amount of pressure on your feet and can lead to lifelong issues and pain. Choosing a shoe that offers support to all parts of the foot, including the arch, is extremely important (**Figure 4-7**).

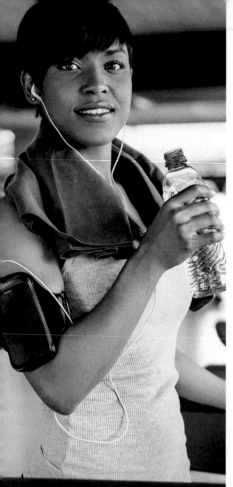

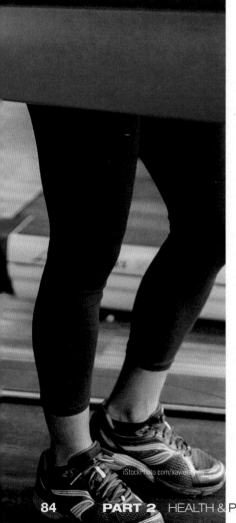

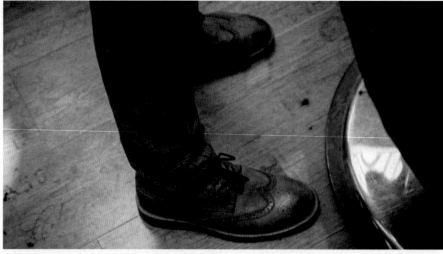

▲ FIGURE 4-7 Wearing sensible shoes goes a long way toward avoiding back, leg, and foot pain.

- Maintaining a healthy weight for your frame is sometimes hard to do but is another joint saver when you are on your feet all day. The joints of your hips, knees, and ankles were not designed to hold extra weight in a largely stationary position for long periods of time.
- Consider support hose/stockings to avoid painful and dangerous varicose veins. These are hereditary for many people; however, even this tendency can be mitigated by use of compression garments.

DEHYDRATION

While everyone knows that staying hydrated is an important component of good health, it is often hard to do on a daily basis. When working in a salon, spa, or barbershop it can be difficult to drink the proper amount of fluid and also find the time to go to the bathroom! Nevertheless, making the decision to restrict fluids to avoid bathroom breaks can have consequences for your health and well-being. In addition, your body relies on the water in the food you eat, so if you are also skipping meals, that adds to your water deficit.

The initial signs of dehydration may be subtle; by the time you feel thirsty, you are already dehydrated. If you let the problem persist, the symptoms will continue to escalate, with dizziness, increased heart rate, and fainting. Remember, your body requires water to function and your clients deserve your best judgment and steady hands when providing a service—things that could be jeopardized by allowing yourself to become dehydrated.

HERE'S A TIP

Consider eating multiple small meals or snacks throughout your day rather than three large meals (or instead of skipping meals entirely). Small, frequent meals maintain the energy your body—and your brain in particular—needs to stay focused and efficient. This goes double for lunch: A large lunch tends to bring with it the dreaded afternoon slump.

DID YOU KNOW?

Never use hydrogen peroxide on a cut. While it is a great disinfectant, it also kills the cells intended to start the healing of tissue, leaving your cut open to secondary infections longer.

HAIR SPLINTERS AND CUTS

Both hair splinters and cuts are common for those who work with hair, even among the most experienced professionals. While these can seem like a minor annoyance at times, they also present the opportunity for infection. A hair splinter should be removed immediately by softening the skin using warm water and removing the splinter with tweezers (**Figure 4-8**). The hands should be washed afterward with soap and water, and an antiseptic and bandage applied to the area. A cut should also be washed immediately with soap and water, and an antiseptic or antibiotic product applied prior to applying a bandage.

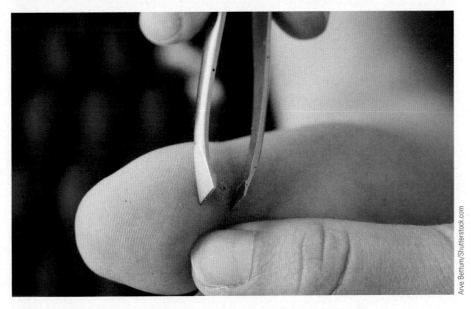

Arve Bettum/Shutterstock.com

▲ FIGURE 4-8 Remove hair splinters with tweezers immediately to avoid infection.

CHECK IN
What can you do to help avoid developing allergies due to overexposure?

PROTECT YOURSELF WITH PROPER BODY MECHANICS

Your muscles and bones work together as a musculoskeletal system, allowing you to walk, raise your arms, and use your fingers. Ergonomics (ur-go-NOM-icks) is the science of designing the workplace as well as its equipment and tools to make specific body movements more comfortable, efficient, and safe.

For example, a hydraulic chair or treatment table can be raised or lowered to accommodate beauty professionals of different heights, allowing each professional to service clients without bending over too far. Certain tools, such as shears, are designed to eliminate hand fatigue because repetitive movements are of particular concern.

Each year, hundreds of beauty professionals report musculoskeletal disorders, including carpal tunnel syndrome (a wrist injury) and back injuries. Beauty professionals may have to stand or sit all day and perform repetitive movements. This makes them susceptible to problems of the hands, wrists, shoulders, neck, back, feet, and legs.

Prevention is the key to avoiding problems. An awareness of your posture and movements, coupled with good work habits, proper tools, and equipment, will enhance your health and comfort.

CAUTION

Wearing inappropriate shoes at work is not only uncomfortable, but it can also be dangerous. Flip-flops and open-toed shoes are not safe to wear around electrical tools and sharp implements.

POSTURE

Good posture conveys an image of confidence and can prevent fatigue and many other physical problems. Sitting or standing improperly can put a great deal of stress on your neck, shoulders, back, and legs. Having good posture allows you to get through your day feeling good and doing your best work.

Practice the following guidelines for maintaining a more stress-free standing posture:

- Hold your head up and chin parallel to the floor.
- Keep your neck elongated and balanced directly above the shoulders.
- Lift your upper body so that your chest is up and out—do not slouch.
- Hold your shoulders level and relaxed.
- Stand with your spine straight (**Figure 4-9**).

Just as there is a mechanically correct posture for standing, there is also a correct sitting posture. Use the following guidelines to learn to sit in a balanced position:

- Keep your hips level and horizontal, not tilted forward or backward.
- Flex your knees slightly and position them over your feet.
- Lower your body smoothly into a chair, keeping your back straight.
- Place the soles of your feet on the floor directly under your knees.
- Keep the seat of the chair even with your knees. This will allow the upper and lower legs to form a 90-degree angle at the knees.
- Distribute your body weight evenly on both hips.

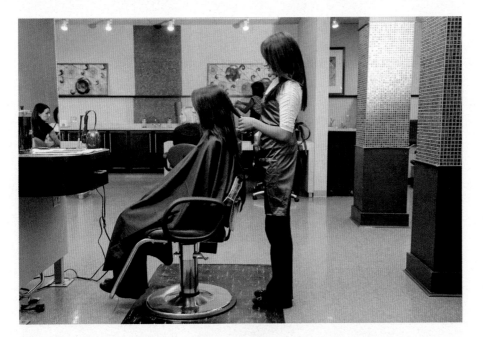

▲ FIGURE 4-9 Good posture both presents you well and protects your joints.

- Keep your torso erect (**Figure 4-10**).
- When sitting at a desk, make sure it is at the correct height so that the upper and lower parts of your arm form a right angle when you are writing.

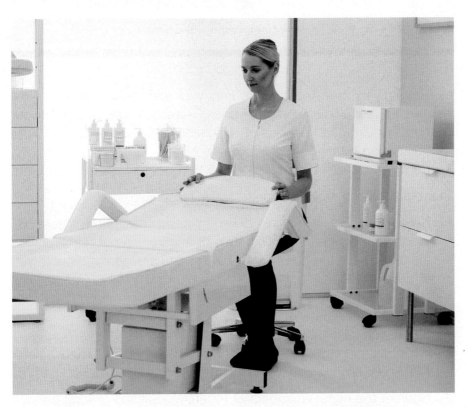

▲ FIGURE 4-10 Practice proper sitting posture in relation to your facial bed.

ERGONOMICS

Ergonomics is important in your ability to work and in your body's wellness. Repetitive motions have a cumulative effect on the muscles and joints. To avoid problems, monitor yourself as you work to see if you are falling into these bad habits:

*   Gripping or squeezing implements too tightly
*   Bending your wrist up or down repeatedly, or contorting your wrist when using the tools of your profession (**Figure 4-11**)

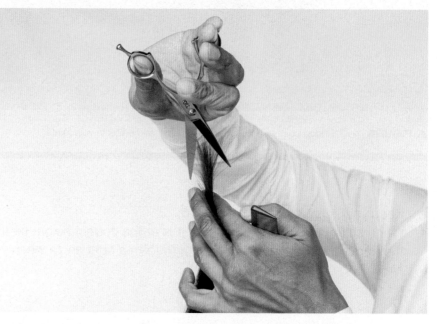

▲ FIGURE 4-11 An improper haircutting position stresses the wrist.

*   Holding your arms too far away from your body as you work
*   Holding your elbows at more than a 60-degree angle away from your body for extended periods of time; elbows should be close to the body when cutting
*   Bending forward and/or twisting your body to get closer to your client

To avoid ergonomic-related injuries, follow these guidelines:

*   Keep your wrists in a straight or neutral position as much as possible.
*   When working on a client's hands or fingers, do not reach across the table; have the client extend their hand across the table to you (**Figure 4-12**).
*   Use ergonomically designed implements.
*   Keep your back and neck straight.
*   Stand on an anti-fatigue mat.
*   When standing to cut hair, position your legs hip-width apart, bend your knees slightly, and align your pelvic area with your abdomen.

Counter the negative impact of repetitive motions or long periods spent in one position by stretching and walking around at intervals. Always put your well-being first.

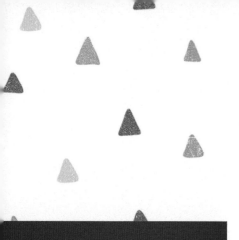

I HAVE A CONFIDENCE ABOUT MY LIFE THAT COMES FROM STANDING TALL ON MY OWN TWO FEET.

— JANE FONDA

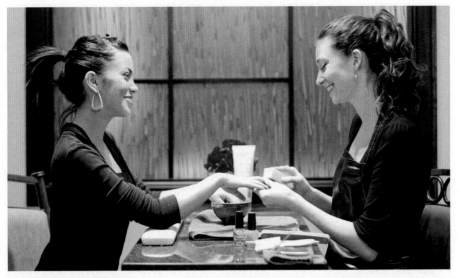

▲ **FIGURE 4-12** Proper ergonomic techniques during nail services include having the client come to you.

LIFTING MECHANICS

Whatever you are lifting, be it patients off of tables in the treatment room or boxes onto shelves in the storeroom, always follow these safe lifting guidelines:

1. Keep feet about shoulder-width apart.
2. Keep chin up and back straight.
3. Bend at the knees, not at the back.
4. Keep objects close to your body.
5. Do not twist your body when lifting or carrying.
6. Exhale when lifting.
7. Lift with the legs, not with the back.
8. Push or pull instead of lifting.
9. Never reach more than 18 inches away from the body.
10. Avoid fast, jerky motions when lifting (**Figure 4-13**).

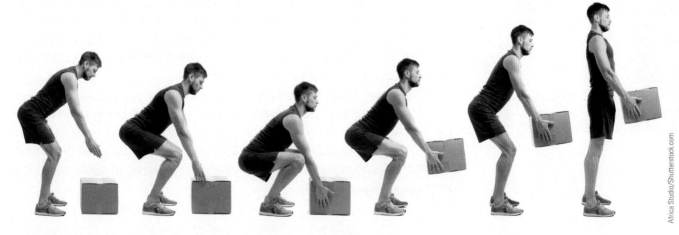

Africa Studio/Shutterstock.com

▲ **FIGURE 4-13** Practice good lifting techniques whenever possible.

ACTIVITY

Ergonomic Exercises

Practice these quick exercises to help you relieve stress from repetitive movements or from standing or sitting in one position for too long:

For Wrists

1. Stand up straight.
2. Raise both of your arms straight out.
3. Bend your wrists so your fingers point upward. Hold for five seconds.
4. Holding your wrists steady, turn your hands so your fingers face the floor. Hold for five seconds.
5. Repeat the cycle five times.

For Fingers

1. Get a ball the size of a tennis or tension ball.
2. Grip it tightly for a count of five. Release.
3. Repeat five times.

For Shoulders

1. Stand up straight and shrug your shoulders upward.
2. Roll your shoulders back. Hold for a count of five.
3. To reverse direction, roll your shoulders forward. Hold for a count of five.
4. Repeat five times.

CHECK IN

What are four ways you can avoid ergonomic-related injuries?

RECOGNIZE THE CHALLENGES POSED BY PREGNANCY

The most critical developments of the fetus—the brain and the heart—are complete within 12 weeks. During this time, exposure to chemicals should be minimal and only when necessary. If you are trying to get pregnant, it is important that you pay attention to chemical labels both at home and at work. Even cleaning chemicals that you use every day have precautionary statements about their use during pregnancy; so as you begin to think about childbearing, reread the labels and understand the safe use of certain products. It is important to remember that everything that touches your skin is absorbed, as is every fume or vapor that you inhale. While this might be a risk you are willing to take for yourself, it is not a safe decision for your unborn baby.

When your clients tell you they are pregnant (or you can see for yourself), it is important to review with them the chemicals being used in their services and allow them an opportunity to read the label or SDS if they wish. When in doubt, direct a client to their physician and give them time to make a decision they are comfortable with in terms of services during pregnancy (**Figure 4-14**).

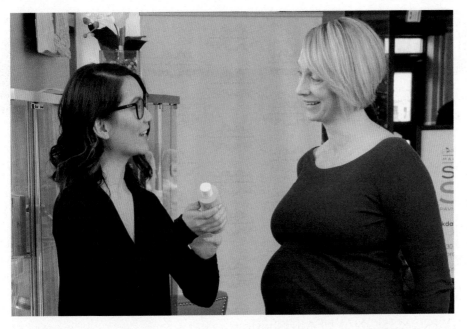

▲ FIGURE 4-14 Pregnancy requires extra care in the salon, spa, or barbershop environment.

PREGNANCY IN THE SALON, SPA, OR BARBERSHOP

Regardless of who is pregnant, the following precautions should be followed:

- Always extend your arm the full length when using a spray and direct the spray away from yourself and your client. When possible, spray with the container held below the waistline.
- Wear gloves during any chemical process, including cleaning. Ensure that the gloves you have chosen are appropriate for the chemicals you are using. For example, gloves made from petroleum products are broken down by products containing petroleum.
- Avoid sitting at a pedicure bowl when the adjacent one is being disinfected. Running disinfectant or bleach through the pedicure jets causes the chemical to become airborne.
- Wash hands frequently.

CHECK IN
How should pregnant individuals handle chemicals?

APPLY THE HEALTHY PROFESSIONAL

Congratulations on completing this chapter! Before you move on, take a moment to think about how these Healthy Professional topics apply to your particular discipline. Discuss with a classmate or study group ways in which you can fit healthy eating into a busy day on the job; specific ergonomic concerns you'll want to watch out for; possible injuries to avoid during your services; and so on.

COMPETENCY PROGRESS

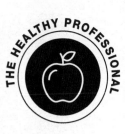

THE HEALTHY PROFESSIONAL

How are you doing with The Healthy Professional? **Check off the Chapter 4 Learning Objectives below that you feel you have mastered; leave unchecked those objectives you will need to return to:**

☐ EXPLAIN THE HEALTHY PROFESSIONAL.

☐ DISCUSS NUTRITIONAL NEEDS IN A BEAUTY CONTEXT.

☐ PRACTICE PROPER HYDRATION.

☐ DESCRIBE HOW IMMUNITY KEEPS THE BODY SAFE.

☐ EXPLAIN WHEN TO TAKE A SICK DAY.

☐ IDENTIFY COMMON BEAUTY PROFESSIONAL HEALTH ISSUES.

☐ PROTECT YOURSELF WITH PROPER BODY MECHANICS.

☐ RECOGNIZE THE CHALLENGES POSED BY PREGNANCY.

GLOSSARY

acquired immunity (uh-KWY-erd im-YOO-net-ee)	p. 80	immunity that is developed after overcoming a disease, through inoculation (such as flu vaccinations) or through exposure to natural allergens (such as pollen, cat dander, and ragweed)
allergies (AL-ur-jees)	p. 83	hypersensitivity disorders of the immune system
antibiotics (ant-ih-by-AHT-iks)	p. 80	substances that kill or slow the growth of bacteria and other microorganisms
carbohydrates (kahr-boh-HY-drayts)	p. 74	nutrients needed for energy to run every function within the body
ergonomics (ur-go-NOM-icks)	p. 85	the science of designing the workplace as well as its equipment and tools to make specific body movements more comfortable, efficient, and safe
fats (FATS)	p. 74	nutrients needed for many body functions, including hormones, sebum production, and absorption of fat-soluble vitamins A, D, E, and K
immunity (im-YOO-net-ee)	p. 79	the ability of the body to resist and destroy pathogens and respond to infection
minerals (MIN-ur-ulz)	p. 75	nutrients used by cells to produce important biochemicals that have many body functions

natural immunity (NATCH- uh-rul im-YOO-net-ee)	p. 80	immunity that is partly inherited and partly developed through healthy living
nutrition (noo-TRISH-un)	p. 74	the processes involved in taking in nutrients and assimilating and utilizing them
patch test (PACH TEST)	p. 81	a test for identifying a possible allergy in a client; also known as a *predisposition test*
proteins (PRO-teens)	p. 75	nutrients important for building muscle and blood tissues and for cell repair and replacement
vitamins (VY-tuh-minz)	p. 74	nutrients required for many body functions to occur, including normal metabolism
vitamin A (VY-tuh-min AYE)	p. 77	supports the overall health of the skin; aids in the health, function, and repair of skin cells; has been shown to improve the skin's elasticity and thickness
vitamin C (VY-tuh-min SEE)	p. 77	an important substance needed for proper repair of the skin and tissues; promotes the production of collagen in the skin's dermal tissues; aids in and promotes the skin's healing process
vitamin D (VY-tuh-min DEE)	p. 77	enables the body to properly absorb and use calcium, the element needed for proper bone development and maintenance. Vitamin D also promotes rapid healing of the skin
vitamin E (VY-tuh-min EE)	p. 77	helps protect the skin from the harmful effects of the sun's UV light
water (WAW-tur)	p. 75	makes up 50 to 70 percent of the body's weight and is necessary for virtually every function of the cells and body

CHAPTER 5
INFECTION CONTROL

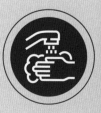

"Growth itself contains the germ of happiness."

-Pearl S. Buck

LEARNING OBJECTIVES

AFTER COMPLETING THIS CHAPTER, YOU WILL BE ABLE TO:

1. EXPLAIN INFECTION CONTROL.
2. DESCRIBE FEDERAL AND STATE REGULATORY AGENCIES.
3. RECOGNIZE THE PRINCIPLES OF INFECTION.
4. IDENTIFY DIFFERENT TYPES OF PATHOGENS.
5. EMPLOY THE PRINCIPLES OF PREVENTION.
6. FOLLOW STANDARD PRECAUTIONS TO PROTECT YOURSELF AND YOUR CLIENTS.
7. DEMONSTRATE SAFE WORK PRACTICES AND SAFETY PRECAUTIONS.

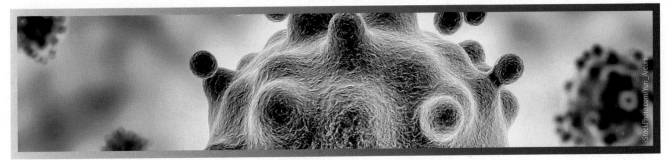

iStockPhoto.com/Yuri_Arcurs

EXPLAIN INFECTION CONTROL

State boards and other regulatory agencies require that infection control measures and safe work practices be applied while serving the public. Infection control (in-FEK-shun con-TROL) refers to the methods used to eliminate or reduce the transmission of infectious (in-FEK-shus) organisms from one individual to another. Since transmission can also occur when using contaminated implements, tools, or equipment, the performance of effective infection control procedures must be a top priority in the salon, spa, and barbershop.

Safe work practices require that implements, tools, and equipment be used safely and that you be aware of situations that can cause accidents. This chapter provides some helpful guidelines to minimize potential risks and accidents.

It is your responsibility as a beauty professional to use proper and effective infection control methods that help safeguard your health and the health of your clients. You are also responsible for employing safe work practices to help prevent accidents and injuries from occurring in the workplace.

FOCUS ON

Infection Control Vocabulary

Before we discuss infection control and safe work practices, the terms *cleaning*, *sanitizing*, *disinfecting*, and *sterilizing* need to be properly differentiated:

- *Cleaning* is a mechanical process using soap and water or detergent and water to remove all visible dirt, debris, and many disease-causing germs. Cleaning also removes invisible debris that interferes with disinfection.
- *Sanitizing* is a chemical process for reducing the number of disease-causing germs on cleaned surfaces to a safe level. Infection control professionals consider sanitation (san-ih-TAY-shun) to be a layperson's term or a product marketing term (as in *hand sanitizers*), preferring *cleaning* to describe the step before disinfecting.
- *Disinfecting* is a chemical process for use with nonporous items that uses specific products to destroy harmful organisms including bacteria, viruses and fungi (except bacterial spores) on implements and environmental surfaces.
- *Sterilizing* is the process that destroys all microbial life, including spores, generally with the use of an autoclave.

Beauty professionals should study and have a thorough understanding of infection control because:

- It is important to know about the pathogens professionals and their clients may be exposed to and their modes of transmission.
- Understanding and practicing proper infection control within the laws and rules will help safeguard professionals' health, the health of their clients, and their business.
- Practicing safety precautions on a daily basis protects their clients and their license.
- A responsible beauty professional is conscientious about infection control and safety.

ACTIVITY

Infection Control on the Home Front

Consider the following questions and then discuss your answers with the rest of the class in comparison to how often you think a salon, spa, or barbershop environment should be cleaned and disinfected.

- How often do you sweep the floors of your home?
- How often do you mop the floors of your home?
- How often do you clean/disinfect the bathroom?
- How often do you clean/disinfect the bathroom doorknob?
- How often do you remove hair and debris from your hairbrush or comb and wash it with soap and water?

DESCRIBE FEDERAL AND STATE REGULATORY AGENCIES

Many federal and state agencies regulate the beauty and wellness professions. Federal agencies set guidelines for the manufacture, sale, and use of equipment and chemical ingredients. These guidelines also monitor safety in the workplace and place limits on the types of services you can perform in a salon, spa, or barbershop. State agencies regulate licensing, enforcement, and your conduct when you are on the job.

FEDERAL AGENCIES

OCCUPATIONAL SAFETY AND HEALTH ADMINISTRATION

The Occupational Safety and Health Administration (OSHA) was created as part of the U.S. Department of Labor to regulate and enforce safety and health standards to protect employees in the workplace. The standards set by OSHA are important to beauty professionals because of the products they use daily. OSHA standards address issues relating to the handling, mixing, storing, and disposing of products; general safety in the workplace; and your right to know about any potentially hazardous ingredients contained in the products and how to avoid these hazards. OSHA does this in part by requiring that chemical manufacturers and importers assess and communicate the potential hazards associated with their products through a Safety Data Sheet (SDS). An SDS is a 16-category, standard-format document that replaces the previously mandated MSDS or PSDS. *Chapter 6: "Chemistry & Chemical Safety" goes into depth on how to read an SDS.*

ENVIRONMENTAL PROTECTION AGENCY

The Environmental Protection Agency (EPA) registers all types of disinfectants sold and used in the United States. Disinfectants (dis-in-FEK-tents) are chemical products that destroy most bacteria (excluding spores), fungi, and viruses on surfaces. It is against federal law to use any disinfecting product in a way contrary to the use indicated on its label. Before manufacturers can sell a product for disinfecting surfaces, tools, implements, or equipment, they must obtain an EPA registration number (indicated on a product label by "EPA Reg. No." near the manufacturer's name) that certifies that the disinfectant, when used correctly, will be effective against the pathogens listed on the label. For example, clipper disinfectants must be approved by the EPA for use with clippers in specific environments (such as a barbershop) or the manufacturer would be breaking federal law by marketing them as clipper disinfectants to the barber market. This also means that if you do not follow the label instructions for mixing, contact time, and the type of surface the disinfecting product can be used on, you are not complying with federal law (**Figure 5-1**). If there were an injury-related lawsuit, you could be held responsible.

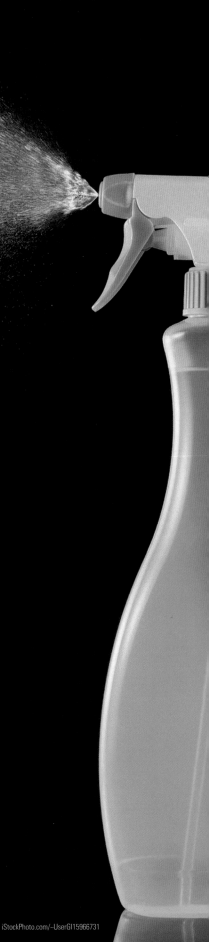

iStockPhoto.com/~UserGI15966731

HERE'S A TIP

You can find a list of disinfectants approved by the EPA by going to the EPA's website at http://www.epa.gov and entering a search on the home page for EPA-registered disinfectants. Disinfectants are not listed as "hospital grade" but instead are listed based on the pathogens they are effective against. Products on list D meet the criteria of most states for hospital disinfectants; products on list E meet the criteria of a tuberculocidal in those states where that is required.

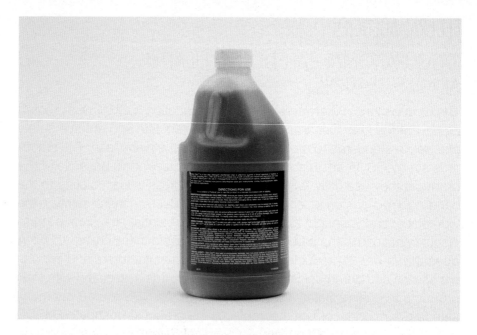

▲ FIGURE 5-1 Follow all label instructions, especially when it comes to disinfectants.

STATE REGULATORY AGENCIES

State regulatory agencies exist to protect beauty professionals' and their customers' health and safety during services. State regulatory agencies include licensing agencies, state boards, commissions, and health departments. Regulatory agencies require that everyone working with clients in a salon, spa, or barbershop follow specific procedures. Enforcement of the rules through inspections and investigations of consumer complaints is also part of an agency's responsibility. An agency can issue penalties against both owners and beauty professional. Penalties vary and include warnings, fines, probation, and suspension or revocation of licenses. It is vital that you understand and follow the laws and rules of your state at all times. Your professional reputation, your license, and your clients' safety depend on it.

LAWS AND RULES—WHAT IS THE DIFFERENCE?

Laws are written by both federal and state legislatures to determine the scope of practice (what each license allows the holder to do) and establish guidelines for regulatory agencies to make rules. Laws are also called *statutes*.

Rules and regulations are more specific than laws. The regulatory agency or the state board writes the rules and determines how the law must be applied. Rules establish specific standards of conduct and can be changed or updated frequently. It is the beauty professional's responsibility to be aware of any changes to the rules and regulations and to comply with them. Ignorance of the law is not an acceptable reason or excuse for noncompliance.

CAUTION

Remember, beauty professionals are not allowed to treat or recommend treatments for infections, diseases, or abnormal conditions. Customers with such problems should be referred to their physicians.

CHECK IN

What are the primary purposes of regulatory agencies?

RECOGNIZE THE PRINCIPLES OF INFECTION

Being a beauty professional is not just rewarding: It is also a great responsibility. One careless action could cause injury or spread **disease** (diz-EEZ), which is any abnormal condition of all or part of the body, its systems, or its organs that makes the body incapable of carrying on normal functions. If your actions hurt a client or make them ill, you could lose your license or ruin your salon, spa, or barbershop's reputation. Fortunately, preventing the spread of **infection** (in-FEK-shun), the invasion of body tissues by disease-causing pathogens, is possible when you know proper procedures and follow them at all times. Prevention begins and ends with you.

Effective infection control also influences the professional image of your establishment. A client's first impression begins the moment they open the door, so a clean environment should extend beyond each professional's immediate work area. All of the sights, sounds, smells, and textures of the salon, spa, or barbershop meld together to form this first impression regardless of the number of times a client has previously visited. A clean and orderly business helps build client confidence and trust that continuous care is being taken to provide a safe and sanitary environment in which to receive personal services.

MODES OF TRANSMISSION

All pathogens are different in terms of where they reside and how they infect humans. Bacteria, viruses, and fungi have different ways of moving from one person to another or from an object to a person. *Transmission* (trans-MISH-uhn) is the process by which pathogens move between individuals and objects—this is *how* we get sick. Merely being exposed to pathogens does not make you sick, as your immune system may be able to put up a good fight. However, transmission is the necessary first step in getting sick, and if you prevent transmission, you prevent illness. The most common types of transmission in the salon, spa, or barbershop environment are direct, indirect (surface), airborne and respiratory droplet.

DIRECT TRANSMISSION

Direct transmission (die-REKT trans-MISH-uhn) is what we most commonly think of in terms of getting sick, as it involves the transmission of pathogens through touching, kissing, coughing, sneezing, and talking. For example, if you shake hands with every customer and one of them has a cold virus, it can be transmitted to you, possibly making you sick if you touch your mouth or nose afterward. If you fail to wash your hands after each handshake, then you risk infecting all of your customers as well as yourself (**Figure 5-2**). Parasitic infections and warts are other examples of diseases spread by direct transmission. Fortunately, diseases spread by direct contact cannot live for long periods of time away from a host.

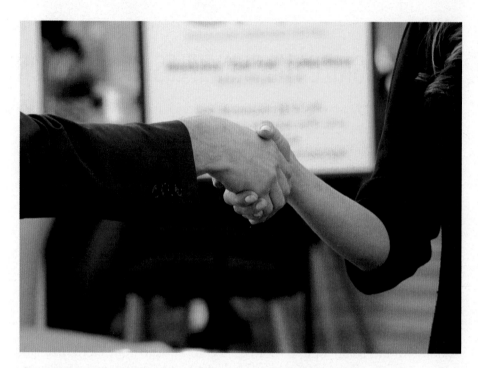

▲ FIGURE 5-2 Shaking hands without washing can directly transmit infections.

INDIRECT TRANSMISSION

Indirect transmission (in-dih-REKT trans-MISH-uhn) occurs through contact with an intermediate contaminated object, such as a razor, extractor, nipper, or an environmental surface upon which the pathogen resides. Doorknobs, phones, food-preparation surfaces, or your implements at work are all possible vectors of indirect transmission. In situations like these, someone has contaminated a surface; the pathogen will attempt to infect anyone who touches that surface, making them their new host. Illnesses transmitted by this method include salmonella, ringworm, and MRSA (**Figure 5-3**).

ACTIVITY

Stopping the Transmission
Look around your classroom and identify all the surfaces, tools, doorknobs, fixtures, etc., that constitute routine sources of contamination. List them as a class, along with possible preventive measures you can take to reduce this transmission.

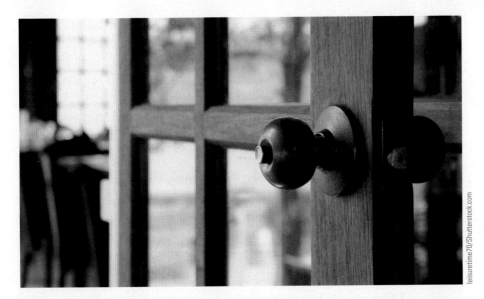

▲ FIGURE 5-3 Doorknobs are a commonly contacted surface ripe for indirect transmission.

AIRBORNE TRANSMISSION AND RESPIRATORY DROPLET

Respiratory droplet and airborne transmission are similar in that transmission occurs when a pathogen living in our respiratory tract is expelled through coughing, sneezing, or even talking. The difference between the two is that respiratory droplets are large particles that do not stay suspended in the air for long – wearing a properly fitted mask should protect you from these pathogens. In airborne transmission, the particles are much smaller and dryer, so they hang in the air longer, allowing for the pathogen to spread further. For an example of respiratory droplet transmission, if you have influenza, every time you exhale your breath carries with it the influenza virus attached to air particles. If you are talking too closely to someone, let alone coughing, sneezing or yelling, you are also projecting those particles into the other person's airspace. This helps explain why we see more influenza in the winter, when people congregate inside and create an environment conducive to spreading the illness through coughing.

PREVENTING TRANSMISSION: INFECTION CONTROL

Under certain conditions, coming into contact with harmful organisms can cause infectious diseases. An infectious disease (in-FEK-shus diz-EEZ) is caused by pathogenic (harmful) organisms that enter the body. An infectious disease, however, may or may not be spread from one person to another, depending on the organism and its method of transmission.

In this chapter, you will learn how to properly clean and disinfect the tools and equipment you use so they are safe for you and your customers. Cleaning (KLEEN-ing) is a mechanical process using soap and water or detergent and water to remove all visible dirt, debris, and many disease-causing germs from tools, implements, and equipment. The process of disinfection (dis-in-FEK-shun) involves the use of a chemical to destroy most, but not necessarily all, harmful organisms on environmental surfaces. Disinfection, however, is not effective against bacterial spores (bak-TEER-ee-ul SPORZ), which are bacteria capable of producing a protective coating that allows them to withstand very harsh environments and to shed the coating when conditions become more favorable to them. Thankfully this type of bacteria is rare and of very little risk in the salon, spa, or barbershop environment.

Cleaning and disinfecting procedures are designed to prevent the spread of infection and disease. At a minimum, disinfectants used in salons, spas, and barbershops must be

- **bactericidal** (bak-TEER-uh-SYD-uhl), capable of destroying bacteria;
- **virucidal** (viy-ruh-SYD-uhl), capable of destroying viruses; and
- **fungicidal** (fun-ji-SYD-uhl), capable of destroying molds and fungi.

HERE'S A TIP

You should know how to look for specific things on the label of any product you use for disinfection in the salon, spa, or barbershop. It should always have the following:

- The list of pathogens against which it is effective; should include HIV (human immunodeficiency virus), HBV (hepatitis B virus), and MRSA (methicillin-resistant staphylococcus aureus); if Pseudomonas aeruginosa is included, the disinfectant will kill other lesser bacteria (**Figure 5-4**)
- EPA registration number
- The words *bactericidal*, *virucidal*, and *fungicidal*
- Mixing and changing instructions

PATHOGEN/PATÓGENO	CONTACT TIME/TIEMPO DE CONTACTO
Clostridium difficile/Clostridium difficile	3 minutes/3 minutos
Bacteria/Bacteria	30 seconds/30 segundos
‡Viruses/‡Virus	1 minute/1 minuto
‡‡Bloodborne Pathogens/ ‡‡Patógenos de Transmisión Sanguinea	1 minute/1 minuto
TB/TB	3 minutes/3 minutos
Parvoviruses/Parvovirus	3 minutes/3 minutos
Fungi/Fungo	3 minutes/3 minutos

ORGANISMS:

Bacteria:
- Acinetobacter baumannii*
- Bordetella pertussis*
- Campylobacter jejuni*
- Carbapenem resistant Klebsiella pneumoniae (CRKP)*
- Clostridium difficile spores***§
- Community Acquired Methicillin resistant Staphylococcus aureus (NARSA NRS123)*
- Community Acquired Methicillin resistant Staphylococcus aureus (NARSA NRS384)*

- Linezolid resistant Staphylococcus aureus (LRSA)*
- Listeria monocytogenes*
- Methicillin resistant Staphylococcus aureus*
- Multi-drug resistant Enterococcus faecium (MDR E. faecium)*
- Proteus mirabilis*
- Pseudomonas aeruginosa*
- Salmonella enterica*
- Serratia marcescens*
- Shigella dysenteriae*
- Staphylococcus aureus*

- ‡Rhinovirus type 37**
- ‡Rotavirus**

Bloodborne Pathogens:
- ‡‡HIV type 1*
- ‡‡Human Hepatitis B**
- ‡‡Human Hepatitis C**

Parvoviruses:
- Canine parvovirus***
- Feline parvovirus***

Fungi:
- Trichophyton mentagrophytes***
- Candida albicans***

Use Sites:
- Ambulances
- BP monitors
- Carts
- Critical care units
- Dialysis clinics
- Emergency rooms
- Examination rooms
- Footboards
- Glucometers
- Headboards
- Hospitals
- Intensive care units
- IV stands
- Nurse-call device
- Nurses' stations
- Nursing homes
- ORs
- Patient restrooms
- Patient rooms
- Radiology rooms
- Recovery rooms
- Sills ledges

Medical Surfaces:
- Bed railings
- Cabinets
- Coated mattresses

- Coated pillows
- Computer keyboards
- Desk tops
- Doorknobs
- Exam tables
- Gurneys
- Hard, nonporous medical surfaces
- High touch surfaces
- Phone cradle
- Pipes
- Showers
- Shower fixtures
- Sinks
- Stretchers
- Support bars
- Tables
- Telephones
- Wheelchairs

Surface Materials:
- Chrome
- Enamel
- Glass
- Glazed ceramic
- Glazed porcelain
- Laminated surfaces
- Plastic

▲ **FIGURE 5-4** Disinfectant labels should include the product's efficacy claims.

Be sure to mix and use these disinfectants according to the instructions on the labels so they are safe and effective (**Figure 5-5**). Remember, in some states, disinfectants may still need to be effective against tuberculosis (tuberculocidal). Check your state board rules and regulations for compliance information.

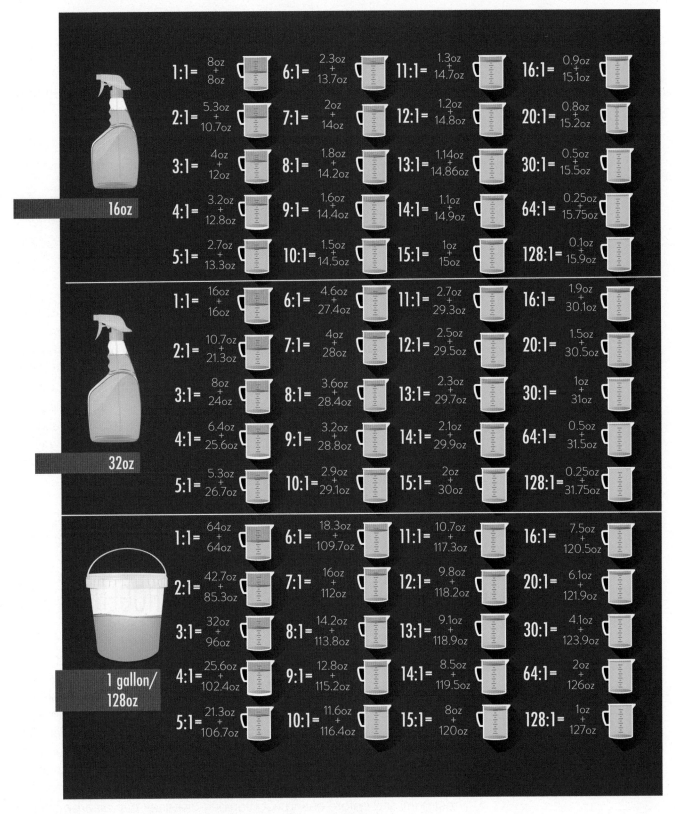

▲ FIGURE 5-5 Understand and follow the mixing instructions on disinfectants.

PREVENTION 101

In general, the risk of infection can be greatly reduced with a few simple steps:

- Eliminate pathogens through proper hand washing, cleaning, and disinfection.
- Clean and disinfect tools and equipment after every service.
- Keep your skin intact to reduce portals of entry for bacteria. Wear gloves when working with chemicals, use lotion to reduce skin drying and cracking, and cover open wounds.
- Be prepared to turn away clients who show signs of illness. Remember, you are not licensed to diagnose illness or infection. Refer ill patients to their doctor for a proper diagnosis and treatment regimen.

PERSONAL HABITS

It is important to think about your personal habits in terms of how they might increase or decrease the risk of transmitting an illness. For example, if you see 50 clients a week and you shake hands with each of them, you are exposing yourself to everything on the hands of those 50 people, every week—it's only a matter of time before you will get sick! However, making a habit of following the rules of proper cleaning and disinfection, both in your home and at work, will help decrease the odds of falling ill. Hand washing, cleaning, and disinfection are all ways in which you can personally combat the spread of disease and safeguard your health and that of your clients.

CHECK IN
What are four modes of pathogen transmission?

IDENTIFY DIFFERENT TYPES OF PATHOGENS

When a disease is capable of being spread from one person to another, it is said to be a contagious disease (kon-TAY-jus diz-EEZ), also known as a communicable (kuh-MYOO-nih-kuh-bul) disease. Some of the more prevalent contagious diseases that prevent a beauty professional from servicing a client are the common cold, ringworm, conjunctivitis (pinkeye), and viral infections. These infections are most often spread through dirty hands, especially under the fingernails and in the webs between the fingers. In many states, you are required to wash your hands prior to every client, but in all states you must wash your hands after using the restroom and before eating. Contagious diseases can also be spread by contaminated implements, cuts, infected nails, open sores, pus, mouth and nose discharges, shared drinking cups, telephone receivers, and towels. Uncovered coughing or sneezing and spitting in public also spread germs. **Table 5-1** lists additional terms and definitions that are important for a general understanding of disease.

TABLE 5-1: ADDITIONAL TERMS RELATED TO DISEASE

TERM	DEFINITION
Contamination (kun-tam-uh-NAY-shun)	The presence, or the reasonably anticipated presence, of blood or other potentially infectious materials on an item's surface, or visible debris or residues such as dust, hair, and skin.
Decontamination	The removal of blood or other potentially infectious materials on an item's surface and the removal of visible debris or residues such as dust, hair, and skin.
Diagnosis (dy-ag-NO-sis)	Determination of the nature of a disease from its symptoms and/or diagnostic tests. Federal regulations prohibit salon professionals from performing a diagnosis.
Germs	Nonscientific synonym for disease-producing organisms.
Occupational Disease (ahk-u-PAY-shun-al diz-EEZ)	Illnesses resulting from conditions associated with employment, such as prolonged and repeated overexposure to certain products or ingredients.
Parasitic Disease (pahr-a-SIT-ick diz-EEZ)	Disease caused by parasites such as lice and mites.
Pathogenic Disease (path-uh-JEN-ick diz-EEZ)	Disease produced by organisms such as bacteria, viruses, fungi, and parasites.
Toxins	Various poisonous substances produced by some microorganisms (bacteria and viruses).

When it comes to preventing the spread of infectious disease, beauty professionals must understand and be prepared to deal with five types of potentially harmful organisms:

- Bacteria
- Viruses
- Fungi
- Parasites
- Biofilms

BACTERIA

Bacteria (bak-TEER-ee-ah) (singular: *bacterium* [bak-TEER-ee-uhm]) are single-celled microorganisms that have both plant and animal characteristics. A microorganism (my-kro-OR-gah-niz-um) is any organism of microscopic or submicroscopic size. Some bacteria are harmful, while others are harmless. Bacteria can exist almost anywhere: on skin, in water, in the air, in decayed matter, on environmental surfaces, in body

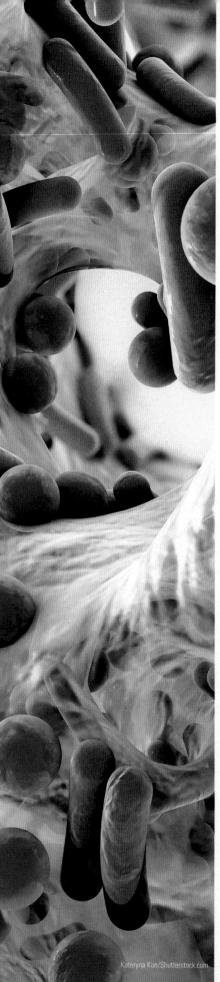

secretions, on clothing, or under the free edge of nails. Bacteria are so small they can be seen only with a microscope.

TYPES OF BACTERIA

There are thousands of different kinds of bacteria, which fall into two primary types: pathogenic and nonpathogenic. Most bacteria are nonpathogenic (nahn-path-uh-JEN-ik); in other words, they are harmless organisms that may perform useful functions. They are safe to come in contact with since they do not cause disease or harm. For example, nonpathogenic organisms are used to make yogurt, cheese, and some medicines. In the human body, nonpathogenic bacteria help the body break down food, protect against infection, and stimulate the immune system.

Pathogenic (path-uh-JEN-ik) bacteria are harmful microorganisms that can cause disease or infection in humans when they invade the body. Salons, spas, and barbershops must maintain strict standards for cleaning and disinfecting at all times to prevent the spread of pathogenic microorganisms. It is crucial that students learn proper infection control practices while in school to ensure that they understand the importance of following them throughout their career.

ACTIVITY

Attacking the Source
Consider where bacteria might grow and reproduce in a salon, spa, barbershop, or school. Keep in mind that bacteria multiply best in warm, dark, damp, or dirty places. Discuss with your classmates how you can help stop the growth and spread of bacteria.

BACTERIAL INFECTIONS

There can be no bacterial infection without the presence of pathogenic bacteria. Therefore, if pathogenic bacteria are eliminated, clients cannot become infected.

Inflammation (in-fluh-MAY-shun) is a condition in which the tissue of the body reacts to injury, irritation, or infection. Inflammation is characterized by redness, heat, pain, and/or swelling.

Pus (PUS) is a fluid containing white blood cells, bacteria, and dead cells, and is the by-product of the infectious process. The presence of pus is a sign of a bacterial infection. A local infection (LOKE-uhl in-FEK-shun), such as a pimple or abscess (**Figure 5-6**), is confined to a particular part of the body and appears as a lesion containing pus. A systemic infection (sis-TEM-ik in-FEK-shun) is an infection where the pathogen has spread throughout the body rather than staying in one area or organ.

Kateryna Kon/Shutterstock.com

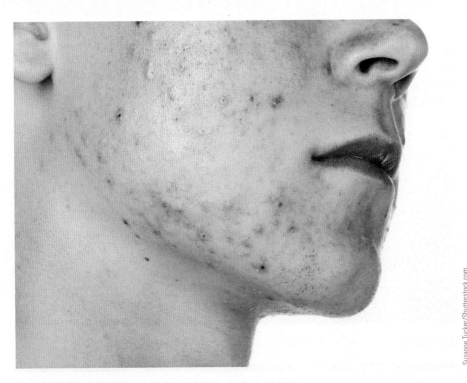

▲ **FIGURE 5-6** Pimples are an example of a local infection.

MRSA

Staphylococci (staf-uh-loh-KOKS-eye) are among the most common bacteria that affect humans and are routinely found in our environment, including on our bodies, although most strains do not make us ill. Staph bacteria can be picked up on doorknobs, countertops, and other surfaces; however, they are more frequently spread in salons, spas, or barbershops through skin-to-skin contact (such as shaking hands), pedicure bowls, or the use of unclean tools or implements, and can be very dangerous.

Staph is responsible for food poisoning and a wide range of diseases, including toxic shock syndrome and some flesh-eating diseases. Some types of infectious staph bacteria are highly resistant to conventional treatments such as antibiotics. An example is the staph infection called methicillin-resistant staphylococcus aureus (meth-uh-SILL-en ree-ZIST-ent staf-uh-loh-KOK-us OR-ee-us) (**Figure 5-7**). Historically, MRSA occurred most frequently among persons with weakened immune systems or who had undergone medical procedures. Today, it has become more common in otherwise healthy people. Clients who appear completely healthy may bring this organism into the shop with them, where it can infect others. Some people carry the bacteria and are not even aware of their infection; however, the people they infect may show more obvious symptoms.

In general, MRSA initially appears as a skin infection, resulting in pimples, rashes, or boils that can be difficult to cure. Without proper treatment, the infection becomes systemic and can have devastating consequences, even resulting in death. Because of these highly resistant bacterial strains, it is important to clean and disinfect all tools and implements used on customers. Additionally, do not perform services if your client's skin, scalp, or neck show visible signs of abrasion or infection.

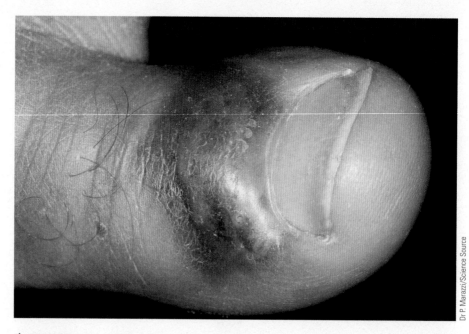

▲ FIGURE 5-7   MRSA infection in a toe.

MYCOBACTERIUM

Mycobacterium (my-co-bac-TEER-ee-um) is the name for a large family of bacteria that is often found in soil and water. In recent years, it has been linked to disfiguring infections associated particularly with pedicure bowls. Because this bacterium may be present in your water supply, it is important to protect your clients by properly disinfecting all implements and bowls. It is also important that both you and your client keep your skin intact and protected. Avoid cracked skin by using lotions frequently, particularly in the winter months. Advise clients not to shave or wax their legs 24 hours prior to a pedicure (**Figure 5-8**).

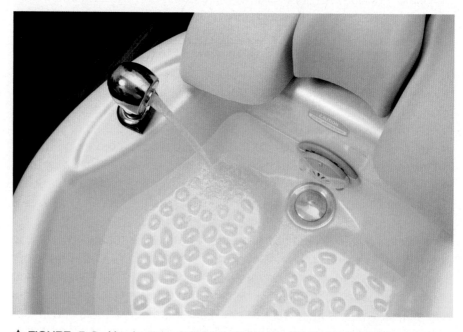

▲ FIGURE 5-8   Mycobacterium infection has been associated with pedicure bowls.

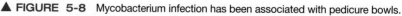

VIRUSES

A virus (VY-rus) is a submicroscopic particle that infects and resides in the cells of a biological organism. A virus is capable of replication only through taking over the host cell's reproductive function. Viruses are so small that they can be seen only under the most sophisticated and powerful microscopes. They cause common colds and other respiratory and gastrointestinal (digestive tract) infections. Some of the viruses that plague humans are measles, mumps, chickenpox, smallpox, rabies, yellow fever, hepatitis, polio, influenza, and HIV (which causes AIDS).

One difference between viruses and bacteria is that a virus can live and reproduce only by taking over other cells and becoming part of them, while bacteria can live and reproduce on their own. Another difference is that while bacterial infections can usually be treated with specific antibiotics, viral infections cannot; also, viruses are hard to kill without harming the host cells in the process (**Figure 5-9**).

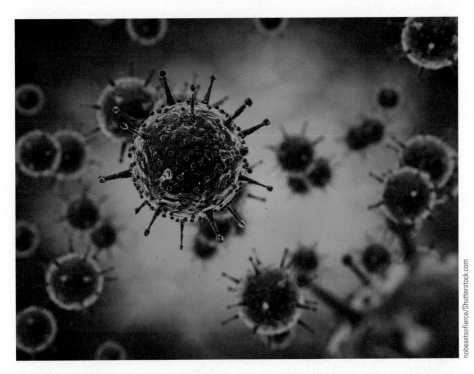

▲ **FIGURE 5-9** Viruses.

PREVENTION

Although we cannot cure viruses, we can often prevent contracting and spreading them through the use of vaccinations. Although there have been several controversies over vaccines in the past, discuss with your physician the vaccines that are recommended for you based on your type of employment, age, and medical history. Along with vaccines, hand washing and disinfection are your best defense against becoming sick with a virus (**Figure 5-10**).

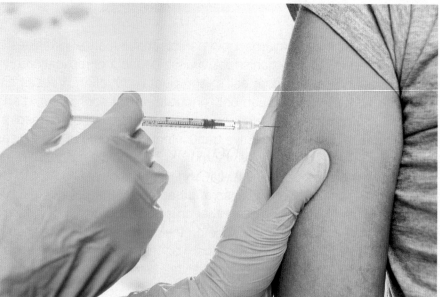

▲ FIGURE 5-10 Vaccines combined with a strong daily infection control regimen are the best way to fight viruses.

INCUBATION AND CONTAINMENT

Many viruses can remain dormant for months to years following exposure, but most produce signs of illness within 10 to 14 days. Unfortunately, in most cases, a person is highly contagious in the days just before symptoms appear. This makes prevention paramount in reducing the spread of illness. Containment is achieved when those who are ill stay home—away from work, school, malls, etc.—until their symptoms resolve to the extent that they are no longer contagious. If you believe you have influenza, for example, it is important to see your doctor as soon as possible, as the medication used to reduce symptoms is only effective if given in the first 48 hours.

HPV AND HSV

Human papilloma virus (HYOO-mun pap-uh-LOW-ma VY-rus) and Herpes simplex virus (HER-peez SIM-pleks VY-rus) are two highly contagious viruses that can be transmitted both directly and indirectly. Both of these viruses can be spread through skin-to-skin contact and are often thought of as sexually transmitted diseases. However, both viruses can also be spread from person to person indirectly through items like a wax pot. Because the majority of people infected with these viruses have no symptoms, it is even more important to follow good infection control procedures with all procedures that may involve contact with blood and fluids (**Figure 5-11**).

HEPATITIS AND HIV/AIDS

Disease-causing microorganisms that are carried in the body by blood or body fluids, such as hepatitis and HIV, are called bloodborne pathogens (BLUD-born PATH-o-genz). In the salon, spa, and barbershop, the

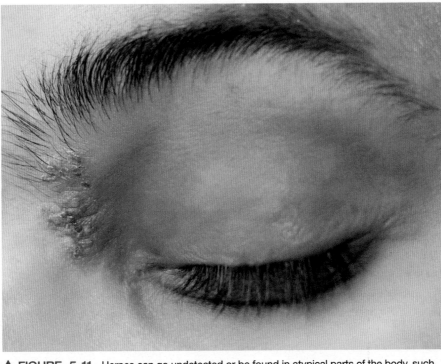

▲ FIGURE 5-11 Herpes can go undetected or be found in atypical parts of the body, such as the eyebrow.

mortalpious/Shutterstock.com

spread of bloodborne pathogens is possible whenever the skin is broken. Use great care to avoid cutting or damaging the customer's skin during any type of service.

Hepatitis (hep-uh-TY-tis) is a bloodborne virus that causes disease and can damage the liver. In general, it is difficult to contract hepatitis. However, it is easier to contract than HIV because it can be present in all body fluids of those who are infected. In addition, unlike HIV, hepatitis can live on a surface outside the body for long periods of time. For this reason, it is vital that all surfaces that a customer comes into contact with are thoroughly cleaned and disinfected.

The human immunodeficiency virus (HYOO-mun ih-MYOO-noh-di-FISH-en-see VY-rus), abbreviated HIV, causes acquired immune deficiency syndrome (uh-KWY-erd ih-MYOON di-FISH-en-see SIN-drome), abbreviated AIDS. AIDS is a disease that breaks down the body's immune system. HIV is spread from person to person through blood and, less often, through other body fluids, such as semen and vaginal secretions. A person can be infected with HIV for many years without showing symptoms; some people who are HIV-positive have never been tested and do not know they have the potential to infect others.

If you accidentally cut a client's skin, the tool will be contaminated with whatever might be in the client's blood, including bloodborne pathogens. You should not continue to use the implement without cleaning and disinfecting it. Continuing to use a contaminated implement without cleaning and disinfecting it puts you and others in the salon, spa, or barbershop at risk of infection.

iStockPhoto.com/ugurhan

FUNGI

Fungi (FUN-ji) (singular: *fungus* [FUN-gus]) are single-celled organisms that grow in irregular masses that include molds, mildews, and yeasts. They can produce contagious diseases, such as ringworm. Mildew (MIL-doo), another fungus, affects plants or grows on inanimate objects but does not cause human infections in the salon, spa, or barbershop.

The most frequently encountered fungal infection resulting from hair services is tinea barbae (TIN-ee-uh BAR-bee), also known as *barber's itch*. A person with tinea barbae may have deep, inflamed or noninflamed patches of skin on the face or the nape of the neck. Tinea barbae is similar to tinea capitis (TIN-ee-uh kap-EYE-tus), a fungal infection of the scalp characterized by red papules, or spots, at the opening of hair follicles. Ringworm (RING-wurm), a fungal infection of the skin that appears in circular lesions, is another fungus that may contraindicate a beauty service (**Figure 5-12**).

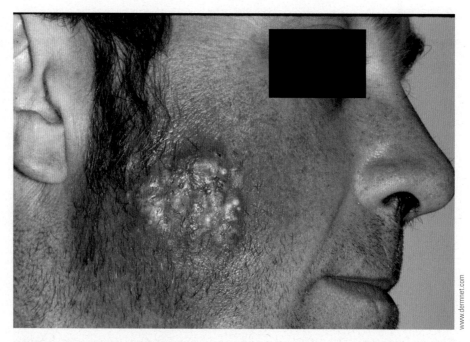

www.dermnet.com

▲ **FIGURE 5-12** Ringworm.

While all beauty professionals must avoid spreading scalp and skin infections, the increased risk for hair services in particular can be reduced by diligently cleaning and disinfecting clippers and similar cutting tools. Always refer to the manufacturer's directions for proper cleaning and disinfecting methods and recommendations.

DID YOU KNOW?

Pathogenic bacteria, viruses, or fungi can enter the body through the following routes:

- *Skin*: broken or inflamed skin, such as a cut or a scratch, or a bruise (weakened tissue) or a rash, but not through intact skin, which is an effective barrier to infection
- *Mouth*: contaminated water, food, fingers, or objects
- *Nose*: inhaling infectious dust or droplets from a cough or sneeze
- *Eyes or ears*: organisms that reside in water that are commonly transmitted when the person is swimming
- *Genitals*: unprotected sex

The body prevents and controls infections through:

- healthy, uncompromised skin—the body's first line of defense
- body secretions, such as perspiration and digestive juices
- white blood cells that destroy bacteria
- antitoxins that counteract toxins (various poisonous substances produced by some microorganisms such as bacteria and viruses)

PARASITES

Parasites (PAYR-uh-sytz) are organisms that grow, feed, and shelter on or inside another organism (referred to as a *host*), while contributing nothing to the survival of that organism. They must have a host to survive. Parasites can live on or inside of humans and animals. They also can be found in food, on plants and trees, and in water. Humans can acquire internal parasites by eating fish or meat that has not been properly cooked. External parasites that affect humans by way of the skin include ticks, lice, fleas, and mites. Services should never be performed on a customer with visible signs of a parasitic infestation. Always refer the client to a physician for treatment.

There are two types of parasites commonly encountered in the salon, spa, and barbershop environment:

- Head lice (**Figure 5-13**) are a type of parasite responsible for contagious diseases and conditions. One condition caused by an infestation of head lice is called pediculosis capitis (puh-dik-yuh-LO-sis kap-EYE-tus).
- Scabies (SKAY-beez) is a contagious skin disease caused by the itch mite, which burrows under the skin.

Contagious diseases and conditions caused by parasites should only be treated by a doctor. Contaminated countertops, tools, and equipment should be thoroughly cleaned and then disinfected with an EPA-registered disinfectant for the time recommended by the manufacturer or with a bleach solution for 10 minutes.

BIOFILMS

Biofilms (BY-o-films) are colonies of microorganisms that adhere to environmental surfaces, as well as the human body. They secrete a sticky,

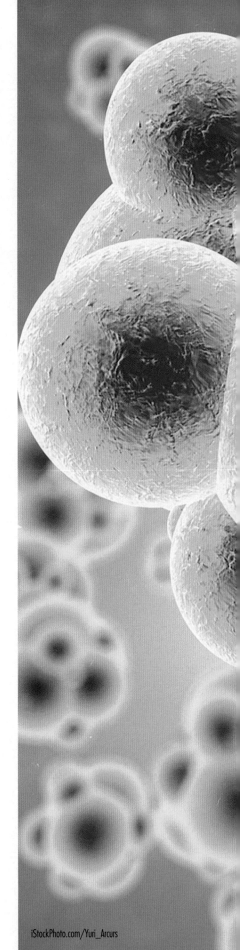

iStockPhoto.com/Yuri_Arcurs

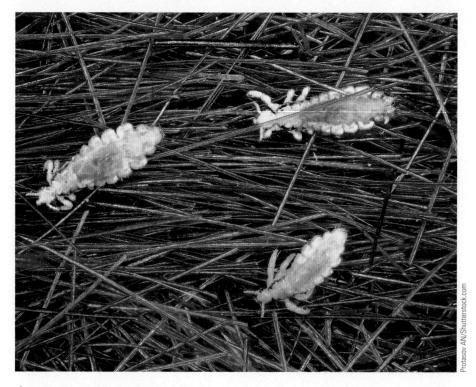

▲ FIGURE 5-13 Head lice.

hard-to-penetrate, protective coating that cements them together. The biofilm grows into a complex structure, with many kinds of microbes. The sticky matrix substance holds communities together, making them very hard to pierce with antiseptics, antimicrobials, and disinfection, ultimately keeping the body in a chronic inflammatory state that is painful and inhibits healing. One action of the biofilm community is to resist the body's defense mechanisms; we are learning that biofilms play a large role in disease and infection.

Biofilms are usually not visible and must grow very large to be seen without a microscope. Dental plaque is an example of a visible human biofilm, and algae colonies on ponds and slime in drains are examples of visible environmental biofilms. In the beauty and wellness world, foot spas can harbor biofilm and require extra attention, especially piped models.

Because biofilms are hard to detect, their presence and effects seem to be underestimated. They are one of the most significant scientific discoveries of the past few decades, though we have much more to learn. Conscientiously using infection control precautions, including Standard Precautions, cleaning, disinfection, and sterilization, is the best method of prevention at the present time.

CHECK IN
List the five types of organisms that are important to a beauty professional.

EMPLOY THE PRINCIPLES OF PREVENTION

Proper infection control can prevent the spread of disease caused by exposure to potentially infectious materials on an item's surface. Infection control will also prevent exposure to blood and visible debris or residue such as dust, hair, and skin.

Proper infection control requires two steps: cleaning and then disinfecting with an appropriate EPA-registered disinfectant. When these two steps are followed correctly, virtually all pathogens of concern in the salon, spa, or barbershop can be effectively eliminated.

Sterilization (ster-ih-luh-ZAY-shun), which is the process that destroys all microbial life including spores, can be incorporated but is rarely mandated. Effective sterilization typically requires the use of an autoclave (**Figure 5-14**)—a piece of equipment that incorporates heat and pressure. For sterilization to be effective, items must be cleaned prior to use and the autoclave must be tested and maintained as instructed in the manufacturer's specifications. The Centers for Disease Control and Prevention (CDC) requires that autoclaves be tested monthly to ensure they are properly sterilizing implements. The accepted method is called a *spore test*. Sealed packages containing test organisms are subjected to a typical sterilization cycle and then sent to a contract laboratory that specializes in autoclave performance testing.

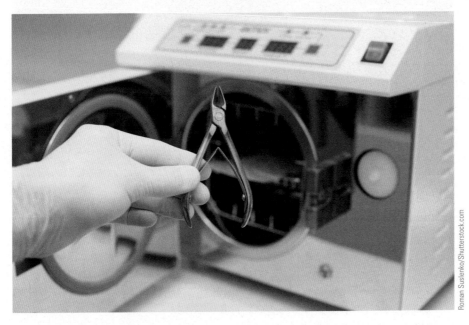

Roman Suslenko/Shutterstock.com

▲ FIGURE 5-14 Sterilization using an autoclave.

STEP 1: CLEANING

The first step in infection control is cleaning. Remember that when you clean, you must remove all visible and surface dirt and debris from tools, implements, and equipment by washing them with liquid soap or detergent and warm water, or a chemical cleaner, and using a clean and disinfected brush to scrub any grooved or hinged portions of the item.

When a surface is properly cleaned, the number of contaminants on the surface is greatly reduced. In addition, proper cleaning removes any oils or residue from items that might interfere with disinfectant being able to work properly. This is why cleaning is an important part of disinfecting tools and equipment. A surface must be properly cleaned before it can be properly disinfected. Using a disinfectant without cleaning first is like using mouthwash without brushing your teeth—it just does not work properly!

Cleaned surfaces can still harbor small amounts of pathogens, but the presence of fewer pathogens means infections are less likely to be spread (**Figure 5-15**). Applying antiseptics to your skin or washing your hands with soap and water will drastically lower the number of pathogens on your hands. Do not underestimate proper cleaning and hand washing. They are the most powerful and important ways to prevent the spread of infection.

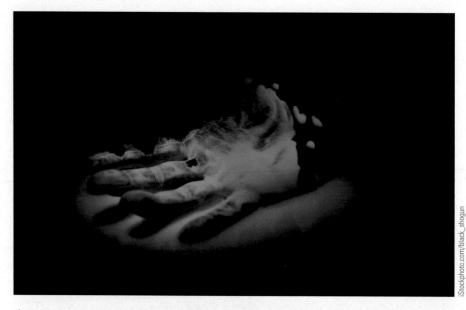

▲ FIGURE 5-15   Unwashed hands can be swarming with pathogens.

There are three ways to clean your tools and implements:

- Washing with soap and warm water and then scrubbing them with a clean and properly disinfected nailbrush
- Using an ultrasonic unit
- Using a chemical cleaner

CAUTION
Read labels carefully. Manufacturers take great care to develop safe and highly effective products. However, when used improperly, many products that are otherwise safe can be rendered dangerous if you do not follow proper guidelines and directions exactly as the label instructs.

HAND WASHING

Properly washing your hands is one of the most important actions you can take to prevent spreading germs from one person to another. Proper hand washing removes germs from the folds and grooves of the skin and from under the free edge of the nail plate by lifting and rinsing germs and contaminants from the surface of your skin. You should wash your hands thoroughly before and after working with each client. Follow the hand washing procedure described in **Procedure 5-1**.

> **CAUTION**
> When washing hands, use liquid soaps in pump containers. Bacteria can grow in bar soaps.

ANTIBACTERIAL SOAPS

While there are many marketing claims on soaps these days, antibacterial and antimicrobial soaps have been under the scrutiny of the FDA since 2014. In 2016, many of the chemicals used in these soaps were banned. What's more, research has shown that repeated use of antibacterial products can actually increase the growth of some of the worst pathogens. The true benefit of hand washing comes from the friction created by the soap bubbles that works to "pull" pathogens off the skin surface. Repeated hand washing can also dry the skin, so using a moisturizing hand lotion after washing is a good practice. Be sure the hand lotion is in a pump container, not a jar.

Avoid using very hot water to wash your hands because this is another practice that can damage the skin. Remember, you must wash your hands thoroughly before and after each service, so do all you can to reduce any irritation that may occur.

WATERLESS HAND SANITIZERS

Antiseptics (ant-ih-SEP-tiks) are chemical germicides formulated for use on skin and are registered and regulated by the Food and Drug Administration. Antiseptics generally contain a high volume of alcohol and are intended to reduce the numbers and slow the growth of microbes on the skin (**Figure 5-16**). When there is visible dirt/debris on the hands, neither waterless hand sanitizers nor antiseptics will work until the dirt/debris is removed; this can be accomplished only with liquid soap, a soft-bristle brush, and water.

Due to the drying effect of alcohol, hand sanitizers should not be overused, but, if allowed by your state, they are an excellent option when hand washing is not possible. Never use an antiseptic to disinfect instruments or other surfaces. It is ineffective for that purpose. Be warned that the high percentage of alcohol can dry the skin to the point of causing openings that allow for infectious agents to infect you. With that in mind, only use hand sanitizers as a secondary option to hand washing.

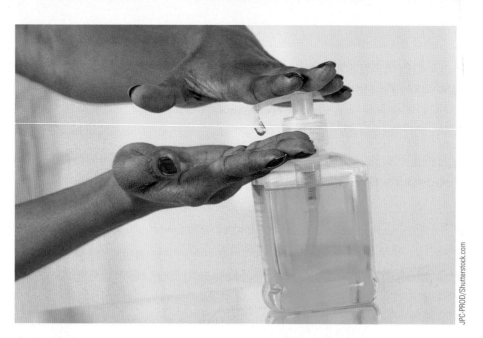

▲ FIGURE 5-16 Hand sanitizers contain a high concentration of alcohol.

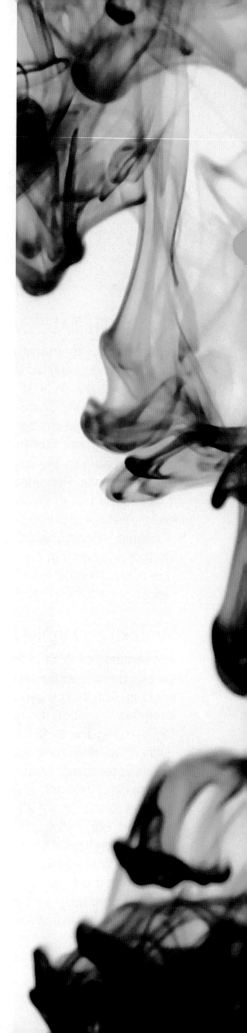

JPC-PROD/Shutterstock.com

> **CAUTION**
> Products and equipment that do not have the word *disinfectant* on the label are merely cleaners. They do not disinfect.

COMMON ANTISEPTICS USED IN THE SALON, SPA, AND BARBERSHOP

- Hydrogen peroxide has been used in homes and the beauty industry virtually forever. It is generally used at 3 percent strength and works well as an antiseptic. However, it should never be used on an open cut, as it destroys the cells that begin the healing process in a wound.

- Isopropyl alcohol is effective in cleaning the skin; however, it can be very drying and cause irritation of the skin. Alcohol is not a disinfectant for surfaces or implements and should be used only as a cleaner or antiseptic.

STEP 2: DISINFECTING

The second step of infection control is disinfection. Remember that disinfection is the process that eliminates most, but not necessarily all, microorganisms on nonporous surfaces. This process, however, is not effective against bacterial spores. In the salon, spa, and barbershop, disinfection is extremely effective in controlling microorganisms on surfaces such as shears, clippers, and other multiuse (mul-tye-YOOS) tools and equipment—multiuse refers to items that can be cleaned, disinfected, and used on more than one person. A disinfectant used in the shop must carry an EPA registration number, and the label should clearly state the specific organisms the solution is effective against when used according to the manufacturer's product instructions.

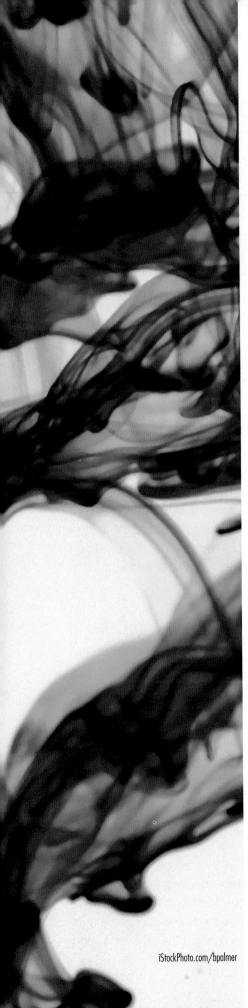

iStockPhoto.com/bpalmer

Remember that disinfectants are products that destroy most bacteria (not including spores), fungi, and viruses on surfaces. Disinfectants are not for use on human skin, hair, or nails. Never use disinfectants as hand cleaners since this can cause skin irritation and allergic reactions. Disinfectants are pesticides and can be harmful if absorbed through the skin.

> **CAUTION**
>
> Improper mixing of disinfectants—to be weaker or more concentrated than the manufacturer's instructions—can significantly reduce their effectiveness. Always add the disinfectant concentrate to the water when mixing and always follow the manufacturer's instructions for proper dilution.
>
> Safety glasses and gloves should be worn while mixing to avoid accidental contact with eyes and skin.

CHOOSING A DISINFECTANT

You must read and follow the manufacturer's instructions whenever you are using a disinfectant. Mixing ratios (dilution) and contact time (the time as listed on the product label required for the disinfectant to be visibly moist to be effective against pathogens) are very important and can vary widely based on manufacturer and delivery method. For example, most concentrates have a 10-minute contact time, whereas most wipes have a 2-minute contact time. In general, as concentration goes up and contact times go down, disinfectants become more corrosive and damaging to implements.

Not all disinfectants have the same concentration, so be sure to mix the correct proportions according to the instructions on the label. If the label does not have the word *concentrate* on it, the product is already mixed and must be used directly from the original container and must not be diluted. All EPA-registered disinfectants, even those sprayed on large surfaces, will specify a contact time in their directions for use. Disinfectants must have efficacy (EF-ih-kuh-see) claims on the label. Efficacy is the ability to produce the intended effect. As applied to disinfectant claims, efficacy means the effectiveness with which a disinfecting solution kills organisms when used according to the label instructions.

PROPER USE OF DISINFECTANTS

Implements must be thoroughly cleaned of all visible matter or residue before being placed in disinfectant solution. This is because residue will interfere with the disinfectant and prevent proper disinfection. Properly cleaned implements and tools, free from all visible debris, must be completely immersed in disinfectant solution. Complete immersion means there is enough liquid in the container to cover all surfaces of the item being disinfected, including the handles, for 10 minutes or for the time recommended by the manufacturer (**Figure 5-17**). When using a spray, wipe, or aerosol disinfectant, you must still look for and adhere to the contact time to ensure that all pathogens on the label are being effectively destroyed.

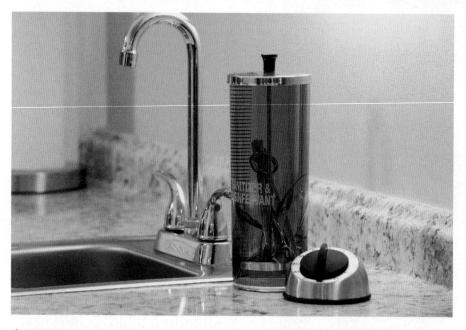
▲ FIGURE 5-17 Implements must be completely immersed in disinfectant solution.

TYPES OF DISINFECTANTS

Disinfectants are not all the same. Some are appropriate for use in the beauty and wellness industry and some are not. As a beauty professional, you will primarily be using disinfectants that are effective for cleaning blood and body fluids from nonporous (nahn-POOR-rus) surfaces. Nonporous items are made of a material that has no pores or openings and that cannot absorb liquids—as opposed to porous (POOR-rus) material that has holes or openings and is absorbent.

QUATS

Quaternary ammonium compounds (KWAT-ur-nayr-ee uh-MO-nee-um KAHM-powndz), also known as *quats* (KWATZ), are disinfectants that are very effective when used properly on nonporous surfaces. The most advanced type of these formulations is called *multiple quats*. Multiple quats contain sophisticated blends of quats that work together to significantly increase the effectiveness of these disinfectants. Quat solutions usually disinfect implements in 10 minutes. As with all disinfectants, leaving tools in a quat solution for prolonged periods can cause dulling or damage. They should be removed from the solution after the specified period, rinsed (if required), dried, and stored in a clean, covered container.

TUBERCULOCIDAL DISINFECTANTS

Tuberculocidal disinfectants (tuh-bur-kyoo-LOH-syd-ahl dis-in-FEK-tents) are proven to kill the bacterium that causes tuberculosis (tuh-bur-kyoo-LO-sus), in addition to other pathogens destroyed through the use of hospital disinfectants. Tuberculosis is a disease caused by a bacterium that is transmitted through coughing or sneezing. It is passed through inhalation only and is not transmitted by the hands or picked up on surfaces.

Phenolic disinfectants (fi-NOH-lik dis-in-FEK-tents) are powerful tuberculocidal disinfectants; however, just because these disinfectants are effective against the pathogen does not mean that you should automatically reach for them. They are a form of formaldehyde, have a very high pH, and can damage the skin and eyes. Phenolic disinfectants can be harmful to the environment if put down the drain. They have been used reliably over the years to disinfect tools; however, they do have significant drawbacks. Phenol can damage plastic and rubber and cause certain metals to rust. Extra care should be taken to avoid skin contact with phenolic disinfectants. Phenolics are known carcinogens and as such should be used only in states that require their use. In those states, you should keep a tuberculocidal disinfectant readily available, but you should use it only when required.

DID YOU KNOW?

While phenolic disinfectants are still required in a handful of states as of this writing, they will be widely unavailable by late 2018. Most states have removed phenolic disinfectants from their requirements, due to the risks outweighing the benefits. Consequently, manufacturers have elected to discontinue the manufacture of these products for the professional beauty industry.

BLEACH

Household bleach, 5.25 percent sodium hypochlorite (SO-dee-um hy-puh-KLOR-eyet), is an effective disinfectant and has been used extensively in salons, spas, and barbershops. Bleach used in the salon, spa, or barbershop must be EPA registered as a disinfectant. Chlorine bleach is the only bleach that disinfects, so it is wise to always look for disinfection instructions on the label to ensure that the bleach you use is actually disinfecting. Bleach is corrosive and can damage metals and plastics (**Figure 5-18**) as well as cause skin irritation and eye damage.

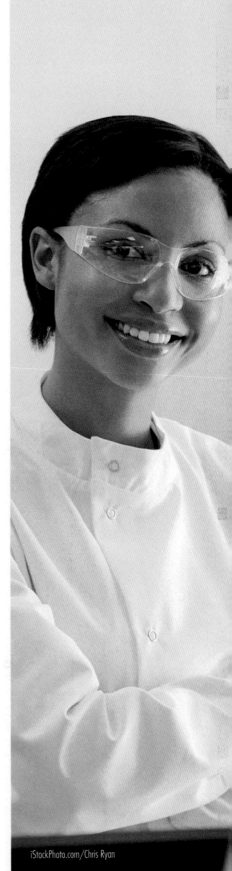

DANGER: POISON:
CORROSIVE. HARMFUL OR FATAL IF SWALLOWED.
PRODUCES CHEMICAL BURNS.
See side panel for precautionary statements and first aid.
NET CONTENTS: 1 Quart / .946 Liters

Product No.: 1730

▲ **FIGURE 5-18** Pay attention to warnings on product labels.

iStockPhoto.com/Chris Ryan

To mix a bleach solution, always follow the manufacturer's directions. Store the bleach solution away from heat and light. A fresh bleach solution should be mixed every 24 hours or when the solution has been contaminated. After mixing the bleach solution, date the container to ensure that the solution is not saved from one day to the next, but rather disposed of daily like other disinfectants. Bleach can be irritating to the lungs, so be careful about inhaling the fumes.

DID YOU KNOW?

Bleach is not a magic potion! All disinfectants, including bleach, are inactivated (made less effective) in the presence of many substances, including oils, lotions, creams, hair, and skin. If bleach is used to disinfect equipment, it is critical to use a soap detergent first to thoroughly clean and rinse the equipment and remove all debris. Never mix detergents with bleach and always use bleach in a well-ventilated area.

Additionally, not all household bleaches are as effective as disinfectants. To be effective, the bleach must have an EPA registration number and contain at least 5 percent sodium hypochlorite and be diluted properly to a 10 percent solution—nine parts water to one part bleach.

DISINFECTANT TIPS AND SAFETY

Never forget that disinfectants are poisonous and can cause serious skin and eye damage. Some disinfectants appear clear while others, especially phenolic disinfectants, are a little cloudy. Always use caution when handling disinfectants, in addition to the tips below.

Always
- Keep the SDS on hand for the disinfectant(s) you use.
- Wear gloves and safety glasses (**Figure 5-19**).

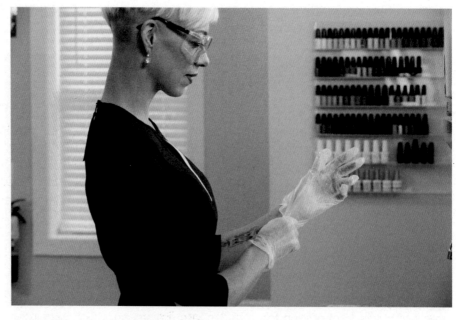

▲ FIGURE 5-19 Wear gloves and safety glasses while handling disinfectants.

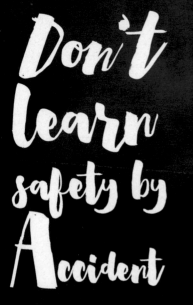

Don't learn safety by Accident

– JERRY SMITH

- Avoid skin and eye contact.
- Add disinfectant to water when diluting (rather than adding water to a disinfectant) to prevent foaming, which can result in an incorrect mixing ratio.
- Use tongs, gloves, or a draining basket to remove implements from disinfectants.
- Keep disinfectants out of reach of children.
- Follow the manufacturer's instructions for mixing, using, and disposing of disinfectants.
- Use disinfectants only on clean, hard, nonporous surfaces.
- Keep an item submerged in the disinfectant for 10 minutes unless the product label specifies differently.
- Immerse the entire implement in disinfectant if the product label calls for "complete immersion."
- To disinfect large surfaces, such as countertops, carefully apply the disinfectant to the clean surface or use a disinfectant spray and allow it to remain moist for 10 minutes, unless state regulations say differently.
- Strictly follow the manufacturer's directions for when to replace the disinfectant solution in order to ensure the healthiest conditions for you and your client. Replace the disinfectant solution every day—more often if the solution becomes soiled or contaminated.

Never
- Let quats, phenols, bleach, or any other disinfectant come in contact with your skin. If you do get disinfectant on your skin, immediately wash the area with liquid soap and warm water. Then rinse and dry the area thoroughly.
- Place any disinfectant or other product in an unmarked container. All containers should be labeled with, at the least, product name, ingredients, date of mixing, and manufacturer's information.
- Mix chemicals together unless specified in the manufacturer's instructions. (For example, mixing together bleach and ammonia products or bleach and vinegar creates potentially fatal toxic vapors!)

DISINFECTING CONTAINERS

In the past, jars or containers used to disinfect implements were often incorrectly called "wet sanitizers." Disinfectant containers contain disinfectant for disinfecting purposes, not for cleaning. The container you choose must be large enough to contain all items to be disinfected and covered, but not airtight. Remember to clean the container every day and to wear gloves when you do. Always follow the manufacturer's label instructions for disinfecting products.

KEEP A LOGBOOK

Salons, spas, and barbershops should always follow manufacturers' recommended schedules for cleaning and disinfecting tools and implements, disinfecting work surfaces, scheduling regular service visits for equipment, and replacing parts when needed. Although your state may

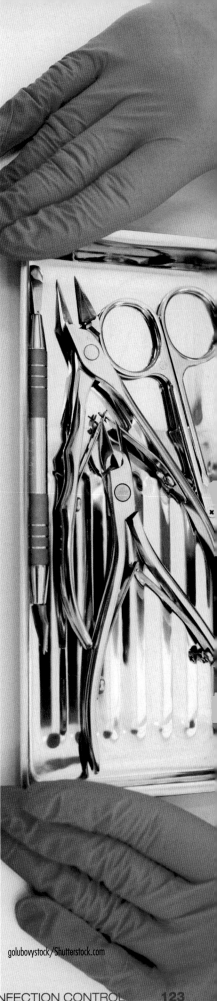

golubovystock/Shutterstock.com

not require you to keep a logbook of all equipment usage, cleaning, disinfecting, testing, and maintenance, it may be advisable to keep one.

CLEANING AND DISINFECTING NONPOROUS, REUSABLE ITEMS

State rules require that all multiuse tools and implements be cleaned and disinfected before every service. Mix all disinfectants according to the manufacturer's directions, always adding the disinfectant to the water, not the water to the disinfectant (**Figure 5-20**). Follow the cleaning and disinfecting nonporous, reusable items procedure described in **Procedure 5-2**.

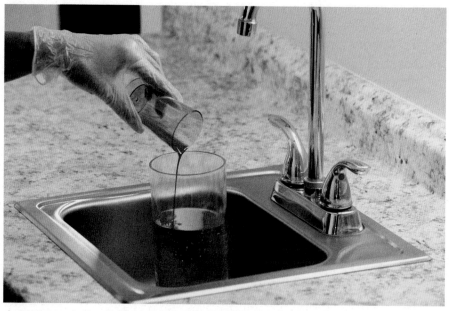

▲ FIGURE 5-20 Carefully pour the disinfectant into the water when preparing disinfectant solution.

DISINFECTING ELECTRICAL TOOLS AND EQUIPMENT

Hair clippers and other types of electrical equipment have contact points that cannot be completely immersed in liquid. These items should be cleaned and disinfected using an EPA-registered disinfectant designed for use on these devices. Follow the procedures recommended by the disinfectant manufacturer for preparing the solution and follow the item's manufacturer directions for cleaning and disinfecting the device.

CAUTION

Electric sterilizers, bead sterilizers, and baby sterilizers should not be used to disinfect or sterilize implements. These devices can spread potentially infectious diseases and should never be used in a salon, spa, or barbershop. Additionally, UV light units will not disinfect or sterilize implements. Most state rules require that you use liquid disinfecting solutions. Autoclaves are effective sterilizers. If you decide to use an autoclave, be sure that you know how to operate and maintain it properly.

DISINFECTING WORK SURFACES

Most states require that all work surfaces be cleaned and disinfected before beginning a service. Be sure to clean and disinfect tables, stations, shampoo sinks, chairs, armrests, and any other surface that a customer's skin may have touched. Clean doorknobs and handles daily to reduce transfer of germs to your hands.

CLEANING TOWELS, LINENS, AND CAPES

Clean towels and linens should be used for each client, and some states require freshly laundered capes for every service. To clean towels, linens, and capes, launder according to the directions on the item's label. Be sure that towels, linens, and capes are thoroughly dried. Items that are not dry may grow mildew and bacteria. Store soiled linens and towels in covered or closed containers, away from clean linens and towels, even if your state regulatory agency does not require that you do so. Whenever possible, use disposable towels, especially in restrooms. Do not allow the neckband of capes to touch the client's skin. All states require the use of a barrier, such as disposable neck strips or towels, to prevent the client's skin from touching the neckline of the cape.

MULTIUSE PRODUCTS

When using creams, lotions, gels, or any other product that is dispensed from a multiuse container, it is important not to contaminate the product. Always use a pump or shaker to dispense products when possible. For products in a tub-type container, always use a clean spatula (disposable or disinfectable) to remove the product—never use your fingers.

SOAPS AND DETERGENTS

Chelating soaps (CHE-layt-ing SOHPS), also known as *chelating detergents*, work to break down stubborn films and remove the residue of products such as scrubs, salts, and masks. The chelating agents in these soaps work in all types of water, are low-sudsing, and are specially formulated to work in areas with hard tap water. Hard tap water reduces the effectiveness of cleaners and disinfectants. If your area has hard water, ask your local distributor for soaps that are effective in hard water. This information will be stated on the product's label.

CHECK IN
What is the difference between cleaning, disinfecting, and sterilizing?

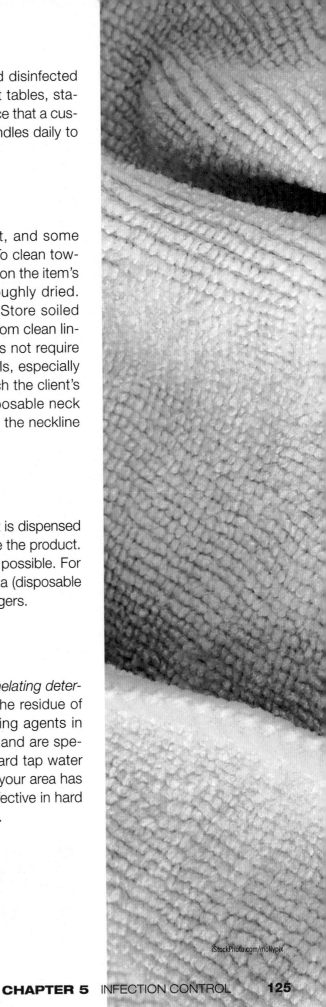

iStockPhoto.com/mollypix

FOLLOW STANDARD PRECAUTIONS TO PROTECT YOURSELF AND YOUR CLIENTS

Standard Precautions (SP) (STAN-derd pruh-CAW-shuns) are guidelines published by the CDC that require the employer and employee to assume that any human blood and body fluids are potentially infectious. Because it may not be possible to identify clients with infectious diseases, whether or not they look sick, strict infection control practices should be used with all clients. In many instances, clients who are just getting sick or are long-term viral carriers are **asymptomatic** (A-simp-toe-MAT-ick), meaning that they show no symptoms or signs of infection.

OSHA and the CDC have set safety standards and precautions that protect employees in situations when they could be exposed to blood-borne pathogens. Precautions include proper hand washing, wearing of gloves, and proper handling and disposing of sharp instruments and any other items that may have been contaminated by blood or other body fluids (**Figure 5-21**). It is important that specific procedures be followed if blood or body fluid is present.

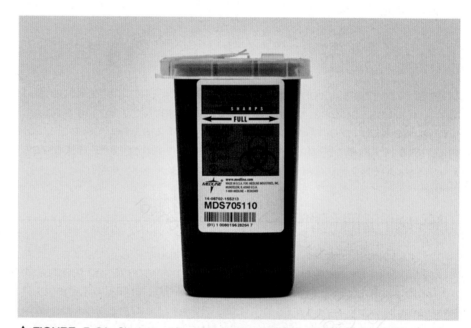

▲ **FIGURE 5-21** Sharps containers are puncture-proof plastic biohazard containers for disposable needles and anything sharp and must be disposed of as medical waste.

CAUTION
Taking the time to conduct a thorough hair and skin analysis will enable you to determine whether a customer has any open wounds or abrasions. If the client does have an open wound or abrasion, do not perform services of any kind.

PERSONAL PROTECTIVE EQUIPMENT (PPE)

Many chemicals used in the salon, spa, or barbershop bear labels that require the use of personal protective equipment, such as gloves and safety glasses, when working with their products. However, some equipment, such as gloves, offer protection from exposure to pathogens and should be worn whenever practical.

GLOVES

OSHA defines PPEs as "specialized clothing or equipment worn by an employee for protection against a hazard." The hazards this particular standard refers to are bloodborne pathogens, such as hepatitis and HIV; however, beauty professionals are required to prevent their occupational exposure to any amount of blood, no matter how miniscule, through the use of gloves, masks, and eye protection.

Gloves are single-use equipment; a new set is used for every client and at times must be changed during the service, according to the protocol. Removal of gloves is performed by inverting the cuffs, pulling them off inside out, and disposing of them into the trash. The glove taken off first is held in the hand with a glove still on it; the glove with the cuff inverted is then pulled over the first glove inside out (**Figure 5-22**). The first glove is then inside the second one, which has the service side now on the inside against the other glove, and they are disposed of together.

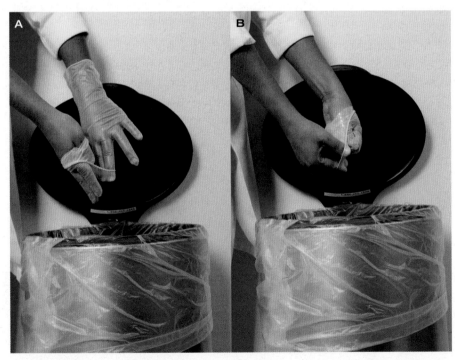

▲ FIGURE 5-22 First remove one glove by inverting the cuff and pulling it off inside out (A). Then, with the cuff inverted, the second glove is pulled off over the inside-out first glove (B). Both are disposed of together.

Olinchuk/Shutterstock.com

If a service requires moving from one place of service to another several times, or working on different body parts—such as when performing a manicure and a pedicure—several sets of gloves will need to be used. The technician is to perform hand washing after removing each set of gloves and before putting on a new set when two services are being performed together, or use antimicrobial gel cleanser between sets of gloves during the same appointment.

CAUTION

When choosing what type of disposable gloves to use, you should avoid latex due to increasingly common allergies to the material. You should also exercise caution when using petroleum-based products, as petroleum-based gloves degrade on contact and cannot maintain a safe barrier. Nitrile gloves are a strong alternative in both instances.

AN EXPOSURE INCIDENT: CONTACT WITH BLOOD OR BODY FLUID

You should never perform a service on any client who comes in with an open wound, a rash, or an abrasion. However, sometimes accidents happen while a service is being performed.

An exposure incident (eks-PO-zhoor IN-sih-dent) is contact with non-intact (broken) skin, blood, body fluid, or other potentially infectious materials that is the result of the performance of a worker's duties. Should the client suffer a cut or abrasion that bleeds during a service, follow the steps outlined in **Procedure 5-3** for the client's safety as well as your own.

As a beauty professional, you will likely work with an array of sharp implements and tools, and cutting yourself is a very real possibility. If you do suffer a cut and blood is present, you must follow the steps for an exposure incident outlined in **Procedure 5-4**. Many of the steps are similar to a client injury, although attending to yourself should hopefully require fewer soft skills!

CHECK IN
What are Standard Precautions?

DEMONSTRATE SAFE WORK PRACTICES AND SAFETY PRECAUTIONS

Most potentially harmful situations in the salon, spa, and barbershop can be avoided by being observant and using common sense. Learn to recognize safety hazards to minimize the occurrence of accidents.

WATER

- At the shampoo bowl, be careful how you handle the spray hose. Position the client's head for comfort and access, being conscious of your own body position as well. Do not bend or twist from the waist unnecessarily. Wipe up any water spills or leaks immediately.
- If the water temperature reaches a scalding level while in the hot position, turn the thermostat on the hot-water tank down to a more acceptable temperature for application to the skin, scalp, and hair. Water heaters should not be set at higher than 130 degrees Fahrenheit.
- As a precaution, always test water temperature on the inside of your wrist before applying to a client's hair or scalp. The same procedure may be used to test steam towels for facials and shaves.

TOOLS AND APPLIANCES

- Tools and equipment should be strategically placed so that items are safely stored when not in use yet are accessible when needed.
- Smaller tools may be placed in countertop receptacles designed for that purpose. Larger equipment may be mounted under the cabinet, attached to a wall, or set on a shelf.
- Disinfecting jars should be set back toward a wall or partition so as not to interfere with other tools. This also limits the risk of accidental spillage of disinfectant solution.
- If a tool or implement is dropped on the floor during a service, it must be replaced with a disinfected tool or you must stop the service and properly disinfect the tool that was dropped prior to continuing the service. This is a good reason to keep an extra set of tools that are ready to use handy.
- All tools and implements should be in good working condition. Replace damaged tools immediately, including worn electrical cords, chipped clipper blades, cracked housings, and broken shears. Do not try to repair tools yourself; send them to the manufacturer for service. Never subject yourself or your client to the risks of faulty or broken equipment.
- Electrical cords can often threaten to become a safety hazard in a busy shop. Cords to clippers, trimmers, curling irons, and blow-dryers tend to become twisted and tangled during use. If the cord is too long, it can get caught on the foot or armrests of a chair or table or even on the foot of a client. Some beauty professionals use cordless tools, such as trimmers, to eliminate the problem altogether. A well-planned workstation with sufficient and conveniently placed outlets can also help minimize "tangled cord syndrome" (**Figure 5-23**).
- Never place any tool or implement in your mouth or pocket.

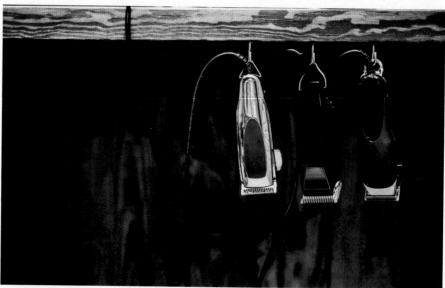

▲ **FIGURE 5-23** Avoid tangled cords, which can be dangerous in addition to unsightly and cumbersome.

EQUIPMENT AND FIXTURES

- Keep all chairs, headrests, tables, heat lamps, and lighting fixtures in good working order. Tighten screws and bolts, grease or oil hinges, and service equipment mechanisms as needed.
- Dust and clean regularly to avoid dust buildup and to maintain clean conditions.
- Maintain lighting fixtures. Change bulbs when necessary to keep workstations well lit.

VENTILATION

- Proper ventilation and air circulation are extremely important in today's salons, spas, and barbershops. Particles from products such as hair sprays and disinfectants can be inhaled and may cause allergic reactions or other health problems.
- Heating and air-conditioning vents should be located to perform their optimum functions without interfering with client services.
- Vents should be vacuumed or cleaned periodically to prevent any buildup of hair that might impede ventilation.
- Fumes from chemical applications and nail care products require sophisticated filtration units that cleanse and detoxify the air. Once installed, air filters should be changed or cleaned regularly.

EXITS

- Exits should be well marked and identifiable. (Check with your local building inspection office for codes and requirements.)
- Employees should know where exits are located and how to evacuate the building quickly in case of fire or other emergencies. Implement fire drills to practice for this contingency.

FIRE EXTINGUISHERS

- Fire extinguishers should be placed where they are readily accessible.
- All employees should be instructed in fire extinguisher use.
- It is a law that fire extinguishers be checked periodically. Be guided by the manufacturer's recommendations and state and local ordinances.

ATTIRE

- Clothing should be comfortable and professional in appearance. Excessively baggy clothes can get in the way of your performance just as easily as tight clothing can restrict it.
- Long hair worn in a loose style may easily get caught in motor vents and other appliances. Keep hair pulled back or short enough to avoid entanglements.
- Necklaces should be of an appropriate length so as not to get caught on equipment or dangle in a client's face during a service. Rings should not be worn on the index and middle fingers as they might interfere with procedure accuracy. In general, rings with stones and elaborate settings are very hard to keep clean. Watches should be waterproof and shock absorbent.
- Shoes should have nonskid rubber soles with good support.
- Electronic devices that may distract you, such as cell phones or tablets, should be kept stored away and checked or answered only between clients.

CHILDREN

- Children can cause serious risk of injury to themselves in the salon, spa, or barbershop environment. Being aware of their inquisitive nature and the speed with which they can move can help prevent accidents from happening.
- Post notices in the reception area advising patrons that children are not to be left unattended.
- Do not allow children to play, climb, or spin on hydraulic chairs.
- Do not allow children to wander freely with access to workstations, storage areas, and so forth.
- When performing a service on a child, try to anticipate the child's sudden moves. Never trust a young child to hold the head or body still while you are wielding tools. Instead, hold the child gently but firmly with one hand while working with the other.

ADULT CLIENTS

- As beauty professionals, many of the things we do to assure client comfort also fall under the category of safety precautions. As you

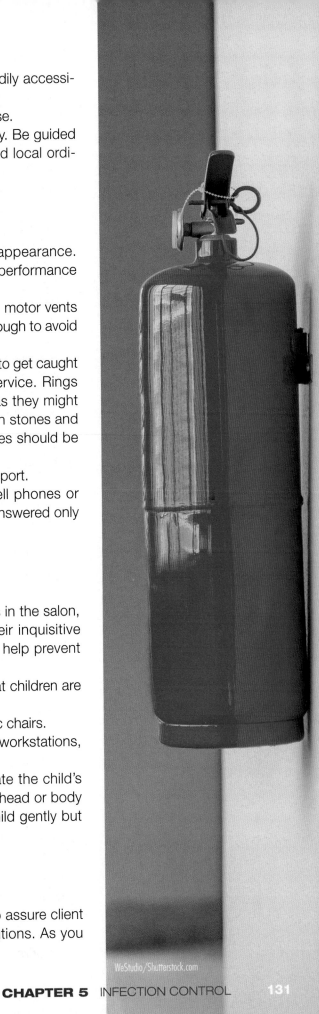

WeStudio/Shutterstock.com

work through your practical skills, you will learn proper protection procedures and chemical application methods to ensure client safety and comfort from the standpoint of avoiding skin irritations, burns, wet or soiled clothing, and so forth; however, there are also several common sense services that should be performed. Using good manners and performing common courtesies will help you gain the reputation of being a safety-conscious and courteous professional.

- Assist clients (especially the elderly) in and out of chairs and onto and off treatment tables. Turn hydraulic chairs so the client may get out of the chair without a risk of feet becoming tangled in any of the cords.
- Always lower a hydraulic chair to its lowest level and lock it in position so that it does not spin before inviting the client to be seated or leave the chair.
- Hold doors open for clients.
- Assist clients in walking whenever necessary.
- Always support the back of the chair, and thus the client, when reclining or raising a chair back. Support the client's head whenever appropriate at the shampoo bowl or during other neck-straining procedures.

HIGH-RISK CLIENTS

- While some customers who know that they have impaired immune systems will share that information with you, many will not because they are embarrassed, do not know it is important, or do not know that they have a compromised immune system. These people are at very high risk of infection should they encounter pathogens. Because you will not always know who these people are, it is important to practice proper infection control with every customer.
- Diabetic customers have immune systems that do not work effectively and have impaired healing. A simple nick from a tool that was not properly disinfected may have devastating effects. While many people will tell you they have diabetes if they do, some type 2 diabetics can be diabetic for years prior to being diagnosed, which means that even if you ask, they may say "no" because they have not yet been diagnosed.
- Lumpectomy/mastectomy patients have had surgical treatment for breast cancer. A part of that surgery involves removing the lymph nodes in the axilla (armpit). With those nodes removed any infectious process in that arm could lead to a permanent condition called *lymphedema*. It is extremely important to these clients that properly disinfected implements be used, particularly in a nail service, to reduce the risk of this very uncomfortable condition (**Figure 5-24**).

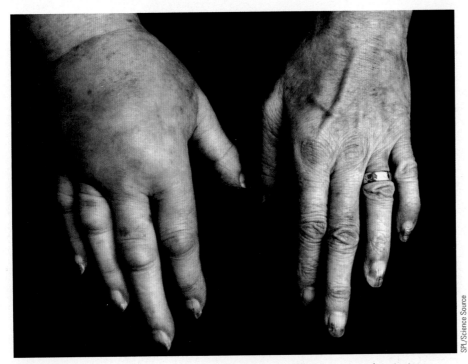

▲ FIGURE 5-24 Lymphedema is a condition that can afflict lumpectomy/mastectomy patients.

SPL/Science Source

- Clients on medication for conditions such as asthma, rheumatoid arthritis, and fibromyalgia are likely to have suppressed immune systems, making them particularly susceptible to infection.
- Clients who are pregnant may be particularly sensitive to harsh smells; their skin may also have unusual reactions to chemicals. Each client must decide for themselves what is safe for their baby during pregnancy; however, allowing a client to read the labels of products prior to using them may help them to decide.

YOUR PROFESSIONAL RESPONSIBILITIES

After studying this chapter, it should be clear that your responsibilities as a beauty professional far exceed the ability to perform a good service; your most important responsibility is to protect your clients' health and safety.

- Never take shortcuts for cleaning and disinfecting. You cannot afford to skip steps in order to save time or money when it comes to safety.
- It is your professional and legal responsibility to follow state and federal laws and rules.
- Keep your license current and notify the licensing agency if you move or change your name.
- Check your state's website monthly for any change or update to the rules and regulations.
- Be aware of your environment so that you can identify and eliminate potential hazards to make your salon, spa, or barbershop safer for you and your clients.

- Be prepared for emergencies. Every salon, spa, and barbershop should have employee and clientele emergency information available.
- An emergency phone number checklist should include the contact numbers for fire, police, poison control, and medical rescue departments; the nearest hospital emergency room; and taxis.
- Utility service companies, such as electricity, water, heat, air-conditioning, and landlord or custodial numbers are also helpful in an emergency or if something breaks down in the shop. Update this information on an annual basis and you will always be prepared.
- Realize that behavior that stems from a knowledgeable and caring manner is what separates a true professional from a nonprofessional. Being a professional is something you can take pride in.

CHECK IN

Why is it of the utmost importance to practice strict infection control protocols with every client?

APPLY INFECTION CONTROL

Congratulations on completing this chapter! Before you move on, take a moment to think about how these Infection Control topics apply to your particular discipline. Discuss with a classmate or study group how you will fit infection control into your daily routine on the job; what special infection control measures you will need to take for specific procedures; what some special needs of your target audience may be; and so on.

PROCEDURE 5-1: PROPER HAND WASHING

Hand washing is one of the most important procedures in your infection control efforts and is required in most states before beginning any service and after eating, smoking, or using the restroom.

MATERIALS, IMPLEMENTS, AND EQUIPMENT

- ❑ Disposable paper towels
- ❑ Liquid soap in a pump container
- ❑ Nail brush

PROCEDURE

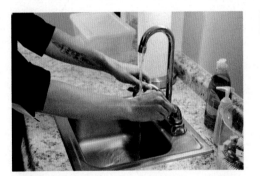

❑ ❶ Turn the water on and wet your hands.

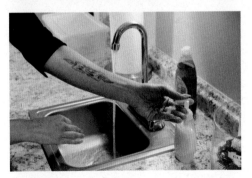

❑ ❷ Pump soap from a pump container onto the palm of your hand.

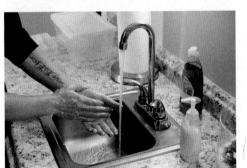

❑ ❸ Rub your hands together, all over and vigorously, until a lather forms. Continue for a minimum of 20 seconds.

4 Scrub your nails with a nail brush if product or debris is visible under your nails or if you are washing your hands following an exposure incident:

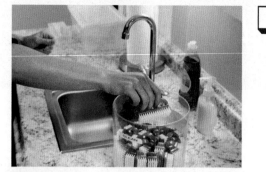

☐ a. Choose a clean and disinfected nail brush.

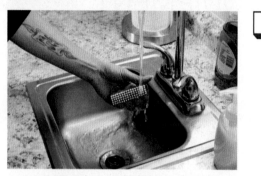

☐ b. Wet the nail brush and pump soap onto the bristles.

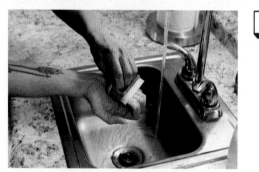

☐ c. Brush your nails horizontally back and forth under the free edges.

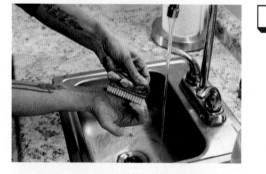

☐ d. Change the direction of the brush to vertical and move the brush up and down along the nail folds of the fingernails. The process for brushing both hands should take about 60 seconds to complete.

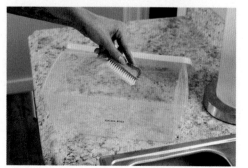

☐ e. Rinse the nail brush and deposit in a labeled container for dirty implements.

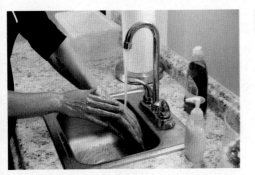

☐ ⑤ Rinse hands in warm running water.

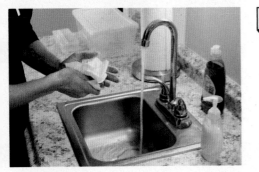

☐ ⑥ Use a clean cloth or paper towel to dry your hands, according to the salon, spa, or barbershop's policies or state rules and regulations.

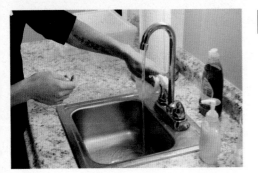

☐ ⑦ After drying your hands, turn off the water with the towel. Use the towel to open the door and then dispose of the towel. Touching a doorknob with your bare fingers can recontaminate your hands.

PROCEDURE 5-2: CLEANING AND DISINFECTING NONPOROUS, REUSABLE ITEMS

Nonporous, reusable items include nonelectrical tools and implements that can be completely submerged, such as combs, brushes, shears, clips, hairpins, tweezers, and nippers, as well as larger equipment that cannot be submerged, all the way up to nonporous work surfaces.

MATERIALS, IMPLEMENTS, AND EQUIPMENT

- ❑ Covered storage container
- ❑ Disinfectant solution, spray, or wipes
- ❑ Disposable gloves
- ❑ Disposable towels
- ❑ Liquid soap or cleaning solution
- ❑ Safety glasses
- ❑ Scrub brush
- ❑ Timer
- ❑ Tongs

PROCEDURE

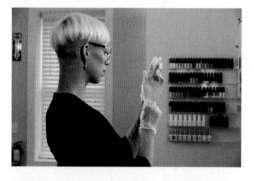

❑ **1** It is important to wear safety glasses and gloves while cleaning and disinfecting to protect your eyes from unintentional splashes of disinfectant, to prevent possible contamination of the implements by your hands, and to protect your hands from the powerful chemicals in the disinfectant solution.

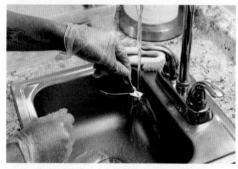

❑ **2** Rinse items with warm running water.

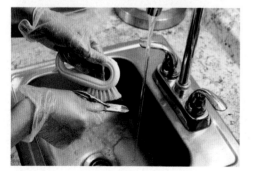

❑ **3** Use a small scrubbing brush to wash items with soap or cleaning solution.

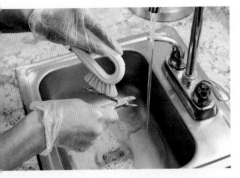

☐ **4** Brush grooved items thoroughly and open hinged implements to scrub the revealed areas clean.

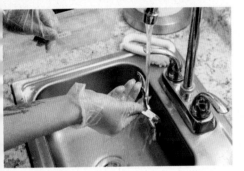

☐ **5** Rinse away all traces of soap or solution with clean running water. Soap is most easily rinsed off in warm, not hot, water.

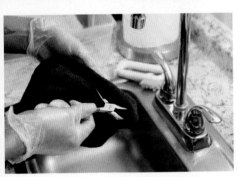

☐ **6** Dry items with a clean or disposable towel.

7 Disinfect items as appropriate or required by your state:
   a. Immersion is used for items that can be safely and effectively immersed in disinfectant.

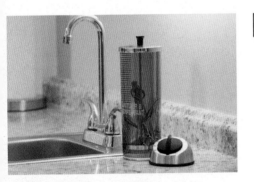

☐ i. Completely immerse cleaned items in an appropriate disinfection container holding an EPA-registered disinfectant approved for use in your state for the required time listed in the manufacturer's instructions. Remember to open hinged implements before immersing them in the disinfectant. If the disinfectant solution is visibly dirty, or if the solution has been contaminated, it must be replaced.

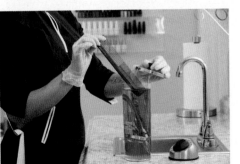

☐ ii. After the required contact time has passed, remove items from the disinfectant solution with tongs or gloved hands, rinse in warm running water, and dry thoroughly with a disposable towel or allow to air dry on a clean towel. Do not store implements with any moisture on them, particularly in the hinges.

b. Sprays are used for larger tools and implements that cannot or should not be immersed.

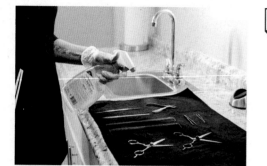

☐ i. Place cleaned items on a disinfected surface or clean towel and spray with disinfectant until thoroughly saturated. Ensure that all surfaces of items stay visibly moist for the full contact time listed on the label.

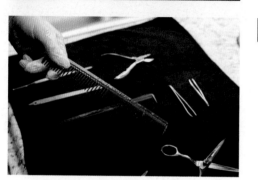

☐ ii. After the required contact time has passed, pick up items with tongs or gloved hands, rinse in warm running water, and pat dry.

c. Wipes are used for surfaces and other nonsubmersible items.

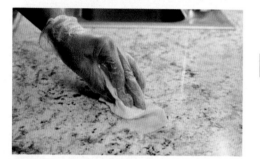

i. Steps #2 through #6 above are not required when using one wipe to clean and a second wipe to disinfect.

☐ ii. Use an EPA-registered wipe to wipe surfaces or items and ensure that all surfaces remain visibly moist for the contact time listed on the label.

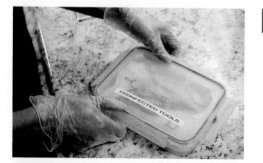

☐ **8** Store items as directed by your state rules. Most states require that dry, disinfected items be stored in a clean, covered container labeled "disinfected" or "ready to use" until needed.

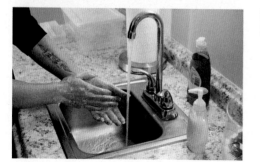

☐ **9** Remove gloves and thoroughly wash your hands with warm running water and liquid soap. Rinse and dry hands with a clean fabric or disposable towel.

PROCEDURE 5-3: HANDLING AN EXPOSURE INCIDENT: CLIENT INJURY

Should you accidentally cut a client during a service, calmly take the following steps:

MATERIALS, IMPLEMENTS, AND EQUIPMENT

- ❑ Antiseptic
- ❑ Bandages
- ❑ Disposable gloves
- ❑ Disposable paper towels
- ❑ Liquid soap
- ❑ Plastic bag
- ❑ Disinfectant solution, spray, or wipes
- ❑ Sharps box (optional)

PROCEDURE

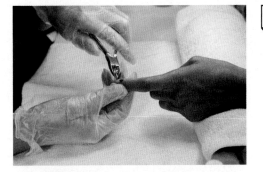

❑ **1** Stop the service immediately.

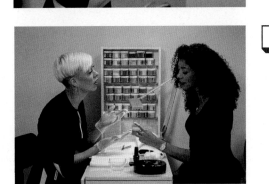

❑ **2** Put on gloves (if you were not already wearing gloves for the procedure).

❑ **3** Face your client and calmly apologize for the incident.

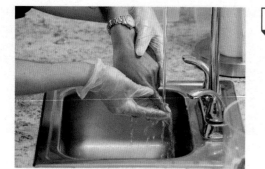

☐ **4** If appropriate, assist your client to the sink, wash the injured area with soap, and rinse under running water.

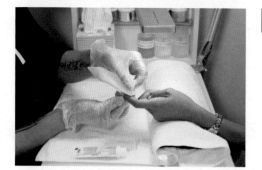

☐ **5** Pat the injured area dry using a new, clean paper towel.

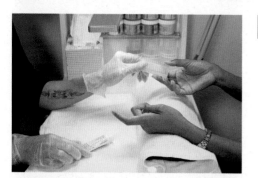

☐ **6** Offer your client antiseptic and an adhesive bandage.

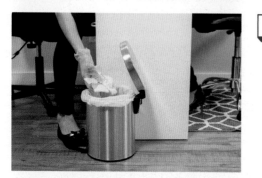

☐ **7** Discard all single-use contaminated objects, such as wipes or cotton balls, in a plastic bag and then place in a trash bag. Deposit sharp disposables in a sharps box. Dispose of double-bagged items and sharps containers as required by state or local law. In general, all of these items (except sharps) may go into the regular trash.

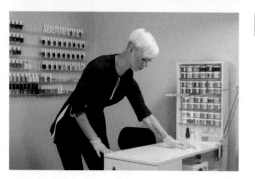

☐ **8** Remove all implements from the workstation and then clean and disinfect workstation surfaces.

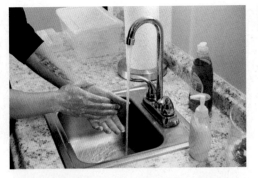

9 Discard gloves and thoroughly wash hands with warm running water and liquid soap. Rinse and dry hands with a clean fabric or disposable towel and then put on fresh gloves.

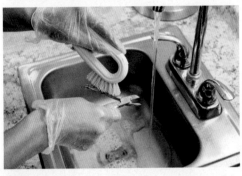

10 Properly clean and disinfect implements.

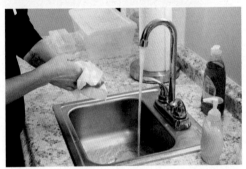

11 Discard gloves and thoroughly wash your hands with warm running water and liquid soap. Rinse and dry hands with a clean fabric or disposable towel and return to the service.

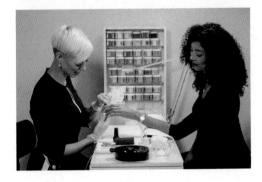

12 Recommend that the client see a physician if any signs of redness, swelling, pain, or irritation develop. Ask if the client would like to continue the service, and return to where you left off if they are willing. If you were working on the client's hands and they have refused a bandage, put on gloves before finishing the service.

PROCEDURE 5-4: HANDLING AN EXPOSURE INCIDENT: EMPLOYEE INJURY

Should you accidentally cut yourself during a service, calmly take the following steps:

MATERIALS, IMPLEMENTS, AND EQUIPMENT

- ❑ Antiseptic
- ❑ Bandages
- ❑ Cotton
- ❑ Disposable gloves
- ❑ Disposable paper towels
- ❑ Liquid soap
- ❑ Plastic bag
- ❑ Disinfectant solution, spray, or wipes
- ❑ Sharps box (optional)

PROCEDURE

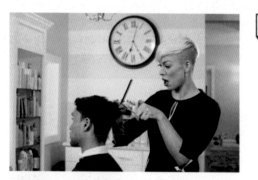

❑ ❶ Stop the service immediately.

❑ ❷ Inform your client of what has happened. Let them know you are taking care of your cut and that the service will be interrupted for a few minutes. If the nature of your cut is severe, ask an employee to assist with the exposure incident.

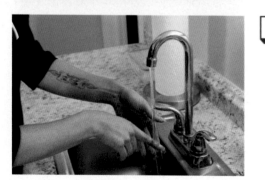

❑ ❸ If appropriate, wash and rinse the injured area under running water.

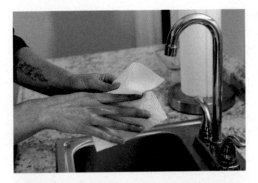

☐ ④ Pat the injured area dry using a new, clean paper towel.

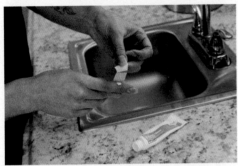

☐ ⑤ Apply antiseptic and an adhesive bandage to the wound.

☐ ⑥ Put on gloves.

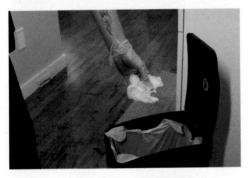

☐ ⑦ Discard all single-use contaminated objects, such as wipes or cotton balls, in a plastic bag and then place in a trash bag. Deposit sharp disposables in a sharps box. Dispose of double-bagged items and sharps containers as required by state or local law. In general, all of these items (except sharps) may go into the regular trash.

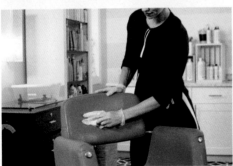

☐ ⑧ Remove all implements from the workstation and then clean and disinfect workstation surfaces.

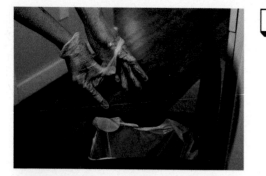

☐ **9** Discard gloves and thoroughly wash hands with warm running water and liquid soap. Rinse and dry hands with a clean fabric or disposable towel and then put on fresh gloves.

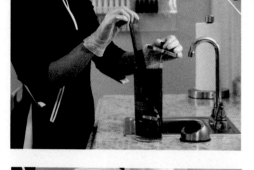

☐ **10** Properly clean and disinfect implements.

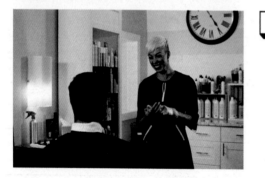

☐ **11** Discard gloves and thoroughly wash your hands with warm running water and liquid soap. Rinse and dry hands with a clean fabric or disposable towel.

☐ **12** Return to where you had left the service.

COMPETENCY PROGRESS

How are you doing with Infection Control? **Check off the Chapter 5 Learning Objectives below that you feel you have mastered; leave unchecked those objectives you will need to return to:**

☐ EXPLAIN INFECTION CONTROL.

☐ DESCRIBE FEDERAL AND STATE REGULATORY AGENCIES.

☐ RECOGNIZE THE PRINCIPLES OF INFECTION.

☐ IDENTIFY DIFFERENT TYPES OF PATHOGENS.

☐ EMPLOY THE PRINCIPLES OF PREVENTION.

☐ FOLLOW STANDARD PRECAUTIONS TO PROTECT YOURSELF AND YOUR CLIENTS.

☐ DEMONSTRATE SAFE WORK PRACTICES AND SAFETY PRECAUTIONS.

GLOSSARY

acquired immune deficiency syndrome (uh-KWY-erd ih-MYOON di-FISH-en-see SIN-drome)	p. 111	abbreviated AIDS; a disease that breaks down the body's immune system; AIDS is caused by the human immunodeficiency virus (HIV)
antiseptics (ant-ih-SEP-tiks)	p. 117	chemical germicides formulated for use on skin; registered and regulated by the Food and Drug Administration
asymptomatic (A-simp-toe-MAT-ick)	p. 126	showing no symptoms or signs of infection
bacteria (bak-TEER-ee-ah)	p. 105	single-celled microorganisms that have both plant and animal characteristics; some bacteria are harmful, some are harmless
bacterial spores (bak-TEER-ee-ul SPORZ)	p. 102	bacteria capable of producing a protective coating that allows them to withstand very harsh environments and to shed the coating when conditions become more favorable to them
bactericidal (bak-TEER-uh-SYD-uhl)	p. 102	capable of destroying bacteria
biofilms (BY-o-films)	p. 113	colonies of microorganisms that adhere to environmental surfaces, as well as the human body
bloodborne pathogens (BLUD-born PATH-o-genz)	p. 110	disease-causing microorganisms carried in the body by blood or body fluids, such as hepatitis and HIV
chelating soaps (CHE-layt-ing SOHPS)	p. 125	break down stubborn films and remove the residue of products such as scrubs, salts, and masks; also known as *chelating detergents*

cleaning (KLEEN-ing)	p. 101	a mechanical process using soap and water or detergent and water to remove all visible dirt, debris, and many disease-causing germs; cleaning also removes invisible debris that interferes with disinfection; cleaning is what beauty professionals are required to do before disinfecting
communicable (kuh-MYOO-nih-kuh-bul)	p. 104	able to be communicated; transferable by contact from one person to another as in a communicable disease
contagious disease (kun-TAY-jus diz-EEZ)	p. 104	also known as *communicable disease*; disease that is capable of being spread from one person to another
contamination (kon-tam-uh-NAY-shun)	p. 105	the presence, or the reasonably anticipated presence, of blood or other potentially infectious materials on an item's surface, or visible debris or residues such as dust, hair, and skin
diagnosis (dy-ag-NO-sis)	p. 105	determination of the nature of a disease from its symptoms and/or diagnostic tests; federal regulations prohibit salon professionals from performing a diagnosis
direct transmission (die-REKT trans-MISH-uhn)	p. 99	transmission of pathogens through touching (including shaking hands), kissing, coughing, sneezing, and talking
disease (diz-EEZ)	p. 99	an abnormal condition of all or part of the body, or its systems or organs, that makes the body incapable of carrying on normal function
disinfectants (dis-in-FEK-tents)	p. 97	chemical products approved by the EPA designed to destroy most bacteria (excluding spores), fungi, and viruses on surfaces
disinfection (dis-in-FEK-shun)	p. 101	a chemical process that uses specific products to destroy harmful organisms (except bacterial spores) on environmental surfaces
efficacy (EF-ih-kuh-see)	p. 119	the ability of a product to produce the intended effect; on a disinfectant label, it indicates specific pathogens destroyed or disabled when used properly
exposure incident (eks-PO-zhoor IN-sih-dent)	p. 128	contact with non-intact (broken) skin, blood, body fluid, or other potentially infectious materials, which is the result of the performance of an employee's duties
fungi (FUN-ji)	p. 112	single-celled organisms that grow in irregular masses and include molds, mildews, and yeasts; they can produce contagious diseases such as ringworm
fungicidal (fun-ji-SYD-uhl)	p. 102	capable of destroying molds and fungi
hepatitis (hep-uh-TY-tis)	p. 111	a bloodborne virus that causes disease and can damage the liver
herpes simplex virus (HER-peez SIM-pleks VY-rus)	p. 110	an inflammatory disease of the skin caused by a viral infection and characterized by small vesicles in clusters
human immunodeficiency virus (HYOO-mun ih-MYOO-noh-di-FISH-en-see VY-rus)	p. 111	abbreviated HIV; virus that causes HIV disease and acquired immune deficiency syndrome (AIDS)
human papilloma virus (HYOO-mun pap-uh-LOW-ma VY-rus)	p. 110	abbreviated HPV; virus that can infect the bottom of the foot and resembles small black dots, usually in clustered groups; also a cutaneous viral infection commonly contracted through sexual transmission and exhibited by genital warts

indirect transmission (in-dih-REKT trans-MISH-uhn)	p. 100	transmission of blood or body fluids through contact with an intermediate contaminated object such as a razor, extractor, nipper, or an environmental surface
infection (in-FEK-shun)	p. 99	the invasion of body tissues by disease-causing pathogens
infection control (in-FEK-shun con-TROL)	p. 95	the methods used to eliminate or reduce the transmission of infectious organisms from one individual to another
infectious (in-FEK-shus)	p. 95	caused by or capable of being transmitted by infection
infectious disease (in-FEK-shus diz-EEZ)	p. 101	disease caused by pathogenic (harmful) microorganisms that enter the body; an infectious disease may or may not be spread from one person to another person
inflammation (in-fluh-MAY-shun)	p. 106	a condition in which the body reacts to injury, irritation, or infection, characterized by redness, heat, pain, and swelling
local infection (LOKE-uhl in-FEK-shun)	p. 106	an infection, such as a pimple or abscess, that is confined to a particular part of the body and appears as a lesion containing pus
methicillin-resistant staphylococcus aureus (meth-uh-SILL-en ree-ZIST-ent staf-uh-loh-KOK-us OR-ee-us)	p. 107	abbreviated MRSA; a type of infectious bacteria that is highly resistant to conventional treatments such as antibiotics
microorganism (my-kro-OR-gah-niz-um)	p. 105	any organism of microscopic or submicroscopic size
mildew (MIL-doo)	p. 112	a type of fungus that affects plants or grows on inanimate objects but does not cause human infections in the barbershop
multiuse (mul-tye-YOOS)	p. 118	also known as *reusable*; items that can be cleaned, disinfected, and used on more than one person, even if the item is accidentally exposed to blood or body fluid
mycobacterium (my-co-bac-TEER-ee-um)	p. 108	a large family of bacteria that is often found in soil and water
nonpathogenic (nahn-path-uh-JEN-ik)	p. 106	harmless microorganisms that may perform useful functions and are safe to come in contact with since they do not cause disease or harm
nonporous (nahn-POOR-rus)	p. 120	an item that is made of a material that has no pores or openings and cannot absorb liquids
occupational disease (ahk-u-PAY-shun-al diz-EEZ)	p. 105	illness resulting from conditions associated with employment, such as prolonged and repeated overexposure to certain products or ingredients
parasites (PAYR-uh-sytz)	p. 113	organisms that grow, feed, and shelter on or inside another organism (referred to as the *host*), while contributing nothing to the survival of that organism. Parasites must have a host to survive
parasitic disease (pahr-a-SIT-ick diz-EEZ)	p. 105	disease caused by parasites, such as lice and mites
pathogenic (path-uh-JEN-ik)	p. 106	harmful microorganisms that can cause disease or infection in humans when they invade the body

pathogenic disease (path-uh-JEN-ick diz-EEZ)	p. 105	disease produced by organisms, including bacteria, viruses, fungi, and parasites
pediculosis capitis (puh-dik-yuh-LO-sis kap-EYE-tus)	p. 113	infestation of the hair and scalp with head lice
phenolic disinfectants (fi-NOH-lik dis-in-FEK-tents)	p. 121	tuberculocidal disinfectants that are a form of formaldehyde, have a very high pH, and can damage the skin and eyes
porous (POOR-rus)	p. 120	made or constructed of a material that has pores or openings; porous items are absorbent
pus (PUS)	p. 106	a fluid created by infection
quaternary ammonium compounds (KWAT-ur-nayr-ee uh-MO-nee-um KAHM-powndz)	p. 120	commonly known as *quats* are products made of quaternary ammonium cations and are designed for disinfection of nonporous surfaces; they are appropriate for use in noncritical (noninvasive) environments and are effective against most pathogens of concern in the salon, spa, or barbershop environment
ringworm (RING-wurm)	p. 112	a fungal infection of the skin that appears in circular lesions
sanitation (san-ih-TAY-shun)	p. 96	also known as *sanitizing*; a chemical process for reducing the number of disease-causing germs on cleaned surfaces to a safe level
scabies (SKAY-beez)	p. 113	a contagious skin disease that is caused by the itch mite, which burrows under the skin
sodium hypochlorite (SO-dee-um hy-puh-KLOR-eyet)	p. 121	common household bleach; an effective disinfectant for the salon, spa, and barbershop
Standard Precautions (STAN-derd pruh-CAW-shuns)	p. 126	are guidelines published by the CDC that require the employer and employee to assume that any human blood and body fluids are potentially infectious
staphylococci (staf-uh-loh-KOKS-eye)	p. 107	pus-forming bacteria that grow in clusters like a bunch of grapes; cause abscesses, pustules, and boils
sterilization (ster-ih-luh-ZAY-shun)	p. 115	the process that completely destroys all microbial life, including spores
systemic infection (sis-TEM-ik in-FEK-shun)	p. 106	an infection where the pathogen has distributed throughout the body rather than staying in one area or organ
tinea barbae (TIN-ee-uh BAR-bee)	p. 112	also known as *barber's itch*, a superficial fungal infection that commonly affects the skin; it is primarily limited to the bearded areas of the face and neck or around the scalp
tinea capitis (TIN-ee-uh kap-EYE-tus)	p. 112	a fungal infection of the scalp characterized by red papules, or spots, at the opening of the hair follicles
tuberculocidal disinfectants (tuh-bur-kyoo-LOH-syd-ahl dis-in-FEK-tents)	p. 120	often referred to as *phenolics*, are proven to kill the bacterium that cause tuberculosis, in addition to other pathogens destroyed through the use of hospital disinfectants

tuberculosis (tuh-bur-kyoo-LO-sus)	p. 120	a disease caused by bacteria that are transmitted through coughing or sneezing
virucidal (viy-ruh-SYD-uhl)	p. 102	capable of destroying viruses
virus (VY-rus)	p. 109	a parasitic submicroscopic particle that infects and resides in cells of biological organisms. A virus is capable of replication only through taking over the host cell's reproductive function

CHEMISTRY & CHEMICAL SAFETY

"Impossible' is not a scientific term."
-Vanna Bonta

LEARNING OBJECTIVES

AFTER COMPLETING THIS CHAPTER, YOU WILL BE ABLE TO:

1. EXPLAIN CHEMISTRY AND CHEMICAL SAFETY.

2. IDENTIFY THE BASICS OF CHEMICAL STRUCTURE.

3. EXPLAIN THE DIFFERENCES BETWEEN SOLUTIONS, SUSPENSIONS, AND EMULSIONS.

4. DESCRIBE POTENTIAL HYDROGEN AND HOW THE PH SCALE WORKS.

5. SUMMARIZE NEUTRALIZATION AND REDOX REACTIONS.

6. PRACTICE CHEMICAL SAFETY.

7. INTERPRET SAFETY DATA SHEETS.

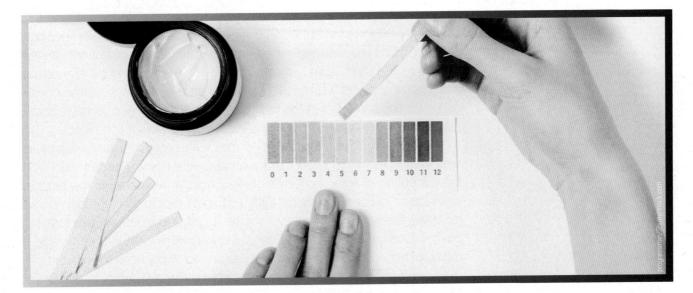

EXPLAIN CHEMISTRY AND CHEMICAL SAFETY

As a beauty professional, you will work with chemistry every day. Chemistry, along with chemicals and chemical changes, makes life on earth possible. The daily functioning of our bodies is based on chemical reactions, and our very hair, skin, and nails are made of chemicals. Creams, lotions, masks, and makeup—whether they come from natural sources like plant extracts or from ingredients manufactured in a laboratory—are made from chemicals.

The effects of cosmetics and beauty products are based on how the body reacts to chemicals. Beauty professionals must have a basic knowledge of chemistry to understand how different chemicals affect the hair, nails, or skin, and to be able to choose the correct products for each client's particular needs.

Beauty professionals should study and have a thorough understanding of chemistry because:

- Without an understanding of basic chemistry, they will not be able to use professional products effectively and safely.
- Every product used in beauty and wellness services contains some type of chemical. Beauty professionals should be able to troubleshoot and solve potential common problems with chemical services.
- It is important to know and follow the procedures for handling chemicals used in the salon, spa, and barbershop by reading labels and following manufactures' instructions to keep their clients and themselves safe.

IDENTIFY THE BASICS OF CHEMICAL STRUCTURE

Chemistry (KEM-uh-stree) is the science that deals with the composition, structures, and properties of matter and how matter changes under different conditions. So then, what is *matter*? Matter (MAT-ur) is any substance that occupies space and has mass (weight). All matter has physical and chemical properties and exists in the form of a solid, liquid, or gas. Since matter is made from chemicals, everything made out of matter is a chemical.

Matter has physical properties that we can touch, taste, smell, or see. In fact, everything you can touch and everything you can see—with the exception of light and electricity—is matter. All matter is made up of chemicals. You can see visible light and light created by electrical sparks; however, these are not made of matter. Light and electricity are forms of energy. Energy is not matter. Everything known to exist in the universe is made of either matter or energy. There are no exceptions to this rule.

Energy does not occupy space or have mass. Energy is discussed further in Chapter 7: Electricity & Electrical Safety.

ELEMENTS

An element (EL-uh-ment) is the simplest form of chemical matter and contains only one type of atom. It cannot be broken down into a simpler substance without a loss of identity.

- There are 118 elements known to science today. Ninety-eight occur naturally on Earth. The remaining elements, known as *synthetic elements*, are produced artificially or through synthesis.

- All matter in the known universe is made up of elements that have their own distinct physical and chemical properties. Each element is identified by a letter symbol, such as *O* for oxygen, *C* for carbon, or *H* for hydrogen.
- Symbols for all the elements can be found on the periodic table of elements in chemistry textbooks or by searching the Internet (**Figure 6-1**).

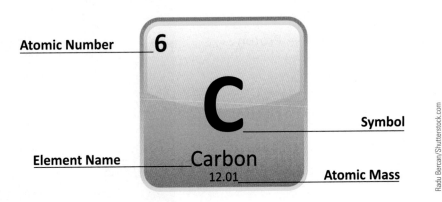

Atomic Number

6

C

Symbol

Element Name

Carbon

12.01

Atomic Mass

Radu Bercan/Shutterstock.com

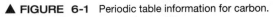

▲ **FIGURE 6-1** Periodic table information for carbon.

DID YOU KNOW?

The use of the word *chemical* to describe something does not mean it is dangerous or harmful. Water and air—and even your body—are completely composed of chemicals. The vast majority of chemicals with which you come in contact every day are safe and harmless. Similarly, the word *organic* simply means that a substance contains the element carbon. Although the term is often used to mean safe or natural because of its association with living things, not all organic substances are natural, healthy, or safe.

ATOMS

Atoms (AT-umz) are the basic unit of matter, with a nucleus at the center surrounded by negatively charged **electrons** (ee-LEK-trahns) that move around the nucleus in orbits. The nucleus consists of **protons** (PRO-tahns) (subatomic particles with a positive charge) and **neutrons** (NEW-trahns) (subatomic particles with no charge), and it is the number of protons that determines the element. Atoms cannot be divided into simpler substances by ordinary chemical means. **Figure 6-2** shows the atomic structure of carbon, with six protons and six neutrons at the nucleus and six electrons in the orbit.

MOLECULES

Just as words are made by combining letters, molecules are made by combining atoms. A **molecule** (MAHL-uh-kyool) is a chemical combination of two or more atoms in definite (fixed) proportions. For example,

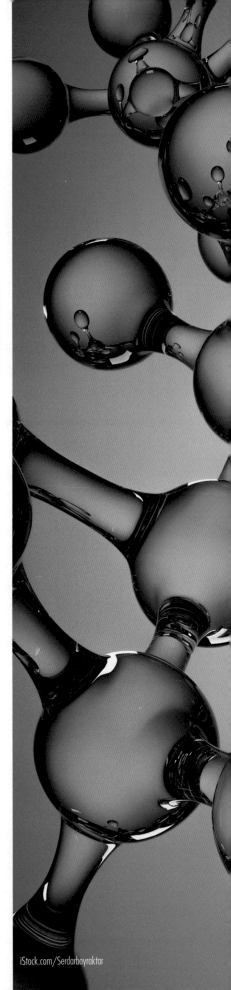

iStock.com/Serdarbayraktar

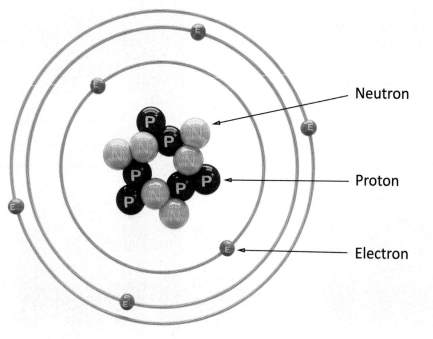

general-fmv/Shutterstock.com

▲ **FIGURE 6-2** Atomic structure of carbon with six protons, six neutrons, and six electrons.

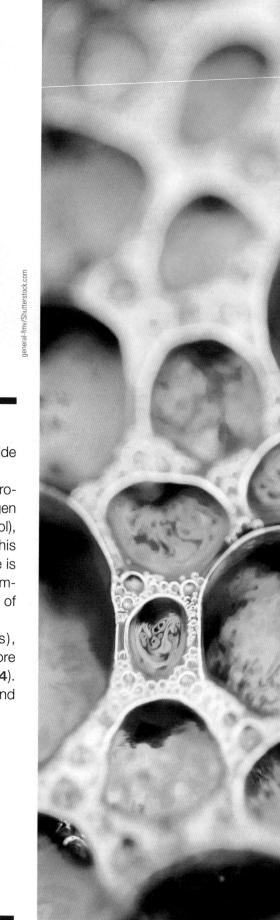

water is made from hydrogen atoms and oxygen atoms. Carbon dioxide is made from carbon atoms and oxygen atoms.

Atmospheric oxygen and other chemical substances, such as nitrogen and water vapor, make up the air you breathe. Atmospheric oxygen is considered an **elemental molecule** (el-uh-MEN-tul MAHL-uh-kyool), a molecule containing two or more atoms of the same element (in this case, oxygen) in definite (fixed) proportions. It is written as O_2. Ozone is another elemental molecule made up of oxygen. Ozone is a major component of smog and can be very dangerous. It contains three atoms of the element oxygen and is written as O_3 (**Figure 6-3**).

Compound molecules (KAHM-pownd MAHL-uh-kyools), also known as *compounds*, are chemical combinations of two or more atoms of different elements in definite (fixed) proportions (**Figure 6-4**). Sodium chloride (NaCl), common table salt, is an example of a compound

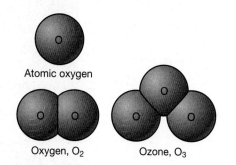

Atomic oxygen

Oxygen, O_2

Ozone, O_3

▲ **FIGURE 6-3** Elemental molecules contain two or more atoms of the same element in definite (fixed) proportions.

Evannovostro/Shutterstock.com

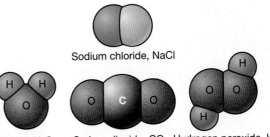

Sodium chloride, NaCl

Water, H_2O Carbon dioxide, CO_2 Hydrogen peroxide, H_2O_2

▲ FIGURE 6-4 Compound molecules contain two or more atoms of different elements in definite (fixed) proportions.

molecule. Each sodium chloride molecule contains one atom of the element sodium (Na) and one atom of the element chlorine (Cl).

PHYSICAL AND CHEMICAL PROPERTIES OF MATTER

Matter can be changed in two different ways. Physical forces cause physical changes and chemical reactions cause chemical changes.

A physical change (FIZ-ih-kuhl CHAYNJ) is a change in the form or physical properties of a substance, without a chemical reaction or the creation of a new substance. No chemical reactions are involved in physical change and no new chemicals are formed. Solid ice undergoes a physical change when it melts into water and then converts into steam when heat is applied (**Figure 6-5**). A physical change occurs when nail polish is applied onto nails and the solvent evaporates, forming a layer or film on the nail.

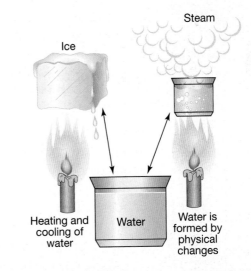

Steam

Ice

Heating and cooling of water

Water

Water is formed by physical changes

▲ FIGURE 6-5 Water changing phases is an example of physical change.

A chemical change (KEM-uh-kul CHAYNJ) is a change in the chemical composition or makeup of a substance. This change is caused by chemical reactions that create new chemical substances, usually by

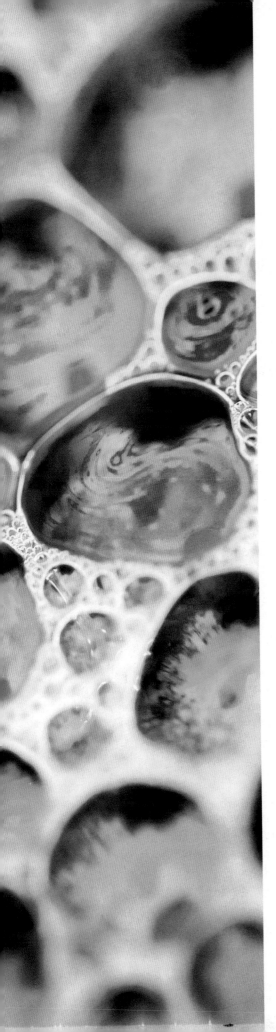

combining or subtracting certain elements. Those new substances have different chemical and physical properties (**Figure 6-6**). In fact, every substance has unique properties that allow us to identify it. As with the two types of changes, the two types of properties are physical and chemical as well.

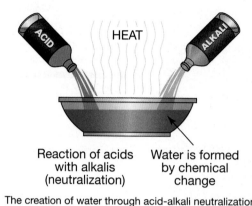

Reaction of acids with alkalis (neutralization)   Water is formed by chemical change

▲ **FIGURE 6-6** The creation of water through acid-alkali neutralization is a chemical change.

Physical properties (FIZ-ih-kuhl PRAH-per-teez) are characteristics that can be determined without a chemical reaction and do not involve a chemical change in the substance. Physical properties include color, solubility, odor, density, melting point, boiling point, hardness, and glossiness. **Chemical properties** (KEM-uh-kul PROP-er-teez) are characteristics that can be determined only by a chemical reaction and involve a chemical change in the substance. Examples include the ability of iron to rust, wood to burn, or hair to change color through the use of haircolor and hydrogen peroxide.

PURE SUBSTANCES AND PHYSICAL MIXTURES

All matter can be classified as either a pure substance or a physical mixture. A **pure substance** (PYOOR SUB-stantz) is a chemical combination of matter in definite (fixed) proportions. Pure substances have unique properties. Water and salt are examples of pure substances, with atoms in set proportion: 2 hydrogen atoms per oxygen atom (H_2O) and 1 sodium atom per chlorine atom (NaCl), respectively. Most substances do not exist in a pure state.

Air contains many substances, including nitrogen, carbon dioxide, and water vapor. This is an example of a physical mixture. A **physical mixture** (FIZ-ih-kuhl MIX-chur) is a physical combination of matter in any proportion. The properties of a physical mixture are the combined properties of the substances in the mixture. Salt water is a physical mixture of salt and water in any proportion. The properties of salt water are the properties contained in salt and in water: salt water is salty and wet. Most of the products that beauty professionals use are physical mixtures (**Figure 6-7**).

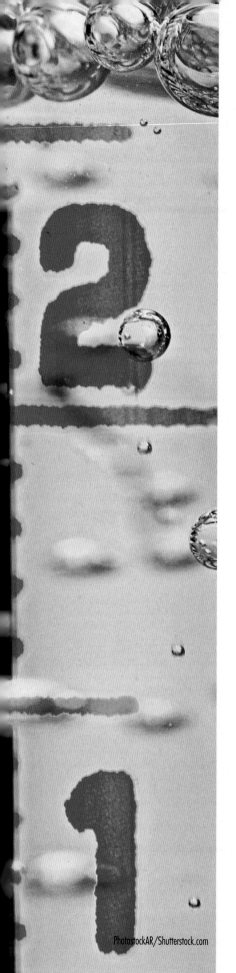

PhotostockAR/Shutterstock.com

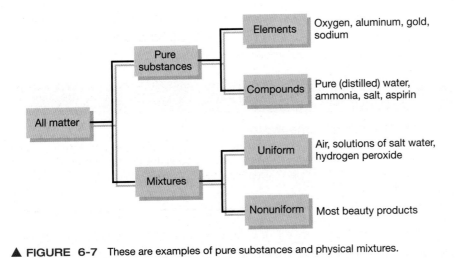

		Elements	Oxygen, aluminum, gold, sodium
Pure substances		Compounds	Pure (distilled) water, ammonia, salt, aspirin
All matter			
Mixtures		Uniform	Air, solutions of salt water, hydrogen peroxide
		Nonuniform	Most beauty products

▲ FIGURE 6-7 These are examples of pure substances and physical mixtures.

CHECK IN
Describe pure substances and physical mixtures. Give examples.

EXPLAIN THE DIFFERENCES BETWEEN SOLUTIONS, SUSPENSIONS, AND EMULSIONS

To better serve their clients, beauty professionals should have an understanding of the chemical composition, preparation, and uses of cosmetics that are intended for the hair, skin, nails, and body in general. Most of the products a beauty professional uses are solutions, suspensions, and emulsions.

Solutions, suspensions, and emulsions are all physical mixtures. The distinction between them depends on the types of substances, the size of the particles, and the solubility of the substances.

- A solution (suh-LOO-shun) is a stable, uniform mixture of two or more substances. The solute (SAHL-yoot) is the substance that is dissolved in a solution. The solvent (SAHL-vent) is the substance that dissolves the solute and makes the solution (**Figure 6-8**).

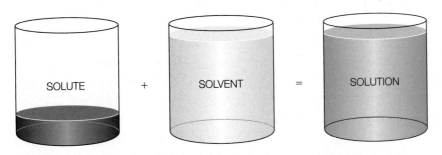

SOLUTE + SOLVENT = SOLUTION

▲ FIGURE 6-8 A solution is created when a solute is dissolved in a solvent.

For example, when salt is dissolved in water, salt is the solute and water is the solvent. Water is known as the universal solvent because it has the ability to dissolve more substances than any other solvent.

ACTIVITY

Evaporation Experimentation
Put an ounce of clear hairstyling spray into a cup. Cover it loosely with a paper towel and set it aside for a week. What happens when the liquid evaporates? What does the residue look like? Touch and feel the residue. In chemistry terms, what is this residue?

All liquids are either miscible or immiscible. Miscible (MIS-uh-bul) liquids are mutually soluble, meaning that they can be mixed together to form solutions. Water and alcohol are examples of miscible liquids, as in a nail polish remover. When these substances are mixed together, they will stay mixed, forming a solution. Solutions contain small particles that are invisible to the naked eye. Solutions are usually transparent, although they may be colored. They do not separate when left still. Again, salt water is an example of a solution with a solid dissolved in a liquid. Water is the solvent that dissolves the salt (solute) and holds it in solution.

Immiscible (im-IS-uh-bul) liquids are not capable of being mixed together to form stable solutions. Water and oil are two examples. They can be mixed together but will separate when they are left sitting still. When immiscible liquids are combined, they form suspensions.

- Suspensions (sus-PEN-shunz) are unstable physical mixtures of undissolved particles in a liquid. Compared with solutions, suspensions contain larger and fewer miscible particles. The particles are generally visible to the naked eye but are not large enough to settle quickly to the bottom. Suspensions are not usually transparent and may be colored. They are unstable and separate over time, which is why some lotions and creams can separate in the bottle and need to be shaken before they are used. An example of a suspension is the glitter in nail polish, which can separate from the polish. Calamine lotion is another example.

- An emulsion (ee-MUL-shun) is an unstable physical mixture of two or more immiscible substances (substances that normally will not stay mixed) plus a special ingredient called an *emulsifier*. An emulsifier (ee-MUL-suh-fy-ur) is an ingredient that brings two normally incompatible materials together and binds them into a uniform and fairly stable mixture. Emulsions are considered to be a special type of suspension because they can separate; however, the separation usually happens very slowly over a long period of time. An example of an emulsion is skin cream (**Figure 6-9**). A properly formulated emulsion, stored under ideal conditions, can be stable for up to three years. Since conditions are rarely ideal, all cosmetic emulsions should be used within one year of purchase. Always refer to the product's instructions and cautions for specific details.

Table 6-1 summarizes the differences between solutions, suspensions, and emulsions.

Picsfive/Shutterstock.com

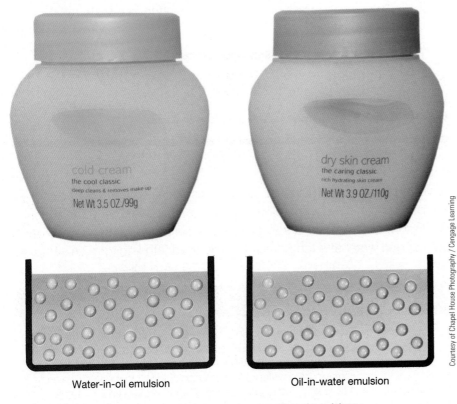

Water-in-oil emulsion   Oil-in-water emulsion

Courtesy of Chapel House Photography / Cengage Learning

▲ FIGURE 6-9 Cold cream and skin cream are examples of emulsions.

TABLE 6-1: DIFFERENCES BETWEEN SOLUTIONS, SUSPENSIONS, AND EMULSIONS

SOLUTIONS	SUSPENSIONS	EMULSIONS
Miscible	Slightly miscible	Immiscible
No surfactant	No surfactant	Surfactant
Small particles	Larger particles	Largest particles
Stable mixture	Unstable, temporary mixture	Limited stability through an emulsifier
Usually clear	Usually cloudy	Usually a solid color
Witch hazel	Nail polish, glitter in nail polish	Shampoos, conditioners, hand lotions

SURFACTANTS

Surfactants (sur-FAK-tants) are substances that allow oil and water to mix, or emulsify. As such, they are one type of emulsifier. A surfactant molecule has two distinct parts (**Figure 6-10**): The head of the surfactant molecule is hydrophilic (hy-druh-FIL-ik), capable of combining with or attracting water (water loving); the tail is lipophilic (ly-puh-FIL-ik), having an affinity for or an attraction to fat and oils (oil loving). Following the like-dissolves-like rule—a chemistry rule of thumb describing how

CHAPTER 6 Chemistry & Chemical Safety   **161**

Oil-loving
tail

Water-loving
head

▲ FIGURE 6-10   A surfactant molecule has two distinct parts.

solvents dissolve chemically similar solutes (for example, water dissolves salt but not oil)—the hydrophilic head dissolves in water and the lipophilic tail dissolves in oil. Thus, a surfactant molecule mixes with and dissolves in both oil and water and temporarily joins them together to form an emulsion.

DID YOU KNOW?

Soaps were the first surfactants. People began making soaps about 4,500 years ago by boiling oil or animal fat with wood ashes. Modern soaps are made from animal fats or vegetable oils. Traditional bar soaps are highly alkaline and combine with the minerals in hard water to form an insoluble film that coats skin and can cause hands to feel dry, itchy, and irritated. Beauty professionals who are performing nail services should be aware that soaps can leave a film on the nail plate, which could contribute to lifting of the nail enhancement. Modern synthetic surfactants have overcome these disadvantages and are superior to soaps; many are milder on the skin than soaps used in the past.

OIL-IN-WATER (O/W) EMULSIONS

In an oil-in-water (O/W) emulsion (OYL-in-WAHT-ur ee-MUL-shun), oil droplets are emulsified in water. The droplets of oil are surrounded by surfactant molecules with their lipophilic tails pointing in and their hydrophilic heads pointing out. Tiny oil droplets form the internal portion of each O/W emulsion because the oil is completely surrounded by water. Oil-in-water emulsions do not feel as greasy as water-in-oil emulsions because the oil is hidden and water forms the external portion of the emulsion. Salons, spas, and barbershops use primarily O/W emulsions.

ACTIVITY

Oil and Water
Have you ever heard the saying "oil and water don't mix"? Pour some water into a glass and add a little cooking oil (or other oil). What happens? Stir the water briskly with a spoon and observe for a minute or two. What does the oil do?

WATER-IN-OIL (W/O) EMULSIONS

In a water-in-oil (W/O) emulsion (WAHT-ur-in-OYL ee-MUL-shun), water droplets are emulsified in oil. The droplets of water are surrounded by surfactants with their hydrophilic heads pointing in and their lipophilic tails pointing out (**Figure 6-11**). Tiny droplets of water form the internal

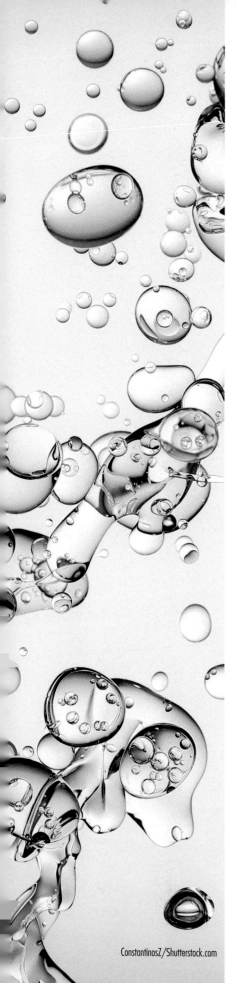

ConstantinosZ/Shutterstock.com

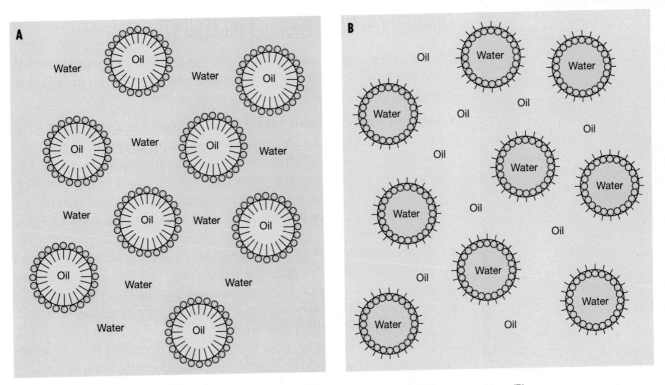

▲ FIGURE 6-11 Compare the structure of oil-in-water emulsions (A) with that of water-in-oil emulsions (B).

portion of a W/O emulsion because the water is completely surrounded by oil. Water-in-oil emulsions feel greasier than oil-in-water emulsions because the water is hidden and oil forms the external portion of the emulsion. Styling creams, cold creams, suntan lotions, and foot balms are examples of W/O emulsions.

OTHER PHYSICAL MIXTURES

Ointments, pastes, pomades, and styling waxes are semisolid mixtures made with any combination of petrolatum (petroleum jelly), oil, and wax.

Powders are a physical mixture of one or more types of solids. Off-the-scalp, powdered hair lighteners are physical mixtures. These mixtures may separate during shipping and storage and should be thoroughly mixed by shaking the container before each use.

DID YOU KNOW?

Mayonnaise is an example of an oil-in-water emulsion of two immiscible liquids. Although oil and water are immiscible, the egg yolk in mayonnaise emulsifies the oil droplets and distributes them uniformly in the water. Without the egg yolk as an emulsifying agent, the oil and water would separate. Most of the emulsions used in a salon, spa, or barbershop are oil-in-water. Haircolor, shampoos, conditioners, hand lotions, and facial creams are oil-in-water emulsions.

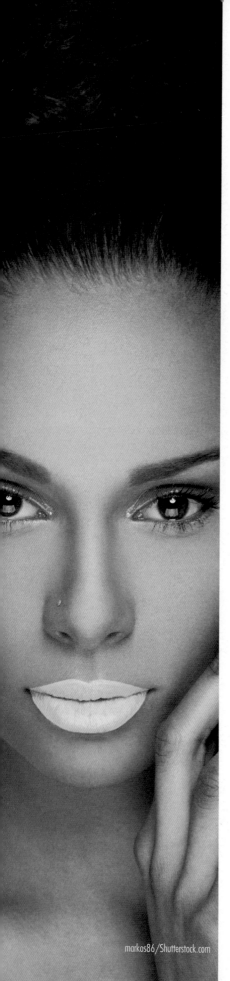

markos86/Shutterstock.com

COMMON CHEMICAL PRODUCT INGREDIENTS

Beauty professionals use many chemical products when performing client services. The following are some of the most common chemical ingredients used in beauty and wellness products:

- Volatile alcohols (VAHL-uh-tul AL-kuh-hawlz) evaporate easily, such as isopropyl alcohol (rubbing alcohol) and ethyl alcohol (hairspray and alcoholic beverages). These chemicals are familiar to most people. However, there are many other types of alcohol, from free-flowing liquids to hard, waxy solids. Fatty alcohols, such as cetyl alcohol and cetearyl alcohol, are nonvolatile alcohol waxes that are used as skin conditioners.
- Alkanolamines (al-kan-AHL-uh-mynz) are alkaline substances used to neutralize acids or raise the pH of many hair products. They are often used in place of ammonia because they produce less odor.
- Ammonia (uh-MOH-nee-uh) is a colorless gas composed of hydrogen and nitrogen that has a pungent odor. It is used to raise the pH in hair products to allow the solution to penetrate the hair shaft. Ammonium hydroxide and ammonium thioglycolate are examples of ammonia compounds that are used to perform chemical services.
- Glycerin (GLIS-ur-in) is a sweet, colorless, oily substance. It is used as a solvent and as a moisturizer in skin and body creams.
- Silicones (SIL-ih-kohnz) are a special type of oil used in hair conditioners, water-resistant lubricants for the skin, and nail polish dryers. Silicones are less greasy than other oils and form a breathable film that does not cause comedones (blackheads). Silicones also give a silky, smooth feeling to skin, and great shine to hair. Certain silicone resins (silicone gums) can withstand high pH environments and can be incorporated into hair relaxers and permanent wave formulations.
- Volatile organic compounds (VOCs) (VAHL-uh-tuhl orr-GAN-ik KAHM-powndz) contain carbon (organic) and evaporate very easily (volatile). For example, a common VOC used in hairspray is SD alcohol (ethyl alcohol). Volatile organic solvents such as ethyl acetate and isopropyl alcohol are used in nail polish, base and top coats, and polish removers.

DID YOU KNOW?

Silicon (Si) is an element, like carbon (C) and oxygen (O), that has a metallic appearance and is widely used in the electronics industry. Do not confuse it with *silicones*, which are compounds made with silicon and other elements. Silicones are used in a variety of personal care products including hair care, skin care, and nail care products.

THE OVEREXPOSURE PRINCIPLE

You may often hear the word *toxic*. People tend to think of a toxic substance as a dangerous poison; however, the toxicity of a substance is related to how it is used, and how much of it is used. The truth is, everything on earth is toxic to some degree—there is nothing in the world that is completely nontoxic. The very word *nontoxic* is a made-up marketing term that has no precise scientific meaning.

Overexposure (OH-var-ex-POH-zur) refers to how prolonged, repeated, or long-term exposure to certain product ingredients can cause sensitivity in some people. The *overexposure principle* is used to describe how overexposure determines toxicity. It holds that it is the dose of a substance that determines whether it will have a negative, poisonous effect on the body. For example, salt water is very toxic to drink yet you can safely swim in the ocean without fear of poisoning. Similarly, rubbing alcohol is quite toxic. A tablespoonful can poison and kill a small child, however it is safe to use on the body (and when kept out of reach of children). Toxicity does not mean a substance is automatically unsafe; instead, it tells you that you must be sure to use it in a safe manner.

To understand how to safely use and handle your products, review the manufacturer's Safety Data Sheet (SDS) for important safety information.

CHECK IN
What are the differences between solutions, suspensions, and emulsions? Give examples.

DESCRIBE POTENTIAL HYDROGEN AND HOW THE PH SCALE WORKS

Although pH (P-H), an abbreviation of *potential hydrogen*, is often mentioned when talking about beauty products, it is one of the least understood chemical properties. Notice that *pH* is written with a small *p* (which represents a quantity) and a capital *H* (which represents the hydrogen ion). The term *pH* represents the quantity of hydrogen ions. Understanding pH and how it affects the hair, skin, and nails is essential to understanding all beauty and wellness services.

WATER AND PH

Before you can understand pH, you need to learn about ions. An ion (EYE-on) is an atom or molecule that carries an electrical charge. Ionization (eye-on-ih-ZAY-shun) is the separation of an atom or molecule into positive and negative ions. An ion with a negative electrical charge is an anion (AN-eye-on). An ion with a positive electrical charge is a cation (KAT-eye-on).

Some water (H_2O) molecules naturally ionize into hydrogen ions and hydroxide ions. The pH scale measures these ions. The hydrogen ion (H^+) is acidic. The more hydrogen ions there are in a substance, the more acidic it will be. The hydroxide ion (OH^-) is alkaline. The more hydroxide ions there are in a substance, the more alkaline it will be. pH is only possible because of this ionization of water. Therefore, only products that contain water can have a pH.

In pure (distilled) water, each water molecule that ionizes produces one hydrogen ion and one hydroxide ion (**Figure 6-12**). Pure water has a neutral pH because it contains the same number of hydrogen ions as hydroxide ions. It is an equal balance of 50 percent acidic and 50 percent alkaline. The pH of any substance is always a balance of both acidity and alkalinity. As acidity increases, alkalinity decreases. The opposite is also true: as alkalinity increases, acidity decreases. Even the strongest acid also contains some alkalinity.

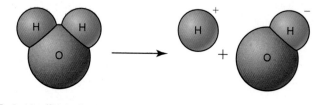

▲ FIGURE 6-12 The ionization of water.

THE PH SCALE

The pH scale (P-H SKAYL) is used to measure the acidity and alkalinity of substances. It has a range of 0 to 14. A pH of 7 is a neutral solution, a pH below 7 indicates an acidic solution (uh-SID-ik suh-LOO-shun), and a pH above 7 indicates an alkaline solution (AL-kuh-line suh-LOO-shun) (**Figure 6-13**). However, one point of pH difference is more than it looks. Because the pH scale is a logarithmic scale, a change of one whole number represents a tenfold change in pH. This means, for example, that a pH of 8 is 10 times more alkaline than a pH of 7. A change of two whole numbers represents a change of 10 times 10, or a 100-fold change. So a pH of 9 is 100 times more alkaline than a pH of 7. Even a small change on the pH scale represents a large change in the pH.

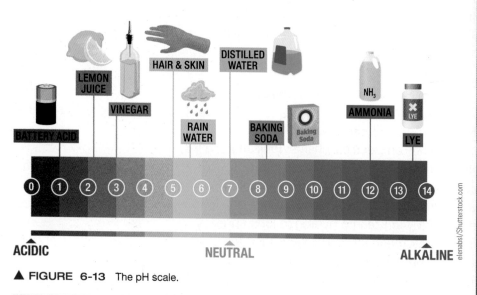

elenabsl/Shutterstock.com

▲ FIGURE 6-13 The pH scale.

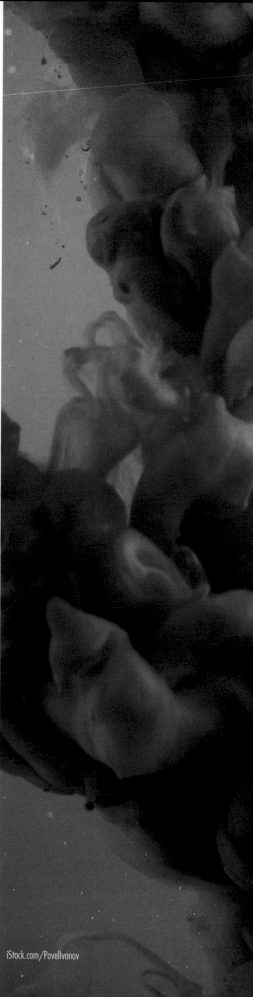

iStock.com/Pavellvanov

pH is always a balance of both acidity and alkalinity. Pure (distilled) water has a pH of 7, which is an equal balance of acid and alkaline. Although a pH of 7 is neutral on the pH scale, it is not neutral compared to the hair and skin, which have an average pH of 5. Pure water, with a pH of 7, is 100 times more alkaline than a pH of 5, so pure water is 100 times more alkaline than your hair and skin. This difference in pH is the reason pure water can cause the hair to swell as much as 20 percent.

PH AND SKIN CARE PRODUCTS

When the skin is exposed to extremes in pH levels, dryness, dehydration, inflammation, and even bacteria can grow if the product is incorrect for a given skin type. It is important to use products that contain the proper pH for a given skin type. For example, if a client has dry, dehydrated skin, giving that client a product that is too acidic could further dry and irritate their skin. Conversely, if a client has an oily skin type, a product that is slightly alkaline may contribute to oil and sebum buildup and possibly create acne. This client may need a product with a more acidic pH.

ACIDS AND ALKALIS

All acids owe their chemical reactivity to the hydrogen ion. Acids have a pH below 7.

Alpha hydroxy acids (AHAs) (AL-fah hy-DROK-see AS-udz), derived from plants (mostly fruit), are examples of acids often used to exfoliate the skin and to help adjust the pH of a lotion, conditioner, or cream. Acids contract and close the hair cuticle. One such acid is thioglycolic acid (thy-oh-gly-KOHL-ik AS-ud), a colorless liquid or white crystals with a strong, unpleasant odor that is used in permanent waving solutions. Glycolic acid (gly-KOHL-ik AS-ud) is an alpha hydroxy acid used in exfoliation and to lower the pH of products.

All alkalis (AL-kuh-lyz), also known as *bases*, owe their chemical reactivity to the hydroxide ion. Alkalis are compounds that react with acids to form salts. Alkalis have a pH above 7. They feel slippery and soapy on the skin. Alkalis soften and swell hair, skin, the cuticle on the nail plate, and calloused skin.

Sodium hydroxide (SO-dee-um hy-DROK-syd), commonly known as lye, is a very strong alkali used in chemical hair relaxers, callous softeners, and drain cleaners. These products must be used according to manufacturers' instructions; it is very important that you do not let these products touch or sit on the skin, as they may cause injury or a burning sensation. Sodium hydroxide products may be especially dangerous if they get into the eyes, so always wear safety glasses to avoid eye contact. Consult the product's SDS for more specific information on safe use.

ACTIVITY

Product pH

For a product to have a pH, it must contain water. Shampoos, conditioners, haircolor, permanent waves, relaxers, lotions, and creams have a pH. Divide into groups and use the Internet to find the pH of these products or of others found in your school. If the information is not available online, contact the manufacturer of the product. Make a chart and compare your findings with your classmates'. How will the pH of these products affect the hair or skin?

Here is a hint to save you some time: Oils, waxes, and nail polish have no pH because they contain no water.

CHECK IN
Define pH and draw a pH scale.

SUMMARIZE NEUTRALIZATION AND REDOX REACTIONS

Two types of chemical reactions are of particular importance to beauty professionals because they explain how major beauty products work. They are acid–alkali neutralization reactions and oxidation–reduction reactions.

NEUTRALIZATION REACTIONS

Acid–alkali neutralization reactions (AS-ud AL-kuh-lye NEW-trah-lyz-A-shun ree-AK-shunz) occur when an acid is mixed with an alkali in equal proportions, balancing the total pH and forming water (H_2O) and a salt (**Figure 6-14**). Neutralizing shampoos and normalizing lotions used to neutralize hair relaxers work by causing an acid-alkali neutralization reaction. This stops the relaxing process and returns the hair to its natural pH level. Similarly, slightly acidic liquid soaps can be used to neutralize alkaline callous softener residues left on the skin after rinsing with water. In both of these examples, the natural pH of the hair or skin is recovered, an important step in beauty services that returns the body to equilibrium.

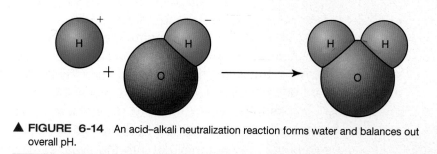

▲ FIGURE 6-14 An acid–alkali neutralization reaction forms water and balances out overall pH.

REDOX REACTIONS

Oxidation–reduction (ahk-sih-DAY-shun ree-AK-shun), also known as redox (REE-docs), is a chemical reaction in which oxidation and reduction take place at the same time. When oxygen is chemically combined with a substance, the substance is oxidized. When oxygen is chemically removed from a substance, the substance is reduced.

An oxidizing agent (ahk-sih-DY-zing AY-jent) is a substance that releases oxygen. Hydrogen peroxide (H_2O_2), which can be thought of as water with an extra atom of oxygen, is an example of an oxidizing agent. A reducing agent (re-DOO-sing AY-jent) is a substance that adds hydrogen to a chemical compound or subtracts oxygen from the compound. When hydrogen peroxide is mixed with an oxidation haircolor, oxygen is subtracted from the hydrogen peroxide and the hydrogen peroxide is reduced. At the same time, oxygen is added to the haircolor and the haircolor is oxidized. In this example, haircolor is the reducing agent.

So far, we have considered oxidation only as the addition of oxygen and reduction only as the loss of oxygen. Although the first known oxidation reactions involved oxygen, many oxidation reactions do not involve oxygen. Oxidation also results from loss of hydrogen and reduction also results from addition of hydrogen (**Figure 6-15**). Redox reactions are also responsible for the chemical changes created by haircolors, hair lighteners, permanent wave solutions, and thioglycolic acid neutralizers. These chemical services would not be possible without oxidation–reduction (redox) reactions.

OXIDATION	REDUCTION
+ Oxygen	– Oxygen
– Hydrogen	+ Hydrogen

▲ **FIGURE 6-15** This chart shows the interconnection of oxidation and reduction reactions.

EXOTHERMIC REACTIONS

When certain chemical reactions release energy in the form of heat, it is called an exothermic reaction (EK-soh-thur-mik ree-AK-shun). An example of this is the heat produced after mixing the activator and waving lotion in an exothermic permanent wave product. When the activator, which contains hydrogen peroxide, is added to the waving lotion, an oxidation reaction occurs that produces heat. The mixing of these chemicals produces a more rapid form of oxidation than the slower oxidation that occurs with permanent wave neutralizers or oxidation haircolor products. In most cases, you can expect to feel a slight warming of the container after mixing the activator with the waving lotion. Another

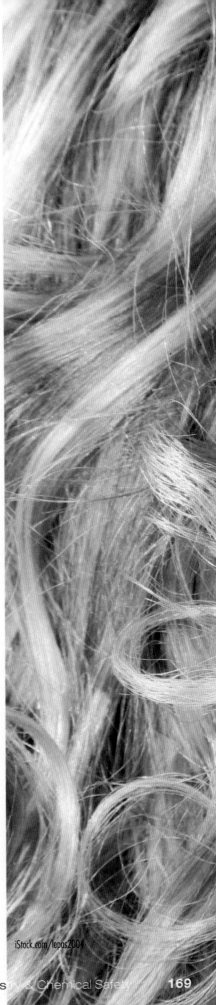

iStock.com/lepas2004

example of an exothermic reaction is a nail product that hardens (polymerizes) to create nail enhancements. In fact, all oxidation reactions are exothermic reactions.

Combustion (kum-BUS-chun) is the rapid oxidation of a substance accompanied by the production of heat and light. Lighting a match is an example of combustion. Oxidation requires the presence of oxygen; this is the reason that there cannot be a fire without air.

ENDOTHERMIC REACTIONS

An endothermic reaction (en-duh-THUR-mik ree-AK-shun) is a chemical reaction that requires the absorption of energy or heat from an external source for the reaction to actually occur. Melting ice is an example of an endothermic reaction: If the ice were not absorbing heat from its surroundings, it would not be melting! Another example, from the world of hair care, is a permanent waving lotion that requires the application of heat from a hood dryer to activate it for processing, rather than processing at room temperature; these are called *endothermic waves*.

CHECK IN
Explain neutralization reactions and why they are an important part of beauty services.

PRACTICE CHEMICAL SAFETY

Considering all of the types of chemicals used daily in the salon, spa, and barbershop, along with all of their potential actions and reactions, practicing chemical safety should be of primary concern. From transporting to disposing of chemicals, you must be aware of the risks involved and the processes needed to ensure safety. Although it may seem time-consuming and complicated, reading the labels of all the products you use and understanding how to safely handle them are important parts of being a beauty professional.

LABELS

Manufacturers of chemicals that are registered with either the EPA or FDA are held to strict standards for their labels. These require that all hazards be disclosed alongside specific cautions and directions for use. It is unfortunate, but many people do not read product labels yet are shocked when they have a bad outcome. For example, using hydrogen peroxide in higher concentrations or applying heat to accelerate a service can cause severe chemical burns. It is vital that you always follow label instructions to avoid dangerous and painful situations (**Figure 6-16**).

Warning Labels

Find and read the labels for three beauty and wellness products (actual labels or from the Internet). What warnings are listed? What active ingredients are listed? What *are* those active ingredients? Do a quick search and report your ingredient and label findings to the class.

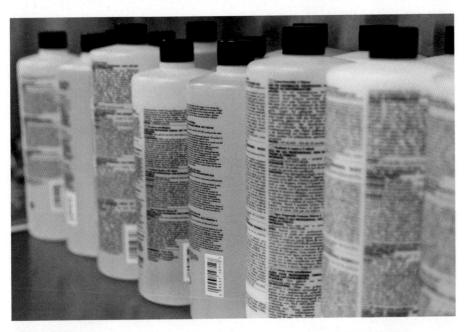

▲ FIGURE 6-16 Be sure to read and follow the directions on all chemical labels.

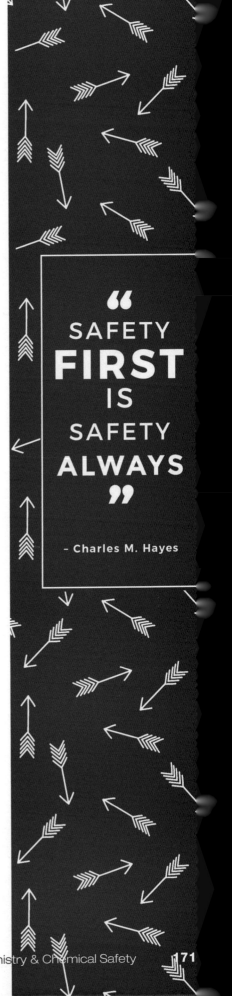

> **" SAFETY FIRST IS SAFETY ALWAYS "**
>
> – Charles M. Hayes

TRANSPORTATION

The first time you enter the beauty supply store as a licensed professional is exciting! Here's an entire store filled with the tools of your trade, and now you are allowed to actually purchase them! It is important that as you shop, you pay attention to product labels. Some may list warnings that will affect how you transport them. For example, if a label says, "Do not store at temperatures above 78 degrees Fahrenheit" or "Avoid direct sunlight," you know that it is not safe to transport this product in your trunk or to let it sit in your car on a hot summer day. In addition, regardless of the temperature outside, a bottle sitting on the back seat with the sun beating through the window could become hot enough to ignite.

Another consideration when transporting chemicals is products that are incompatible (in-com-PAT-uh-bul), meaning that they should not be mixed or even stored near each other. For example, hydrogen peroxide is a common chemical in hair developer (oxidizer); however, when it is mixed with bleach, it creates chlorine gas, which can be deadly. With this in mind, driving with developer and bleach rolling around in the backseat might not be the best idea. All chemicals should be transported upright and in their original containers; because many of these chemicals become more dangerous as they decompose, opened or partially used containers should not be transported at all.

STORAGE

The storage of chemicals in the salon, spa, or barbershop is also an area where safety and strict processes should be followed to prevent injury and fire. Having designated places to store specific chemicals and never allowing chemicals to sit out, even in a dispensing area, can mean the difference between a safe and an unsafe environment for you and your clients. In particular, chemicals should be locked up at all times—if an adult can get to them, so can a child!

All chemicals should be stored and disposed of in their original containers. Even if two chemicals are similar, they should never be haphazardly combined together or stored mixed. When storing chemicals next to each other, it is critical to know how the two would react if they somehow came into contact with each other. For example, an oxidizer such as hydrogen peroxide mixed with a flammable solvent such as acetone results in fire, so placing those types of products next to each other could potentially be disastrous (**Figure 6-17**).

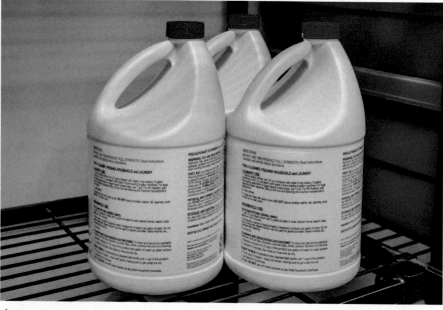

▲ **FIGURE 6-17** Store chemicals – especially bleach! – in a secure, designated space, following manufacturer guidelines.

CAUTION

Despite being an extremely common chemical in the salon, spa, and barbershop (and home), bleach can pose unforeseen safety risks because of its chemical composition and reactivity. Bleach should never be mixed with any cleaning product unless expressly instructed on the manufacturer's label, as even just vinegar and bleach creates chlorine gas. In fact, bleach should always be stored away from other chemicals because of the possibility of harmful gases inadvertently being created.

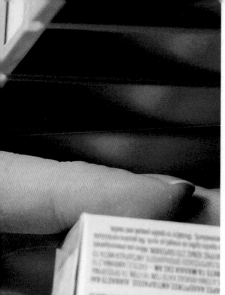

Ravil Sayfullin/Shutterstock.com

MIXING

Mixing chemicals can create dangerous gases, such as chlorine, nitrogen trichloride, chloramine vapor, and hydrazine. Because these gases can be life threatening, processes concerning the mixing of chemicals should be clear to everyone who works in a salon, spa, or barbershop, and should never be compromised. Consider these guidelines when mixing or preparing to mix chemicals:

- The location you use for mixing chemicals must be well ventilated and have protective equipment available, including an eyewash bottle.
- Always read chemical labels thoroughly before mixing. If there are potential reactions listed and you are uncertain if the chemicals should be mixed, do not mix them. For example, bleach has a warning on the label that it should not be mixed with any acids or ammonia products; however, it can be hard to tell which ingredients are acids. When in doubt, do not mix!
- Use a measuring device, such as a measuring cup or spoon, and make sure that it is cleaned thoroughly between uses.
- Always add the chemical to the water, not the other way around, when using concentrated chemicals like disinfectants.
- When concentrates are mixed and used in a secondary container, such as a spray bottle, that container should be labeled to indicate the product name, ingredients, and any hazards listed by the manufacturer.

DISPOSAL

Many of the chemicals that go down the sink drain every day in a salon, spa, or barbershop are dangerous to the environment and create burdens on our wastewater systems. Unfortunately, although many products have instructions for disposal of the container, few address disposal of the chemical itself. In many parts of the country, however, programs that recycle the chemical waste from beauty services exist and will likely continue to grow.

While most states and counties do not currently regulate the disposal of chemicals in the salon, spa, or barbershop, it is highly likely that such rules *will* be enacted over the next few years. For this reason, it is important to review your state's rules periodically to see if changes have occurred.

CHECK IN
What are four guidelines for properly storing chemicals?

INTERPRET SAFETY DATA SHEETS

The OSHA Hazard Communication Standard requires that employees be notified of any chemical in their workplace that could be hazardous. Prior to 2015, the Material Safety Data Sheet (MSDS) was the document used to provide this information to workers and first responders. In 2015 these were replaced by the Safety Data Sheet (SDS) (SAYF-tee DAY-tuh SHEET);

while they contain essentially the same information, there are some significant differences between the two. While both sheets provide valuable safety information about chemicals, the organization and ease of understanding has been greatly improved in the SDS.

All SDS are formatted into sixteen categories, with nine accepted pictograms, and are provided for free from the manufacturer of the chemical. Having an SDS available for every chemical used in the salon is a requirement of OSHA. Additionally, it is required that SDSs be immediately available to all employees, so storing them on a computer that only managers can access or keeping them in a locked office is not acceptable (**Figure 6-18**). Remember, these sheets are for use in emergencies, which are often chaotic situations where every second counts.

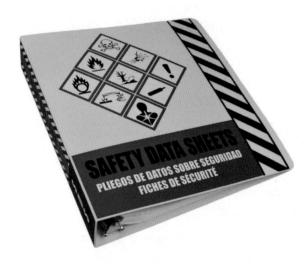

▲ FIGURE 6-18 Safety Data Sheets must be immediately available to all employees in the event of an emergency.

SDS CATEGORIES

The categories on the SDS are in a uniform format and order that must be followed by all manufacturers:

1. **Identification**: Includes the name of the product and contact information for the manufacturer or distributor. It also contains recommended use and restrictions on use.
2. **Hazard(s) Identification**: List all hazards associated with the product and include hazard classification (flammable, etc.), precautionary statements, and hazard pictograms (**Figure 6-19**).
3. **Composition/Information on Ingredients**: Identifies the ingredients of the product, including concentrations used in mixtures and when chemicals have been withheld due to a trade secret.
4. **First-Aid Measures**: Includes short- and long-term symptoms and first-aid instructions.
5. **Fire-Fighting Measures**: Lists suitable (and unsuitable) fire extinguishers, any chemical hazards associated with a fire, and recommended protective equipment or precautions.

iStock.com/Gwengoat

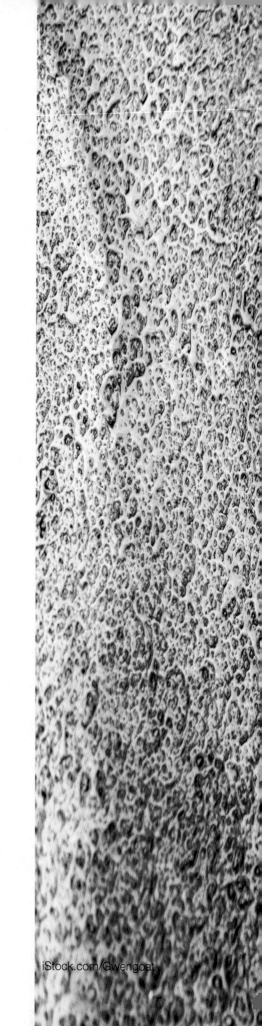

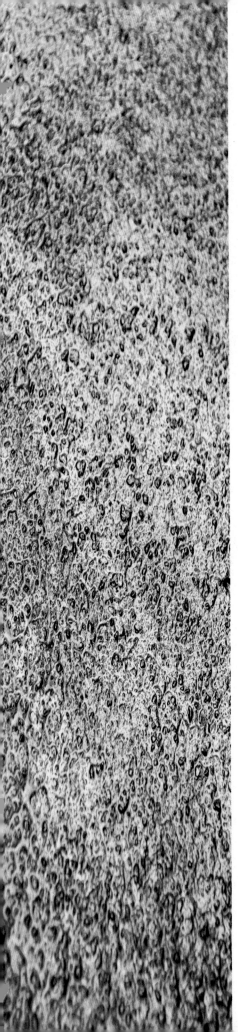

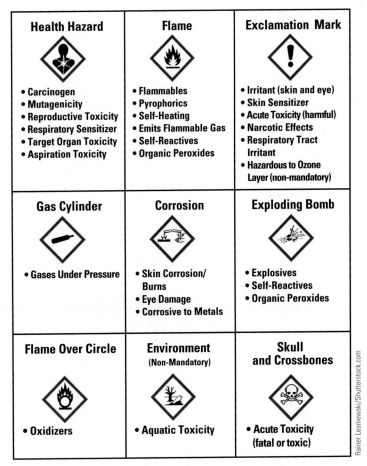

Health Hazard	Flame	Exclamation Mark
• Carcinogen • Mutagenicity • Reproductive Toxicity • Respiratory Sensitizer • Target Organ Toxicity • Aspiration Toxicity	• Flammables • Pyrophorics • Self-Heating • Emits Flammable Gas • Self-Reactives • Organic Peroxides	• Irritant (skin and eye) • Skin Sensitizer • Acute Toxicity (harmful) • Narcotic Effects • Respiratory Tract Irritant • Hazardous to Ozone Layer (non-mandatory)
Gas Cylinder	**Corrosion**	**Exploding Bomb**
• Gases Under Pressure	• Skin Corrosion/ Burns • Eye Damage • Corrosive to Metals	• Explosives • Self-Reactives • Organic Peroxides
Flame Over Circle	**Environment** (Non-Mandatory)	**Skull and Crossbones**
• Oxidizers	• Aquatic Toxicity	• Acute Toxicity (fatal or toxic)

Rainer Lesniewski/Shutterstock.com

▲ FIGURE 6-19 Safety Data Sheet hazard pictograms dictated by the international Globally Harmonized System of Classification and Labelling of Chemicals (GHS).

6. **Accidental Release Measures**: Provides instruction for proper cleanup of a spill, protective equipment needed, and emergency measures to follow.

7. **Handling and Storage**: Includes guidelines for safe handling and storage of chemicals, including incompatible chemicals.

8. **Exposure Controls/Personal Protection**: Provides recommended limits on exposure and methods to reduce exposure, such as personal protective equipment and proper ventilation.

9. **Physical and Chemical Properties**: Consists of a minimum of 18 properties, from color to pH to viscosity. Unknown or irrelevant properties for a product must be noted.

10. **Stability and Reactivity**: Provides information on the environmental, stability, and reaction risks associated with the product.

11. **Toxicological Information**: Details the risks of exposure, including symptoms like skin irritation, and measure of toxicity.

12. **Ecological Information**: Covers the impact of the chemical on the environment, such as groundwater absorption or danger to plants and animals.

13. **Disposal Considerations**: Lists any procedures for disposal.

14. **Transport Information**: Provides guidelines and restrictions for safe transportation.

15. **Regulatory Information**: Includes any specific safety, health, or environmental regulations.
16. **Other Information**: Indicates when the SDS was created or last updated[i].

SDS VOCABULARY

Safety Data Sheets make use of a wide range of scientific, medical, and specialized vocabulary to describe chemical properties and hazards. While it is well beyond the scope of this book to tackle SDS vocabulary as a whole, it is important to make a distinction between two pairs of related terms:

- A **carcinogen** (car-SIN-oh-jen) is a substance that causes or is believed to cause cancer. A **mutagen** (MEW-tah-jen), on the other hand, is a substance that *may* cause cancer but not always. Mutagens cause an increase in cellular mutations (changes), some of which are harmful; others have little or no effect on the body's function.
- **Combustible** (kum-BUS-tah-bul) material is capable of igniting and burning. Compared to this, **flammable** (FLA-ma-bul) material is even easier to ignite—combustible liquid has a flash point between 100 and 200 degrees Fahrenheit, while flammable liquid has a flash point below 100 degrees. The term *inflammable* is an older term, meaning flammable; *nonflammable* signifies something that is not flammable.

CHECK IN
List all of the categories found on a Safety Data Sheet.

APPLY CHEMISTRY AND CHEMICAL SAFETY

Congratulations on completing this chapter! Before you move on, take a moment to think about how these Chemistry and Chemical Safety topics apply to your particular discipline. Discuss with a classmate or study group how chemical reactions will come into play on the job; what processes you will need to follow when transporting and storing products; any special safety measures you may need to take during a service in order to protect yourself and your clients; and so on.

COMPETENCY PROGRESS

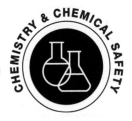

How are you doing with Chemistry and Chemical Safety? **Check off the Chapter 6 Learning Objectives** below that you feel you have mastered; leave unchecked those objectives you will need to return to:

☐ EXPLAIN CHEMISTRY AND CHEMICAL SAFETY.

☐ IDENTIFY THE BASICS OF CHEMICAL STRUCTURE.

☐ EXPLAIN THE DIFFERENCES BETWEEN SOLUTIONS, SUSPENSIONS, AND EMULSIONS.

☐ DESCRIBE POTENTIAL HYDROGEN AND HOW THE PH SCALE WORKS.

☐ SUMMARIZE NEUTRALIZATION AND REDOX REACTIONS.

☐ PRACTICE CHEMICAL SAFETY.

☐ INTERPRET SAFETY DATA SHEETS.

GLOSSARY

acidic solution uh-SID-ik suh-LOO-shun	p. 166	a solution that has a pH below 7 (neutral)
acid—alkali neutralization reactions AS-ud AL-kuh-lye NEW-trah-lyz-A-shun ree-AK-shunz	p. 168	when acids are mixed with alkalis in equal proportions, balancing the total pH and forming water (H_2O) and a salt
alkaline solution AL-kuh-line suh-LOO-shun	p. 166	a solution that has a pH above 7 (neutral)
alkalis AL-kuh-lyz	p. 167	also known as *bases*; compounds that react with acids to form salts
alkanolamines al-kan-AHL-uh-mynz	p. 164	alkaline substances used to neutralize acids or raise the pH of many hair products
alpha hydroxy acids AL-fah hy-DROK-see AS-udz	p. 167	abbreviated AHAs; acids derived from plants (mostly fruit) that are often used to exfoliate the skin
ammonia uh-MOH-nee-uh	p. 164	colorless gas with a pungent odor that is composed of hydrogen and nitrogen

anion AN-eye-on	p. 165	an ion with a negative electrical charge
atoms AT-umz	p. 155	the smallest chemical components (often called particles) of an element; structures that make up the element and have the same properties of the element
carcinogen car-SIN-oh-jen	p. 176	a substance that causes or is believed to cause cancer
cation KAT-eye-on	p. 165	an ion with a positive electrical charge
chemical change KEM-uh-kul CHAYNJ	p. 157	a change in the chemical composition or make-up of a substance
chemical properties KEM-uh-kul PROP-er-teez	p. 158	characteristics that can be determined only by a chemical reaction and a chemical change in the substance
chemistry KEM-uh-stree	p. 154	science that deals with the composition, structures, and properties of matter and how matter changes under different conditions
combustible kum-BUS-tah-bul	p. 176	material that is capable of igniting and burning
combustion kum-BUS-chun	p. 170	rapid oxidation of a substance accompanied by the production of heat and light
compound molecules KAHM-pownd MAHL-uh-kyools	p. 156	also known as compounds; a chemical combination of two or more atoms of different elements in definite (fixed) proportions
electrons ee-LEK-trahns	p. 155	subatomic particles with a negative charge
element EL-uh-ment	p. 154	the simplest form of chemical matter; an element cannot be broken down into a simpler substance without a loss of identity
elemental molecule el-uh-MEN-tul MAHL-uh-kyool	p. 156	molecule containing two or more atoms of the same element in definite (fixed) proportions
emulsifier ee-MUL-suh-fy-ur	p. 160	an ingredient that brings two normally incompatible materials together and binds them into a uniform and fairly stable mixture
emulsion ee-MUL-shun	p. 160	an unstable physical mixture of two or more immiscible substances (substances that normally will not stay mixed) plus a special ingredient called an emulsifier
endothermic reaction en-duh-THUR-mik ree-AK-shun	p. 170	chemical reaction that requires the absorption of energy or heat from an external source for the reaction to occur
exothermic reaction EK-soh-thur-mik ree-AK-shun	p. 169	chemical reaction that releases a significant amount of heat

flammable FLAH-ma-bul	p. 176	material that is capable of igniting and burning, and easier to ignite than combustible material
glycerin GLIS-ur-in	p. 164	sweet, colorless, oily substance used as a solvent and as a moisturizer in skin and body creams
glycolic acid gly-KOHL-ik AS-ud	p. 167	an alpha hydroxy acid used in exfoliation and to lower the pH of products
hydrophilic hy-druh-FIL-ik	p. 161	capable of combining with or attracting water (water-loving)
immiscible im-IS-uh-bul	p. 160	liquids that are not capable of being mixed together to form stable solutions
incompatible in-com-PAT-uh-bul	p. 171	substances that should not be mixed or even stored near each other
ion EYE-on	p. 165	an atom or molecule that carries an electrical charge
ionization eye-on-ih-ZAY-shun	p. 165	the separation of an atom or molecule into positive and negative ions
lipophilic ly-puh-FIL-ik	p. 161	having an affinity for or an attraction to fat and oils (oil-loving)
matter MAT-ur	p. 154	any substance that occupies space and has mass (weight)
miscible MIS-uh-bul	p. 160	liquids that are mutually soluble, meaning that they can be mixed together to form stable solutions
molecule MAHL-uh-kyool	p. 155	a chemical combination of two or more atoms in definite (fixed) proportions
mutagen MEW-tah-jen	p. 176	a substance that causes an increase in cellular mutations, some of which are harmful but others which have little or no effect on the body's function; *may* cause cancer but not always
neutrons NEW-trahns	p. 155	subatomic particles with no charge
oil-in-water emulsion OYL-in-WAHT-ur ee-MUL-shun	p. 162	abbreviated O/W emulsion; oil droplets emulsified in water
overexposure OH-var-ex-POH-zur	p. 165	prolonged, repeated, or long-term exposure that can cause sensitivity
oxidation—reduction ahk-sih-DAY-shun ree-AK-shun	p. 169	also known as *redox*; a chemical reaction in which the oxidizing agent is reduced (by losing oxygen) and the reducing agent is oxidized (by gaining oxygen)

oxidizing agent ahk-sih-DY-zing AY-jent	p. 169	a substance that releases oxygen
pH P-H	p. 165	the abbreviation used for potential hydrogen. pH represents the quantity of hydrogen ions
pH scale P-H SKAYL	p. 166	a measure of the acidity and alkalinity of a substance; the pH scale has a range of 0 to 14, with 7 being neutral. A pH below 7 is an acidic solution; a pH above 7 is an alkaline solution
physical change FIZ-ih-kuhl CHAYNJ	p. 157	a change in the form or physical properties of a substance without a chemical reaction or the creation of a new substance
physical mixture FIZ-ih-kuhl MIX-chur	p. 158	a physical combination of matter in any proportion
physical properties FIZ-ih-kuhl PRAH-per-teez	p. 158	characteristics that can be determined without a chemical reaction and that do not cause a chemical change in the substance
protons PRO-tahns	p. 155	subatomic particles with a positive charge
pure substance PYOOR SUB-stantz	p. 158	a chemical combination of matter in definite (fixed) proportions
reducing agent re-DOO-sing AY-jent	p. 169	a substance that adds hydrogen to a chemical compound or subtracts oxygen from the compound
Safety Data Sheet SAYF-tee DAY-tuh SHEET	p. 173	required by law for all products sold; SDSs include safety information about products compiled by the manufacturer, including hazardous ingredients, safe use and handling procedures, proper disposal guidelines, and precautions to reduce the risk of accidental harm or overexposure
silicones SIL-ih-kohnz	p. 164	special type of oil used in hair conditioners, water-resistant lubricants for the skin, and nail polish dryers
sodium hydroxide SO-dee-um hy-DROK-syd	p. 167	a very strong alkali used in chemical products and cleaners; commonly known as *lye*
solute SAHL-yoot	p. 159	the substance that is dissolved in a solution
solution suh-LOO-shun	p. 159	a stable, uniform mixture of two or more substances
solvent SAHL-vent	p. 159	the substance that dissolves the solute and makes a solution
surfactants sur-FAK-tants	p. 161	a contraction of surface active agents; substances that allow oil and water to mix, or emulsify
suspensions sus-PEN-shunz	p. 160	unstable physical mixtures of undissolved particles in a liquid

thioglycolic acid thy-oh-gly-KOHL-ik AS-ud	p. 167	a colorless liquid or white crystals with a strong unpleasant odor that is used in permanent waving solutions
volatile alcohols VAHL-uh-tuhl ALkuh-hawlz	p. 164	alcohols that evaporate easily
volatile organic compounds VAHL-uh-tuhl orr-GAN-ik KAHM-powndz	p. 164	abbreviated VOCs; compounds that contain carbon (organic) and evaporate very easily (volatile)
water-in-oil emulsion WAHT-ur-in-OYL ee-MUL-shun	p. 162	abbreviated W/O emulsion; water droplets emulsified in oil

CHAPTER 7

ELECTRICITY & ELECTRICAL SAFETY

"Enthusiasm is the electricity of life."
-Gordon Parks

LEARNING OBJECTIVES

AFTER COMPLETING THIS CHAPTER, YOU WILL BE ABLE TO:

1. EXPLAIN ELECTRICITY AND ELECTRICAL SAFETY.

2. OUTLINE ELECTRICAL THEORY.

3. PRACTICE ELECTRICAL EQUIPMENT SAFETY.

4. IDENTIFY ELECTROTHERAPY MODALITIES.

5. DISCUSS LIGHT ENERGY.

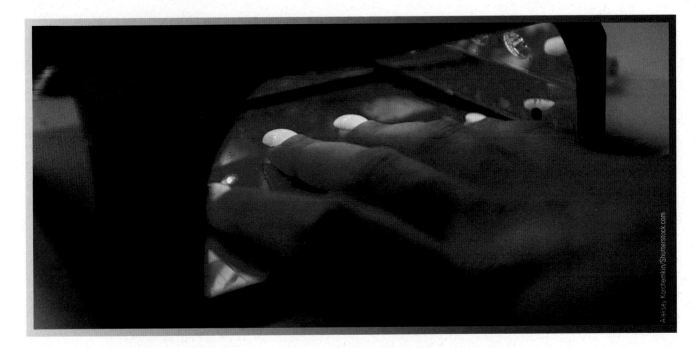

Aleksej Korchemkin/Shutterstock.com

EXPLAIN ELECTRICITY AND ELECTRICAL SAFETY

You decided to enter this field because you love beauty and wellness and all of the services it offers to clients, from hairstyling and haircoloring, to facials, massages, and nail wraps. How many of these services could you offer without using electricity? As you study this chapter, you will learn how important it is for beauty professionals to have a basic working knowledge of electricity.

Beauty professionals should study and have a thorough understanding of electricity because:

- Beauty professionals rely upon a variety of electrical appliances. Knowing what electricity and electrical safety devices are and how they work will allow professionals to use their tools wisely and safely.
- A basic understanding of electricity will enable them to properly use and care for their equipment and tools.
- Electricity use impacts other aspects of the salon, spa, or barbershop environment, such as lighting and the temperature of heating tools. It impacts all of the services beauty professionals offer their clients.
- Advanced electrical and light therapy machines require a foundational understanding of electrical theory to be operated safely and effectively.

OUTLINE ELECTRICAL THEORY

If you look at lightning on a stormy night, what you see are the effects of electricity. If you plug in a poorly wired appliance and sparks fly out of the socket, you will also see the effects of electricity. You are not really seeing electricity, however; instead, you are seeing its *visual* effects on the surrounding air. Electricity does not occupy space or have mass (weight), so it is not matter. If it is not matter, then what is it? Electricity (ee-lek-TRIS-ih-tee) is the movement of electrons from one atom to another along a conductor. Electricity is a form of energy that, when in motion, exhibits magnetic, chemical, or thermal effects.

An electric current (ee-LEK-trik KUR-unt) is the flow of electricity along a conductor. All materials can be classified as conductors or nonconductors depending on the ease with which an electric current can be transmitted through them.

A conductor (kahn-DUK-tur) is any material that conducts electricity. Most metals are good conductors. This means that electricity will pass through the material easily. Copper is a particularly good conductor and is used in electric wiring and electric motors. Pure (distilled) water is a poor conductor, but the ions usually found in ordinary water, such as tap water or a river or a lake, make it a good conductor. This explains why you should not swim in a lake during an electrical storm.

A nonconductor (nahn-kun-DUK-tur), also known as an *insulator* (IN-suh-layt-ur), is a material that does not transmit electricity. Rubber, silk, wood, glass, and cement are good insulators. Electric wires are composed of twisted metal threads (the conductor) covered with a rubber or plastic coating (the nonconductor or insulator). A complete electric circuit (kahm-PLEET ee-LEK-trik SUR-kit) is the path that negative and positive electric currents take from the generating source through the conductors and back to the generating source.

TYPES OF ELECTRIC CURRENT

There are two types of electric current:

- Direct current (dy-REKT KUR-unt), abbreviated as DC, is a constant, even-flowing current that travels in one direction only and is produced by chemical means. Flashlights, cell phones, and cordless tools use the direct current produced by batteries. The battery in your car stores electric energy. Without it, your car would not start. An inverter (in-VUR-tur) is an apparatus that changes direct current to alternating current. Inverters usually have a plug and a cord. They allow you to use appliances outside of your salon, spa, barbershop, or home that normally would have to be plugged into an electric wall outlet. The phone charger in a car is an example of an inverter (**Figure 7-1**).

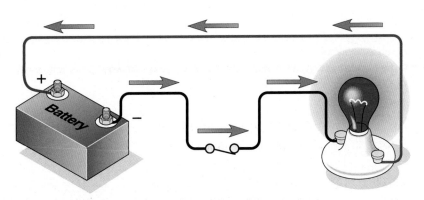

▲ **FIGURE 7-1** A complete direct current (DC) electric current.

- Alternating current (AWL-tur-nayt-ing KUR-rent), abbreviated as AC, is a rapid and interrupted current, flowing first in one direction and then in the opposite direction; it is produced by mechanical means and changes directions 60 times per second. Corded hair dryers, curling irons, electric files, and table lamps that plug into a wall outlet use alternating current. A rectifier (REK-ti-fy-ur) is an apparatus that changes alternating current to direct current. Cordless electric clippers and phone chargers use a rectifier to change the AC from an electric wall outlet to the DC needed to recharge their batteries.

Table 7-1 outlines the differences between direct current and alternating current.

TABLE 7-1: DIRECT CURRENT AND ALTERNATING CURRENT

DIRECT CURRENT (DC)	ALTERNATING CURRENT (AC)
Constant, even flow	Rapid and interrupted flow
Travels in one direction	Travels in two directions
Produced by chemical means	Produced by mechanical means

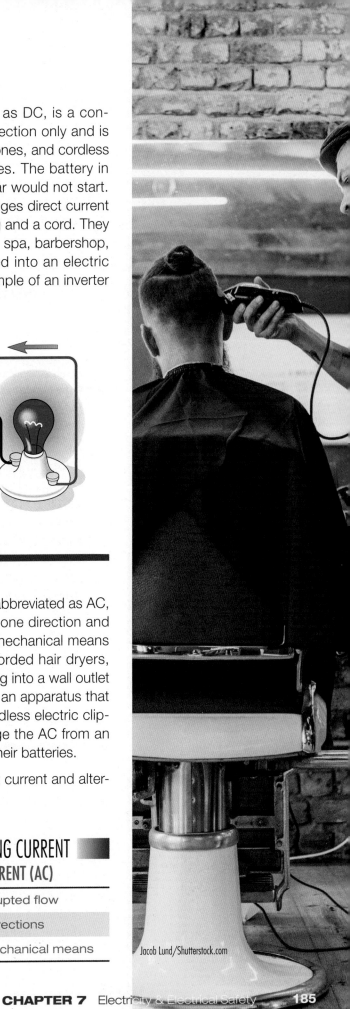

Jacob Lund/Shutterstock.com

ELECTRICAL MEASUREMENTS

The flow of an electric current can be compared to water flowing through a hose. Without pressure, neither water nor electricity would flow.

- A **volt** (VOLT), abbreviated as V and also known as *voltage* (VOL-tij), is the unit that measures the pressure or force that pushes electric current forward through a conductor (**Figure 7-2**). Car batteries are 12 volts. Normal electric wall sockets that power your tools are 120 volts. Most air conditioners and clothes dryers run on 240 volts. A higher voltage indicates more power.

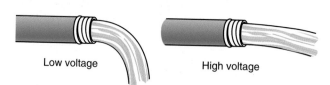

Low voltage   High voltage

▲ **FIGURE 7-2**   Volts measure the pressure or force that pushes the electric current forced through a conductor.

- An **ampere** (AM-peer), abbreviated as A and also known as *amp* (AMP), is the unit that measures the strength of an electric current. Just as a hose must be large enough to carry the amount of water flowing through it, a wire must be large enough to carry the amount of electricity (amps) flowing through it. A hair dryer rated at 12 amps must have a cord that is twice as thick as one rated at 6 amps; otherwise, the cord might overheat and start a fire. A higher amp rating indicates a greater number of electrons and a stronger current (**Figure 7-3**).

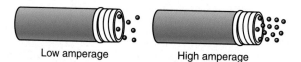

Low amperage   High amperage

▲ **FIGURE 7-3**   Amps measure the strength of the electric current.

- A **milliampere** (mil-ee-AM-peer), abbreviated as mA, is 1/1,000 of an ampere. The current used for facial and scalp treatments is measured in milliamperes; an ampere current would be much too strong. If used for facials and scalp treatments, an ampere current would damage the skin or body.
- An **ohm** (OHM), abbreviated as O, is a unit that measures the resistance of an electric current. Current will not flow through a conductor unless the force (volts) is stronger than the resistance (ohms).

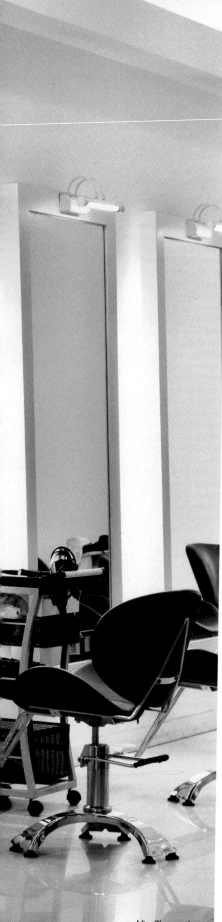

Adisa/Shutterstock.com

One kilowatt-hour will power a television for 3 hours, run a 100-watt bulb for 12 hours, and keep an electric clock ticking for three months.

- A watt (WAHT), abbreviated as W, is a unit that measures how much electric energy is being used in one second. A 40-watt light bulb uses 40 watts of energy per second.
- A kilowatt (KIL-uh-waht), abbreviated as kw, is 1,000 watts. The electricity in your house is measured in kilowatts per hour (kwh). A 1,000-watt (1-kilowatt) hair dryer uses 1,000 watts of energy per second.

CHECK IN
Define the two types of electric current.

PRACTICE ELECTRICAL EQUIPMENT SAFETY

When working with electricity, you must always be concerned with your own safety, as well as the safety of your clients. All electrical equipment should be inspected regularly to determine whether it is in safe working order. Careless electrical connections and overloaded circuits can result in an electrical shock, a burn, or even a serious fire.

SAFETY DEVICES

A wire that is not large enough to carry the electrical current passing through it will overheat. The heating element in a hair dryer or curling iron heats up because it is not large enough to carry the electric current. Heating elements are designed to overheat and are safe when used properly; however, when the electrical wires in a wall overheat, they can cause a fire. If excessive current passes through a circuit or a fuse, the circuit breaker turns off the circuit to prevent overheating.

These are the electrical safety devices that you may encounter when working in a salon, spa, or barbershop:

- A fuse (FYOOZ) prevents excessive current from passing through a circuit. It is designed to blow out or melt when the wire becomes too hot from overloading the circuit with too much current, such as when faulty equipment or too many appliances are connected to an electric source. To re-establish the circuit, disconnect the appliance, check all connections and insulation, insert a new fuse, then reconnect the appliance. Fuses are often found in older buildings that have not been renovated or modernized.
- A circuit breaker (SUR-kit BRAYK-ar) is a switch that automatically interrupts or shuts off an electric circuit at the first indication of an overload. Circuit breakers have replaced fuses in modern electric circuits. They have all the safety features of fuses but do not require

replacement and can simply be reset by switching the circuit breaker back on. A hair dryer has a circuit breaker located in the electric plug that is designed to protect both professional and client in case of an overload or short circuit. When a circuit breaker shuts off, you should disconnect the appliance and check all connections and insulation before resetting it (**Figure 7-4**).

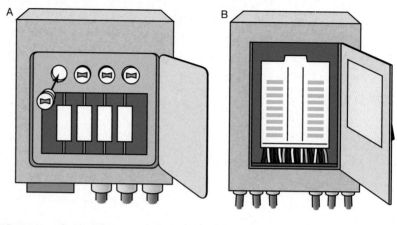

▲ **FIGURE 7-4** Fuse box (A) and circuit breakers (B).

GROUNDING

Grounding (GROWND-ing) completes an electric circuit and carries the current safely away. It is another important way to promote electrical safety. All electrical appliances must have at least two rectangular electrical connections, or prongs, on the plug. This is called a two-prong plug. The two prongs supply electric current to the circuit. If you look closely at the two prongs, you will see that one is slightly larger than the other. This guarantees that the plug can be inserted into an outlet only one way and protects you and your client from an electric shock in the event of a short circuit.

For added protection, some appliances (especially ones with metal casings) have a third circular electric connection that is a grounding pin. This is called a three-prong plug. The grounding pin is designed to guarantee a safe path for electricity and protect the user from electrical shock even if a wire comes loose. Appliances with a third circular grounding pin offer the most protection for you and your clients (**Figure 7-5**).

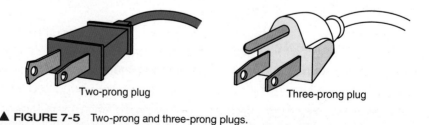

Two-prong plug   Three-prong plug

▲ **FIGURE 7-5** Two-prong and three-prong plugs.

GROUND FAULT INTERRUPTERS

A **ground fault interrupter** (GROWND fallt int-er-UP-ter) (GFI) is designed to protect from electrical shock by interrupting a household circuit when there is a leak in the circuit. GFIs are required by the electrical code for receptacles in bathrooms, kitchens, and some outside receptacles. A GFI is designed to detect currents of a few milliamperes and trip a breaker at the receptacle or at the breaker panel to avoid a shock hazard. When it is working properly, a GFI has a green light that turns red when it trips. Once the appliance is removed from the socket, it can be reset with a "reset" button on the panel (**Figure 7-6**).

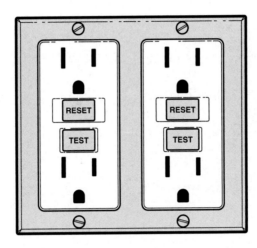

▲ **FIGURE 7-6** GFI outlets.

UNDERWRITERS LABORATORIES

Underwriters Laboratories (UL) certifies the safety of electrical appliances. Curling irons, hair dryers, electric clippers, UV lamps, pedicure chairs, heating mitts, electric files, and more should be UL approved. This certifies that they are safe when used according to the manufacturer's directions. Always look for the UL symbol on electric appliances and take the time to read and follow the manufacturer's directions (**Figure 7-7**).

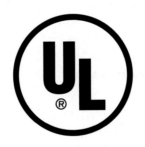

▲ **FIGURE 7-7** UL symbol, as it appears on electrical devices.

ACTIVITY

Gadget Inspection
Inspect any electric items in your kit or equipment in the classroom for UL approval. Also look for any labels, precautions, and warnings on these tools and take notes on what you find. Discuss your observations as a class.

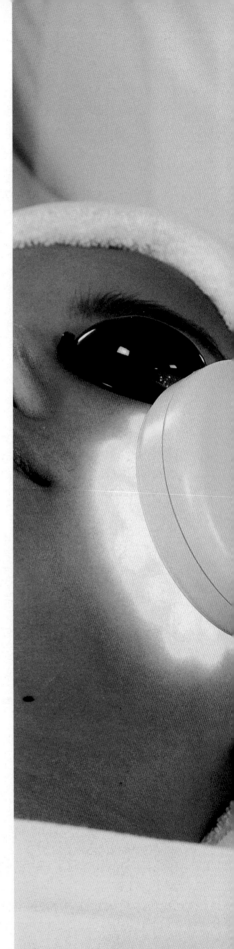

GUIDELINES FOR SAFE USE OF ELECTRICAL EQUIPMENT

Shop fires are often caused by electrical problems, such as shorts in the wiring of the building or improper use of appliances, extension cords, and plugs. Careful attention to electrical safety involves following recommended UL guidelines, manufacturer's directions, and the safety instructions and policies of your establishment. The guidelines below will help you use electricity and electrical equipment safely.

- All the electrical appliances you use should be UL certified.
- Read all instructions carefully before using any piece of electrical equipment.
- Always register electrical appliances with the manufacturer so that you will be notified of any safety recalls immediately.
- Disconnect all appliances when not in use; pull on the plug, not the cord, to disconnect.
- Disconnect all electrical appliances prior to cleaning them.
- Never poke hairpins or wires through any part of an appliance, including lint screens.
- Inspect all electrical equipment regularly.
- Keep all wires, plugs, and electrical equipment in good repair. Do not use cords that have exposed wiring in any part of the cord or where it attaches to the appliance.
- Use only one plug in each outlet; overloading may cause the circuit breaker to pop. If more than one plug is needed in an area, use a power strip with a surge protector (**Figure 7-8**).

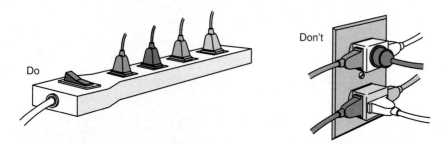

▲ FIGURE 7-8 Use only one plug per outlet on a power strip or on the wall.

- Avoid contact, for both you and your client, with water and metal surfaces when using electricity and do not handle electrical equipment with wet hands or while standing on a wet floor.
- Keep electrical cords off the floor and away from everyone's feet; getting tangled in a cord could cause you or your client to trip.
- Do not leave your client unattended while the client is connected to an electrical device.
- Do not attempt to clean around electric outlets while equipment is plugged in.
- Do not touch two metal objects at the same time if either is connected to an electric current.

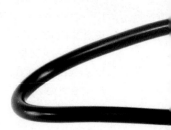
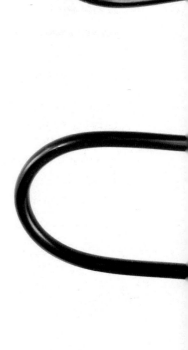
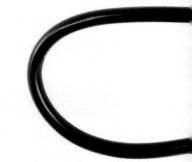

Daniel Hixon/Shutterstock.com

- Do not step on or place objects on electrical cords.
- Do not allow electrical cords to become twisted; this can cause a short circuit.
- Do not alter a three-prong plug to fit into a two-prong outlet.
- Do not attempt to repair electrical appliances. If you have a problem with electric wiring or an electrical device or appliance, tell your supervisor immediately, take the device to a repair store, or call a certified electrician or repair representative to resolve the issue.
- If you see sparks when plugging or unplugging an appliance, do not use the appliance or outlet until it has been approved by a certified electrician as safe to use.
- Verify regularly that fire extinguishers are appropriate for electrical fires, are not expired, and that you are comfortable with using one.
- Remove lint from clothes dryers before each load to reduce the chance of fire.

ACTIVITY

Hazard Sweep

Evaluate the electrical safety of your home or classroom. What safety devices can you find (GFI, circuit breakers, surge protectors, etc.)? What are some potential hazards? How might you address or minimize these electrical hazards? Share your findings as a class.

WHAT TO DO IN AN ELECTRICAL EMERGENCY

Virtually all electrical incidents in a salon, spa, or barbershop environment will be related to low voltage (less than 500 watt) appliances. Low voltage shocks are rarely critical, but they can be quite painful and dangerous to some individuals. It is important that you take signs of wear and tear seriously and replace or discontinue using appliances or outlets as soon as you notice these signs.

If you receive a light shock sensation while using, turning on or off, or plugging or unplugging an electrical appliance:

- Stop using the appliance immediately and turn it completely off.
- Unplug it from the wall or turn off the circuit breaker to that outlet.
- Replace the appliance or have it repaired by an authorized repair representative.
- If similar issues occur with other appliances in the same outlet, discontinue use of that outlet until approved for use by a certified electrician.

If you drop an electrical appliance in water:

- If the outlet is GFI protected, it will kill the circuit immediately and you may unplug the appliance from the wall, after releasing the appliance. Do NOT have one hand in the water and one at the outlet – if the outlet is still live, your body will conduct the electricity.

- If the outlet is not GFI protected, go to the breaker box and flip the circuit off. If you are unsure which circuit controls that outlet, it is better to momentarily shut off power to the entire shop while you fix the situation. Once the power is off, unplug the item and then restore power.
- Never use an appliance that has been dropped in water.

When to seek medical care after an electrical shock:

- Anytime during pregnancy
- If you have burns on the skin, particularly those that are open or do not heal well over time
- If you are not current on your tetanus immunizations (given every five years to adults)

CHECK IN
What are at least five steps to take for electrical safety?

IDENTIFY ELECTROTHERAPY MODALITIES

The use of electrical currents to treat the skin is commonly referred to as electrotherapy (ee-lek-troh-THAYR-uh-pee). Currents used in electrical facial and scalp treatments are called modalities (moh-DAL-ih-tees). Each modality produces a different effect on the skin.

An electrode (ee-LEK-trohd), also known as a *probe*, is an applicator for directing electric current from an electrotherapy device to the client's skin. It is usually made of carbon, glass, or metal. Each modality requires two electrodes—one negative and one positive—to conduct the flow of electricity through the body. The only exception to this rule is the Tesla high-frequency current, which uses a single electrode.

CAUTION
Older buildings and homes may have two-prong wall outlets. Some equipment and tools have three-prong plugs. Never tamper with the wiring of a building or home, wall outlets, or plugs to make them fit your equipment and tools. Adapters are available, if it is appropriate for you to use one. Consult the manufacturer and your local hardware store about whether you can use an adapter and, if so, what type of an adapter is recommended.

POLARITY

Polarity (poh-LAYR-uh-tee) refers to the poles of an electric current, either positive or negative. The electrodes on many electrotherapy devices have one negatively charged pole and one positively charged pole. The positive electrode is called an anode (AN-ohd); the anode is usually red and is marked with a P or a plus (+) sign. The negative electrode is called a cathode (KATH-ohd); it is usually black and is marked with an N or a minus (–) sign (**Figure 7-9**). The negatively charged electrons from the cathode flow to the positively charged anode. If the electrodes are not marked, ask your instructor, manager, or supervisor to help you determine the positive and negative poles.

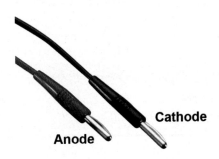

▲ **FIGURE 7-9**   Anode (+) and cathode (–).

MODALITIES

The main modalities used in beauty and wellness services are galvanic current, microcurrent, and Tesla high-frequency current.

GALVANIC CURRENT

Galvanic current (gal-VAN-ik KUR-unt) is a constant and direct current, having a positive and negative pole, that produces chemical changes when it passes through the tissues and fluids of the body.

> ### DID YOU KNOW?
>
> Galvanic current is named after Luigi Galvani, an Italian physician, physicist, biologist, and philosopher (1737–1798). His studies about electric charges and how they affected the muscles of animals helped others to develop the galvanic current machines that are used in salons and spas today.

Two different chemical reactions are possible with galvanic current, depending on the polarity (positive or negative) that is used (**Table 7-2**). The **active electrode** (AK-tiv ee-LEK-trohd) is the electrode used on the area to be treated. The **inactive electrode** (in-AK-tiv ee-LEK-trohd) is the opposite pole from the active electrode. The effects produced by the positive pole are the exact opposite of those produced by the negative pole. Galvanic current is used to infuse water-soluble products into unbroken skin (the scientific term for this is *phoresis*) (**Figure 7-10**).

Iontophoresis (eye-ahn-toh-foh-REE-sus) is the process of infusing water-soluble products into the skin with the use of electric current, such as the use of the positive and negative poles of a galvanic machine.

Cataphoresis (kat-uh-foh-REE-sus) infuses an acidic (positive) product into deeper tissues, using galvanic current from the positive pole toward the negative pole.

Yulai Studio/Shutterstock.com

TABLE 7-2: EFFECTS OF GALVANIC CURRENT

POSITIVE POLE (ANODE) CATAPHORESIS	NEGATIVE POLE (CATHODE) ANAPHORESIS
Produces acidic reactions	Produces alkaline reactions
Closes the pores	Opens the pores
Soothes nerves	Stimulates and irritates the nerves
Decreases blood supply	Increases blood supply
Contracts blood vessels	Expands blood vessels
Hardens and firms tissues	Softens tissues

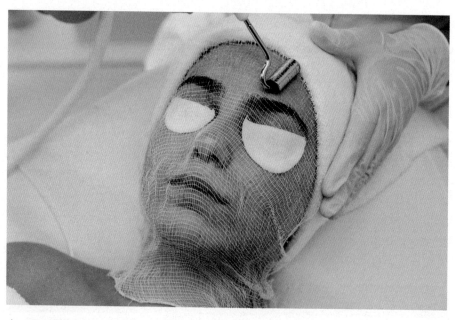

▲ FIGURE 7-10   A treatment using galvanic current.

CAUTION
Do not use negative galvanic current on skin with broken capillaries or pustular acne conditions or on clients with high blood pressure or metal implants.

Anaphoresis (an-uh-foh-REE-sus) infuses an alkaline (negative) product into the tissues from the negative pole toward the positive pole. Desincrustation (des-in-krus-TAY-shun), a form of anaphoresis, is a process used to soften and emulsify grease deposits (oil) and blackheads in the hair follicles. Desincrustation is frequently used to treat acne, milia (small, white cyst-like pimples), and comedones (blackheads and whiteheads).

MICROCURRENT

Microcurrent (MY-kroh-kur-unt) is an extremely low level of electricity that mirrors the body's natural electrical impulses. Microcurrent can be used for iontophoresis, firming, toning, and soothing skin. It also can help heal inflamed tissue, such as acne. Newer microcurrent devices have negative and positive polarity in one probe, not two probes. This allows the client to relax rather than having to hold on to a probe during the service or treatment.

Microcurrent does not travel throughout the entire body; it serves only the specific area being treated. Microcurrent can be effective in the following ways:

- Improves blood and lymph circulation
- Produces acidic and alkaline reactions
- Opens and closes hair follicles and pores
- Increases muscle tone
- Restores elasticity
- Reduces redness and inflammation
- Minimizes healing time for acne lesions
- Improves the natural protective barrier of the skin
- Increases metabolism

When microcurrent is used during aging-skin treatments, it may give your client's skin a softer, firmer, more hydrated appearance.

CAUTION

As with all electric current devices, microcurrent should not be used on clients who have a pacemaker, epilepsy, cancer, phlebitis, or thrombosis or who are pregnant. It also should not be used on anyone under a physician's care for a condition that may exclude them from using certain ingredients or products or from having treatments. If you are unsure about whether it is appropriate to treat clients, ask them to obtain a physician's consent for the service.

TESLA HIGH-FREQUENCY CURRENT

The Tesla high-frequency current (TES-luh HY FREE-kwen-see KUR-ent), also known as *violet ray*, is a thermal or heat-producing current with a high rate of oscillation or vibration that is commonly used for scalp and facial treatments. Tesla current does not produce muscle contractions, and the effects can be either stimulating or soothing, depending on the method of application. The electrodes are made from either glass or metal, and only one electrode is used to perform a service (**Figure 7-11**).

The benefits of the Tesla high-frequency current are:

- Stimulates blood circulation
- Increases elimination and absorption
- Increases skin metabolism
- Improves germicidal action
- Relieves skin congestion

As you learn more about specific treatments, you will become familiar with the term contraindication (con-tra-in-dih-KAY-shun), referring to a condition that requires avoiding certain treatments, procedures, or products to prevent undesirable side effects. For example, Tesla high-frequency current should not be used on clients who are pregnant

vlastas/Shutterstock.com

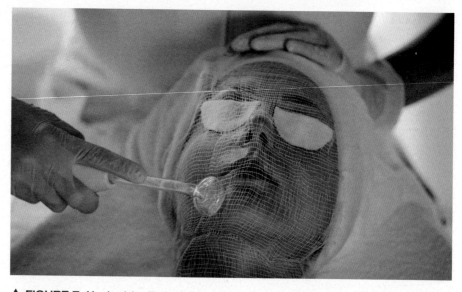

▲ FIGURE 7–11   Applying Tesla high-frequency current with a facial electrode.

or who have epilepsy or any other seizure disorder, asthma, high blood pressure, a sinus blockage, a pacemaker, or metal implants. Additionally, clients should avoid contact with metal, such as chair arms, jewelry, and metal bobby pins, during the treatment, as a burn may occur if contact is made.

DID YOU KNOW?

The Tesla high-frequency current is named after electrical engineer Nikola Tesla, who was born in 1856 in Croatia. He moved to the United States in 1884, where he did the majority of his work on alternating current. Tesla died in New York City in 1943.

 CHECK IN
Briefly describe three electrical modalities used in beauty and wellness services.

DISCUSS LIGHT ENERGY

The electromagnetic spectrum (ee-lek-troh-mag-NEH-tik SPEK-trum), also known as *electromagnetic spectrum of radiation*, is the name given to all of the forms of energy (or radiation) that exist. The forms of energy in the electromagnetic spectrum are radio waves (used by radios and televisions), microwaves (used in microwave ovens), light waves (infra-red light, visible light, and ultraviolet light used for light therapy services), X-rays (used by physicians and dentists), and gamma rays (used for nuclear power plants) (**Figure 7-12**).

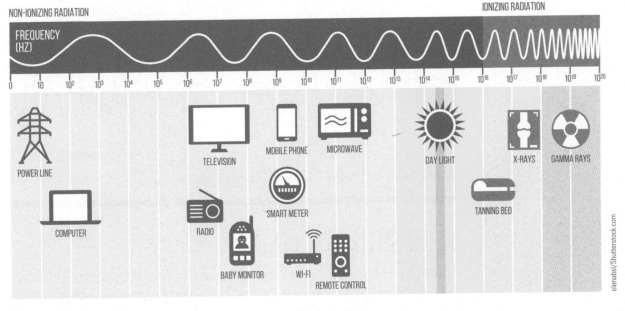

▲ **FIGURE 7–12** The electromagnetic spectrum.

elenabsl/Shutterstock.com

DID YOU KNOW?

Although the electric lighting in your salon, spa, or barbershop is not a form of light therapy, the quality of this light can have an effect on your work and on your client's satisfaction. Fluorescent light is produced by fluorescent lamps and may be cooler (green-blue) than natural sunlight. Incandescent light is produced by standard (tungsten) light bulbs and is warmer (yellow-gold) than either natural sunlight or fluorescent light. Your client's hair, skin, and nails will appear more green-blue when viewed with fluorescent lighting and more golden when viewed with incandescent lighting.

Be careful when handling fluorescent light bulbs; they contain dangerous substances, including mercury. Avoid breaking fluorescent bulbs and dispose of used bulbs properly.

Energy moves through space in waves. These waves are similar to the waves caused when a stone is dropped on the surface of water. Each type of energy has its own wavelength (WAYV-length), the distance between successive peaks of electromagnetic waves. A waveform (WAYV-form) is the measurement of the distance between two wavelengths. Some wavelengths are long and some are short (**Table 7-3**). Long wavelengths have low frequency, meaning that the number of waves is less frequent (fewer waves) within a waveform pattern. Short wavelengths have higher frequency because the number of waves is more frequent (more waves) within a waveform pattern (**Figure 7-13**).

TABLE 7-3: LONG WAVELENGTHS COMPARED WITH SHORT WAVELENGTHS

LONG WAVELENGTHS	SHORT WAVELENGTHS
Low frequency	High frequency
Deeper penetration	Less penetration
Less energy	More energy

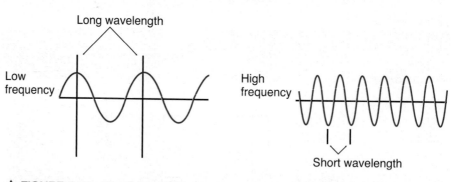

▲ FIGURE 7–13   Waveform patterns of long and short wavelengths.

VISIBLE SPECTRUM OF LIGHT

Visible light (VIS-ible LYT) is the part of the electromagnetic spectrum that can be seen. The visible spectrum of light makes up only 35 percent of natural sunlight. Within the visible spectrum of light, violet has the shortest wavelength and red has the longest. The wavelength of infrared light is just below that of red light and the wavelength of ultraviolet light is just above that of violet light.

DID YOU KNOW?

Natural sunlight is made up of three types of light:

- Visible light = 35 percent
- Invisible infrared light = 60 percent
- Invisible ultraviolet light = 5 percent

Although they are referred to as *light*, infrared light and ultraviolet light are not really light. Ultraviolet light and infrared light are also forms of electromagnetic energy but are invisible because their wavelengths are beyond the visible spectrum of light. Invisible light makes up 65 percent of natural sunlight (**Figure 7-14**).

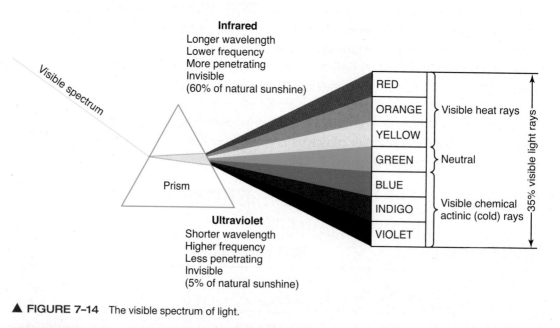

▲ FIGURE 7–14   The visible spectrum of light.

INVISIBLE LIGHT

Invisible light (in-VIS-ible LYT) is the light at either end of the visible spectrum of light that is invisible to the naked eye. Before the visible violet light of the spectrum is ultraviolet light; it is the shortest and least-penetrating light of the spectrum. Beyond the visible red light of the spectrum is infrared light, which produces heat.

DID YOU KNOW?

If light from the sun is passed through a glass prism (a glass or plastic prism usually resembles a pyramid shape after it is cut), it will appear in the seven different colors of the rainbow, in the following order: violet (the shortest wavelength), indigo, blue, green, yellow, orange, and red (the longest wavelength). These colors, which are visible to the eye, constitute visible light.

Ultraviolet light (ul-truh-VY-uh-let LYT), abbreviated as UV light and also known as *cold light* or *actinic light* (ak-TIN-ik LYT), is invisible light that has a short wavelength (giving it higher energy), is less penetrating than visible light, causes chemical reactions to happen more quickly than visible light, produces less heat than visible light, and kills some germs.

UV light prompts the skin to produce vitamin D, a fat-soluble vitamin that is good for bone growth and health. We need sunlight to survive on the planet; however, overexposure to UV light can cause premature aging of the skin and skin cancer. Incidence of skin cancer has reached a near-epidemic level, with over one million new cases being diagnosed each year. It is estimated that one in five Americans will develop skin cancer, and that 90 percent of those cancers will be the result of exposure to UV radiation from natural sunlight, sun lamps, and tanning beds.

There are three types of UV light:

- **Ultraviolet A (UVA).** Ultraviolet A light has the longest wavelength of the UV light spectrum and penetrates directly into the dermis of the skin, damaging the collagen and elastin. UVA light is the light that is often used in tanning beds.
- **Ultraviolet B (UVB).** Ultraviolet B light is often called the *burning light* because it is most associated with sunburns. Excessive use of both UVA and UVB light can cause skin cancers.
- **Ultraviolet C (UVC).** Ultraviolet C light is blocked by the ozone layer. If the Earth loses its protective layer of ozone, life as we know it will no longer exist. UVC is effective at killing bacteria, viruses, mold and other pathogens.

CAUTION

Although the application of UV light can be beneficial, it must be done with the utmost care in a proper manner by a qualified professional—overexposure can lead to skin damage and skin cancer. UV light has been used to kill bacteria on the skin and to help the body produce vitamin D and is used in a weaker form to cure UV gel nails. Dermatologists also use UV therapy in addition to drugs for the treatment of psoriasis.

Subbotina Anna/Shutterstock.com

Infrared light (in-fruh-RED LYT) has longer wavelengths, penetrates more deeply, has less energy, and produces more heat than visible light. Infrared light makes up 60 percent of natural sunlight.

Infrared lamps are used mainly during hair conditioning treatments and to process haircolor. They are also used in spas and saunas for relaxation and for warming up muscles. Infrared light has been used to diminish signs of aging such as wrinkles, to heal wounds, and to increase circulation.

DID YOU KNOW?

We need to strike a delicate balance with sunlight exposure. Keep in mind that tanned skin is damaged skin. Tanning will eventually cause photoaging (premature aging due to sun exposure) and irreversibly damage the skin's collagen-building properties

LIGHT INTO CHEMICAL ENERGY

Catalysts (CAT-a-lists) are substances that speed up chemical reactions. Some catalysts use heat as an energy source while others use light. Whatever the energy source, catalysts absorb energy like a battery. At the appropriate time, they pass this energy to the initiator and the reaction begins. Like other chemicals, a catalyst will not get consumed in a chemical reaction. For example, in hair coloring services, hydrogen peroxide (developer) is the catalyst that allows the hair color to penetrate the cortex of the hair, creating a permanent color. In acrylic nails, the monomers used are the catalyst that solidify the nails; in the application of gel nails, the UV light is the catalyst for hardening.

LIGHT THERAPY

Light therapy (LYT THAYR-ah-pee), also known as *phototherapy*, is the application of light rays to the skin for the treatment of wrinkles, capillaries, or pigmentation or for hair removal. Lasers and light therapy devices have been used for decades; and yet, some of the original techniques are still valid today. Lasers are designed to focus all light power to a specific depth and in one direction within the skin, using the same color of light (**Figure 7-15**). In contrast, other light therapies have multiple depths, colors, and wavelengths, and the light may be scattered. The most important point to remember about light therapy is that the equipment you use is selected based on the skin type and condition you are treating.

I Have NOT Failed I've just found 10,000 ways that won't work.

— THOMAS EDISON

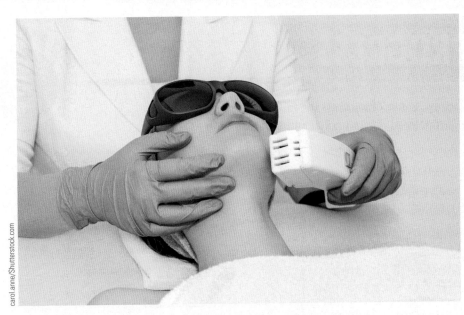
carol.anne/Shutterstock.com

▲ FIGURE 7–15   Light therapy devices are used to treat a variety of skin conditions.

CHECK IN
Explain the difference between electromagnetic radiation, visible light, and invisible light.

APPLY ELECTRICITY AND ELECTRICAL SAFETY

Congratulations on completing this chapter! Before you move on, take a moment to think about how these Electricity and Electrical Safety topics apply to your particular discipline. Discuss with a classmate or study group how electrical theory might come into play on the job; what machine you are looking forward to working with; any special safety measures you may need to take with particular services; and so on.

COMPETENCY PROGRESS

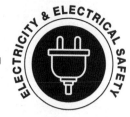

How are you doing with Electricity and Electrical Safety? **Check off the Chapter 7 Learning Objectives** below that you feel you have mastered; leave unchecked those objectives you will need to return to:

- ☐ EXPLAIN ELECTRICITY AND ELECTRICAL SAFETY.
- ☐ OUTLINE ELECTRICAL THEORY.
- ☐ PRACTICE ELECTRICAL EQUIPMENT SAFETY.
- ☐ IDENTIFY ELECTROTHERAPY MODALITIES.
- ☐ DISCUSS LIGHT ENERGY.

GLOSSARY

active electrode AK-tiv ee-LEK-trohd	p. 193	electrode of an electrotherapy device that is used on the area to be treated
alternating current AWL-tur-nayt-ing KUR-rent	p. 185	abbreviated as AC; rapid and interrupted current, flowing first in one direction and then in the opposite direction; produced by mechanical means and changes directions 60 times per second
ampere AM-peer	p. 186	abbreviated as A and also known as *amp* (AMP); unit that measures the strength of an electric current
anaphoresis an-uh-foh-REE-sus	p. 194	process of infusing an alkaline (negative) product into the tissues from the negative pole toward the positive pole
anode AN-ohd	p. 192	positive electrode of an electrotherapy device; the anode is usually red and is marked with a *P* or a plus (+) sign
catalysts CAT-a-lists	p. 200	substances that speed up chemical reactions
cataphoresis kat-uh-foh-REE-sus	p. 193	process of fusing an acidic (positive) product into deeper tissues using galvanic current from the positive pole toward the negative pole
cathode KATH-ohd	p. 192	negative electrode of an electrotherapy device; the cathode is usually black and is marked with an *N* or a minus (–) sign
circuit breaker SUR-kit BRAYK-ar	p. 187	switch that automatically interrupts or shuts off an electric circuit at the first indication of overload

complete electric circuit kahm-PLEET ee-LEK-trik SUR-kit	p. 184	the path of negative and positive electric currents moving from the generating source through the conductors and back to the generating source
conductor kahn-DUK-tur	p. 184	any material that conducts electricity
contraindication con-tra-in-dih-KAY-shun	p. 196	a condition that requires avoiding certain treatments, procedures, or products to prevent undesirable side effects
desincrustation des-in-krus-TAY-shun	p. 194	a form of anaphoresis; process used to soften and emulsify grease deposits (oil) and blackheads in the hair follicles
direct current dy-REKT KUR-unt	p. 185	abbreviated as DC; constant, even-flowing current that travels in one direction only and is produced by chemical means
electric current ee-LEK-trik KUR-unt	p. 184	flow of electricity along a conductor
electricity ee-lek-TRIS-ih-tee	p. 184	the movement of electrons from one atom to another along a conductor
electrode ee-LEK-trohd	p. 192	also known as *probe*; applicator for directing electric current from an electrotherapy device to the client's skin
electromagnetic spectrum ee-lek-troh-mag-NEH-tik SPEK-trum	p. 196	also known as *electromagnetic spectrum of radiation*; name given to all of the forms of energy (or radiation) that exist
electrotherapy ee-lek-troh-THAYR-uh-pee	p. 192	use of electrical currents to treat the skin
fuse FYOOZ	p. 187	prevents excessive current from passing through a circuit
galvanic current gal-VAN-ik KUR-unt	p. 193	constant and direct current, having a positive and negative pole, that produces chemical changes when it passes through the tissues and fluids of the body
grounding GROWND-ing	p. 188	completes an electric circuit and carries the current safely away
ground fault interrupter GROWND fallt int-er-UP-ter	p. 188	protects from electrical shock by interrupting a household circuit when there is a leak in the circuit
inactive electrode in-AK-tiv ee-LEK-trohd	p. 193	opposite pole from the active electrode
infrared light in-fruh-RED LYT	p. 199	invisible light with longer wavelengths, deeper penetration, less energy, and more heat production than visible light; makes up 60 percent of natural sunlight
inverter in-VUR-tur	p. 185	apparatus that changes direct current to alternating current

invisible light in-VIS-ible LYT	p. 198	light at either end of the visible spectrum of light that is invisible to the naked eye
iontophoresis eye-ahn-toh-foh-REE-sus	p. 193	process of infusing water-soluble products into the skin with the use of electric current, such as the use of the positive and negative poles of a galvanic machine
kilowatt KIL-uh-waht	p. 187	abbreviated as kw; 1,000 watts
light therapy LYT THAYR-ah-pee	p. 200	also known as *phototherapy*; the application of light rays to the skin for the treatment of wrinkles, capillaries, pigmentation, or hair removal
microcurrent MY-kroh-kur-unt	p. 194	an extremely low level of electricity that mirrors the body's natural electrical impulses
milliampere mil-ee-AM-peer	p. 186	abbreviated as mA; 1/1,000 of an ampere
modalities moh-DAL-ih-tees	p. 192	currents used in electrical facial and scalp treatments
nonconductor nahn-kun-DUK-tur	p. 184	also known as *insulator*; a material that does not transmit electricity
ohm OHM	p. 187	abbreviated as O; unit that measures the resistance of an electric current
polarity poh-LAYR-uh-tee	p. 192	positive or negative poles of an electric current
rectifier REK-ti-fy-ur	p. 185	apparatus that changes alternating current to direct current
Tesla high-frequency current TES-luh HY FREE-kwen-see KUR-ent	p. 195	also known as *violet ray*; thermal or heat-producing current with a high rate of oscillation or vibration that is commonly used for scalp and facial treatments
ultraviolet light ul-truh-VY-uh-let LYT	p. 199	abbreviated as UV light and also known as *cold light* or *actinic light*; invisible light that has a short wavelength (giving it higher energy), is less penetrating than visible light, causes chemical reactions to happen more quickly than visible light, produces less heat than visible light, and kills germs
visible light VIS-ible LYT	p. 198	the part of the electromagnetic spectrum that can be seen; visible light makes up only 35 percent of natural sunlight
volt VOLT	p. 186	abbreviated as V and also known as *voltage*; unit that measures the pressure or force that pushes electric current forward through a conductor

watt			
WAHT	p. 187	abbreviated as W; unit that measures how much electric energy is being used in one second

waveform		
WAYV-form	p. 197	measurement of the distance between two wavelengths

wavelength		
WAYV-length	p. 197	distance between successive peaks of electromagnetic waves

PART 3

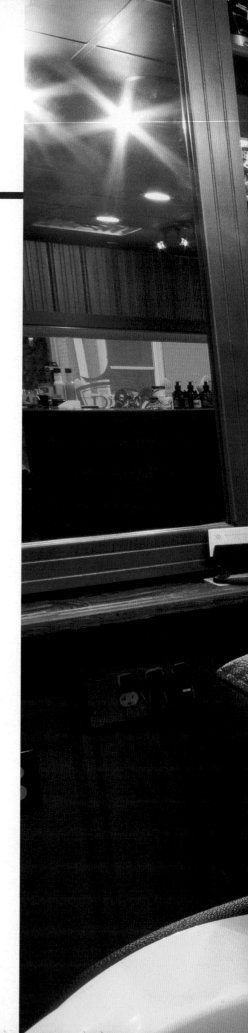

BUSINESS SKILLS

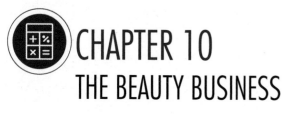

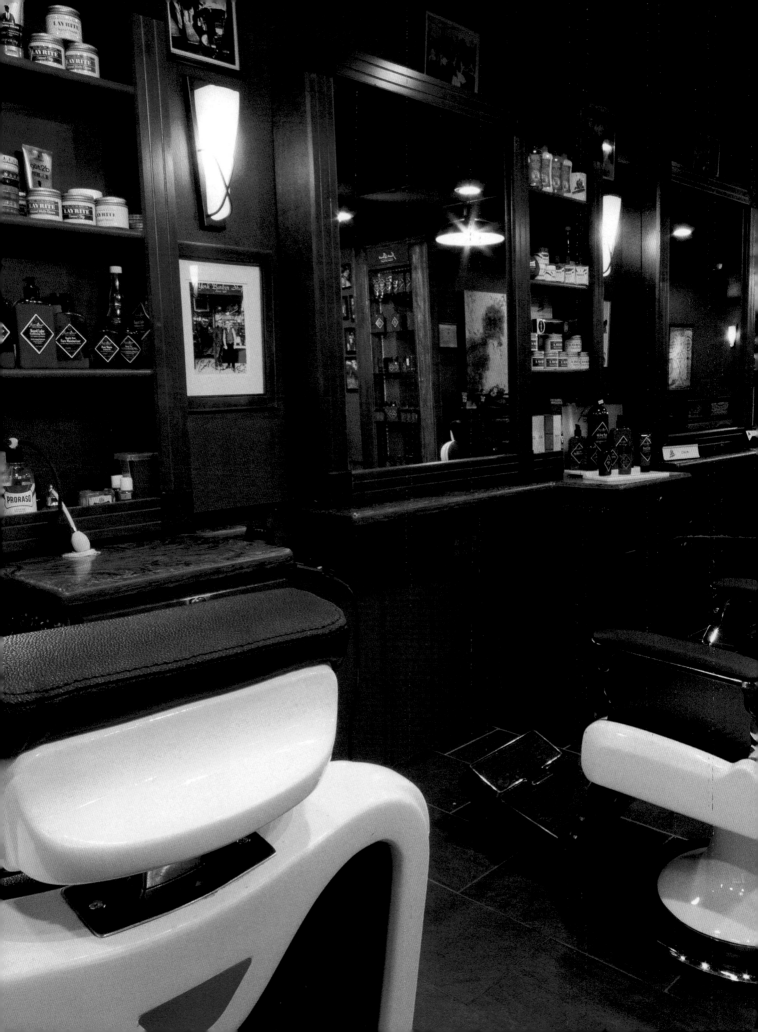

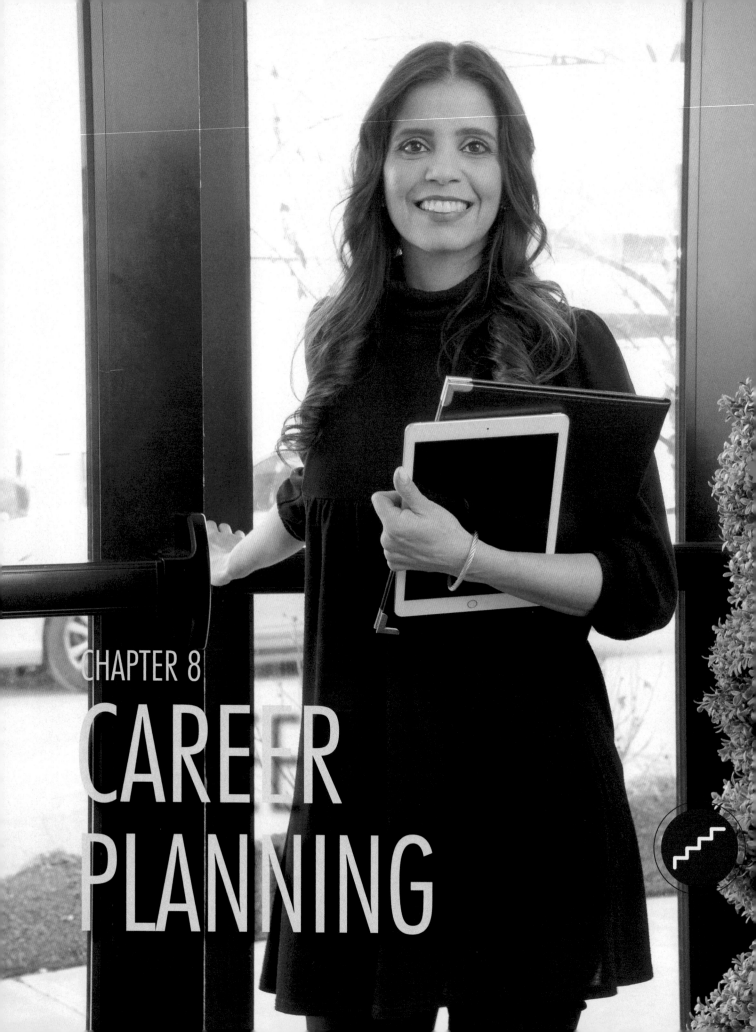

CHAPTER 8
CAREER
PLANNING

"My life didn't please me,
so I created my life."
-Coco Chanel

AFTER COMPLETING THIS CHAPTER, YOU WILL BE ABLE TO:

1. EXPLAIN CAREER PLANNING.

2. REVIEW THE STATE LICENSING EXAMINATION PROCESS.

3. DISCOVER POTENTIAL EMPLOYERS.

4. DEVELOP AN EFFECTIVE RESUME.

5. PREPARE FOR A JOB INTERVIEW IN THE BEAUTY INDUSTRY.

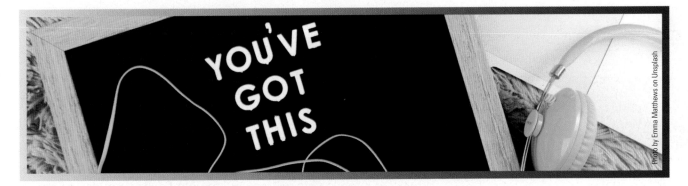

Photo by Emma Matthews on Unsplash

EXPLAIN CAREER PLANNING

There are plenty of great jobs out there for energetic, hardworking, talented people. If you look at the top professionals in the beauty and wellness industry, you will find they were not born successful; they achieved success through self-motivation, energy, and persistence. Like you, these beauty professionals began their careers by enrolling in school. They were the ones who used their time wisely, planned for the future, went the extra mile, and drew on a reservoir of self-confidence to meet challenges. They owe their success to no one but themselves, because they created it. If you want to enjoy similar success, you must prepare for the opportunities that await you.

No matter what changes occur in the economy, there are often more jobs available for entry-level beauty professionals than there are people to fill them. This is a tremendous advantage for you. However, you still must thoroughly research the job market in your geographical area before committing to your first job (**Figure 8-1**). If you make the right choice, your career will be on the road to success. If you make the wrong choice, it will not be a tragedy, but it may cause unnecessary delay.

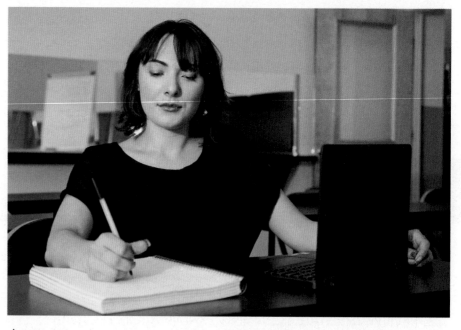

▲ FIGURE 8-1 Job listings are posted online at various job boards.

Beauty professionals should study and have a thorough understanding of career planning because:

- They must pass a state board exam to be licensed and must be licensed to be hired; therefore, preparing for licensure and passing the exam is the first step to employment success.
- A successful employment search is a job in itself. There are many tools that can give beauty professionals the edge—as well as mistakes that can cost them an interview or a job.
- The ability to pinpoint the right salon, spa, or barbershop and target it as a potential employer is vital for career success.
- Proactively preparing the right materials, such as a great resume, and practicing interviewing will provide the confidence needed to secure a job in an establishment they will love.

REVIEW THE STATE LICENSING EXAMINATION PROCESS

Before you can land that professional position you are hoping for, you must pass your state licensing examinations (usually a written and a practical exam) and secure the required credentials from your state's licensing board by filling out an application and paying a fee. For details on fees, testing dates, requirements, and more, visit the website of your state board or your state's department of licensing.

Many factors will affect how well you perform during that licensing examination and on tests in general. They include your physical and psychological state; your memory; your time management skills; and your academic skills, such as reading, writing, note taking, test taking, and general learning.

Above all, the most important of these factors is your mastery of course content. However, even if you feel that you have truly learned the material, it is still very beneficial to have strong test-taking skills. Being test-wise (TEST-whys) means understanding the strategies for successfully taking tests.

PREPARING FOR THE WRITTEN EXAM

A test-wise student begins to prepare for a test by practicing good study habits and time management. These habits include the following:

- Have a planned, realistic study schedule.
- Read content carefully and become an active studier.
- Keep well-organized notes.
- Develop a detailed vocabulary list.
- Take effective notes during class.
- Organize and review handouts.
- Review past quizzes and tests.
- Listen carefully in class for cues and clues about what could be expected on the test.

More holistic or "whole you" hints to keep in mind include the following:

- Make yourself mentally ready and develop a positive attitude toward taking the test.
- Get plenty of rest the night before the test.
- Dress comfortably and professionally.
- Anticipate some anxiety (feeling concerned about the test results may actually help you do better).
- Avoid cramming the night before an examination.
- Find out if your state uses computers for the written portion of the test. If so, make certain you are comfortable with computerized test taking.
- If possible, do a "test drive" to the site before test day if you are unsure of the location. Some exams may be administered at your school and some may be given in alternate locations.

DID YOU KNOW?

If you have a physician-documented disability, such as a learning disability, your state may allow you extra time to take the written exam or even provide a special examiner. Ask your instructor and check with your state licensing board. Be certain to make any special arrangements well in advance of the test date.

CANDIDATE INFORMATION BULLETINS

Although the extent of information made available to exam candidates varies from state to state, most states now maintain candidate information

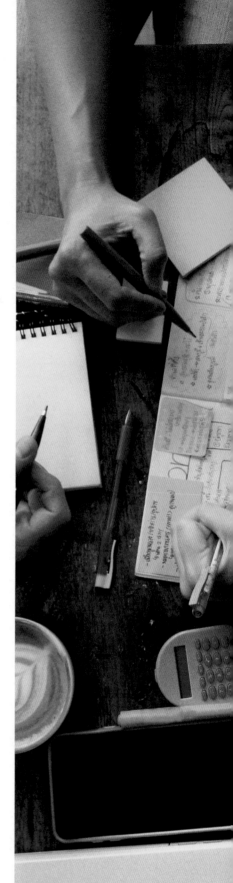

rawiwano/Shutterstock.com

online for easy access. Be sure to review these valuable test-taking tools as you begin to familiarize yourself with all parts of your licensing exam. In most cases, candidate information booklets or materials will contain the following:

- Introduction to written and practical exams
- Examination rules
- Location and contact information for exams
- Manner of testing (computer based, paper and pencil, etc.)
- Requirements, procedures, and reservation information for computer-based testing, if applicable
- Content overview—written (number of questions, subject areas, sample questions, etc.)
- Content overview—practical (specific procedures to be tested, possible points, etc.)
- Model requirements (practical)
- Tool and equipment requirements (practical)
- What to bring and what not to bring (written and practical)
- References used to write or develop the examinations
- Grading and scoring policies (reexamination information, notification of results, etc.)
- Administrative policies (late arrivals, cancellations, exam review process, etc.)

ON TEST DAY

After you have taken all the necessary steps to prepare for your test, there are a number of strategies you can adopt on the day of the exam that may be helpful (**Figure 8-2**):

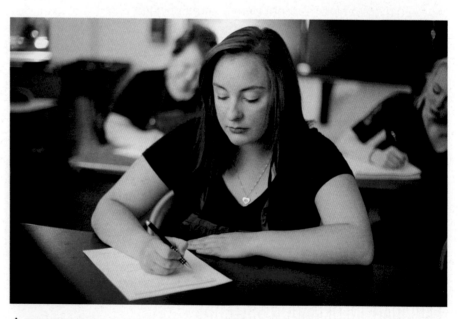

▲ FIGURE 8-2 Candidates taking an in-house school exam.

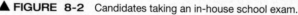

THE MORNING OF

- Eat breakfast.
- Relax and try to slow down physically.
- Review the material lightly.
- Arrive early with a self-confident attitude; be alert, calm, and ready for the challenge.

THINGS TO BRING

- Required documentation and identification(s)
- Your model and their identification
- Practical exam kit (prepared well in advance)
- Equipment and material too large to fit in kit
- A watch so that you can monitor the time
- Clean professional clothing and good shoes

DURING THE TEST

- Read all written directions and listen carefully to all verbal directions before beginning.
- If there are things you do not understand, do not hesitate to ask the examiner questions.
- Do not talk to other participants or your model; ignore other test takers if they speak to you.
- If possible, skim the entire test before beginning.
- Budget your time to ensure that you have plenty of opportunity to complete the test; do not spend too much time on any one question.
- Begin work as soon as possible; mark the answers in the test carefully but quickly.
- Answer the easiest questions first in order to save time for the more difficult ones. Quickly scanning all the questions first may clue you in to the more difficult questions.
- Make a note of the questions you skip so that you can find them again later. If the test is administered online you may not be given this option. Some software prevents you from moving forward without answering all questions on the page first. Discuss this with your instructor or the testing facility before taking the exam.
- Read each question carefully to make sure that you know exactly what the question is asking and that you understand all parts of the question.
- Answer as many questions as possible. For questions that cause uncertainty, guess or estimate.
- Look over the test when you are done to ensure that you have read all questions correctly and that you have answered as many as possible.
- Make changes to answers only if there is a good reason to do so.
- Check the test carefully before turning it in. (For instance, you might have forgotten to put your name on it!)

BELIEVE YOU CAN AND YOU'RE HALFWAY THERE.

THEODORE ROOSEVELT

UNDERSTANDING THE TEST FORMAT

There are a few additional tips that all test-wise learners should know, especially with respect to the format of the written state licensing examination. Keep in mind, of course, that the most important strategy of test taking is to know your material. Beyond that, consider the following tips on taking a multiple-choice exam.

THE MULTIPLE-CHOICE FORMAT

Multiple-choice questions are no doubt very familiar to you at this point, given their prevalence in education at many levels. Luckily for you, the characteristics that make the format attractive to educators and testers also mean that there are a number of tactics you can use when taking this type of test:

- Read the entire question carefully, including all the choices.
- Look for the best answer; more than one choice may be true.
- Eliminate incorrect answers by crossing them out (if taking the test on the test form).
- When two choices are close or similar, one of them is probably right.
- When two choices are identical, both must be wrong.
- When two choices are opposites, one is probably wrong and one is probably correct, depending on the number of other choices.
- "All of the above" and similar responses are often the correct choice.
- Pay special attention to words such as *not*, *except*, and *but*.
- Guess if you do not know the answer (provided that there is no penalty).
- The answer to one question may be in the stem of another.

DEDUCTIVE REASONING

Deductive reasoning (dee-DUCK-tiv REE-son-ing) is the process of reaching logical conclusions by employing logical reasoning. Deductive reasoning used as a test-taking technique very often leads to better test results, regardless of the exam format.

Some strategies associated with deductive reasoning include the following:

- Eliminate options known to be incorrect. The more incorrect answers you can eliminate, the better your chances are of identifying the correct answer.
- Watch for key words or terms. Look for any qualifying conditions or statements. Keep an eye out for phrases and words such as *usually*, *commonly*, *in most instances*, *never*, and *always*.
- Study the stem (STEM), which is the basic question or problem. It will often provide a clue to the correct answer. Look for a match between the stem and one of the choices.
- Watch for grammatical clues. For instance, if the last word in a stem is *an*, the answer must begin with a vowel rather than a consonant.
- Look at similar or related questions. They may provide clues.

eakasarn/Shutterstock.com

- When questions include paragraphs to read and questions to answer, read the questions first. This will help you identify the important information as you read the paragraph.

Remember that even though you may understand test formats and effective test-taking strategies, this does not take the place of having a complete understanding of the material on which you are being tested. In order to be successful at taking tests, you must follow the rules of effective studying and be thoroughly knowledgeable of the exam content for both the written and the practical examination.

THE PRACTICAL EXAM

After completing their school curriculum, examination candidates should be competent in their technical skills and ready for state board **practical exams** (PRAC-ti-cal ex-AMZ) where required. Although performance criteria for practical examinations vary from state to state, there are basic skills or procedures that are usually evaluated for each discipline. (You can bet infection control is in there!) Review your state board rules and candidate information literature for details about what you will be tested on at the practical exam.

Practical exams require a different approach than written exams. After all, performing services is what your license is for and practical exams are the best way to evaluate a person's technical competency.

Basic preparation for practical exams should always include practice on the model that you will be taking to the examination. To feel confident about your performance, you must be familiar with the model's hair/skin/nails and the service that you will be performing. This preparation will help eliminate some nervousness and stress during the practical exam.

In order to be better prepared for the practical portion of the examination, follow these tips:

- Practice the correct skills required in the test as often as you can.
- Participate in mock licensing examinations, complete with timed sections.
- Familiarize yourself with the content contained in the examination bulletins sent by the licensing agency.
- Make a list of equipment and implements you are expected to bring to the examination.
- Make certain that all equipment and implements are clean and in good working order prior to the exam (**Figure 8-3**).
- If allowed by the regulatory or licensing agency, observe other practical examinations prior to taking yours.
- As with any exam, listen carefully to the examiner's instructions and follow them explicitly.
- Focus on your own knowledge and do not allow yourself to be concerned with what other test candidates are doing.
- Follow all infection control and safety procedures throughout the entire examination.
- Look the part: neat, clean, and professional.

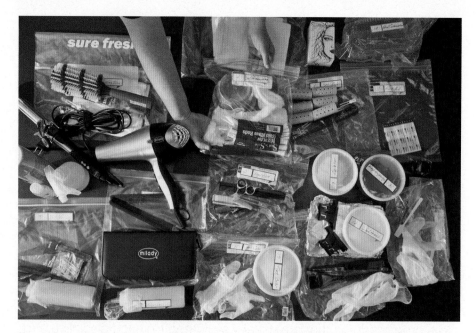

▲ FIGURE 8-3   Pack and be familiar with your practical exam kit well before exam time.

ACTIVITY

Personal Test Scheduling

As soon as you know the date and time of your exam, whip out your phone or calendar app—or flip through your tried and true paper planner—and add them in. Most exam sites require you to arrive 15 to 30 minutes ahead of time, so you may as well build that in right now. Don't forget to add an alarm (or three)!

You'll want to make some important notes on the event as well:

- Required prior arrival time
- Exam site address
- Directions to site
- Your model's name and number
- Hotel name, phone number, reservation confirmation number and cost (if you have to travel some distance)
- Everything you will need to bring with you (practical kit, ID, etc.)

CHECK IN
What are three habits of test-wise students?

DISCOVER POTENTIAL EMPLOYERS

When you chose to enter your field, your primary goal was to find a good job after being licensed. Now you need to narrow that goal into reality by answering a number of important questions.

- What do you really want out of a career in the beauty industry?
- What particular areas within the industry are the most interesting to you?

- What are your strongest practical skills? In what ways do you wish to use these skills?
- What clientele do you want to work with? What level of style do they demand?
- Where do you want to work, geographically speaking? What part of the world, the nation, or the city (downtown or suburbs)?

These questions will help specify your goal and provide guidance for future training and growth. In addition, you should be getting a better idea of what type of establishment would best suit you for your eventual employment.

During your training, you may have the opportunity to network with various industry professionals who are invited to the school as guest speakers. Be prepared to ask them questions about what they like least and most in their current positions. Ask them for any tips they might have that will assist you in your search for the right salon, spa, or barbershop. In addition, be sure to take advantage of your institution's in-house placement assistance program if available when you begin your employment search (**Figure 8-4**).

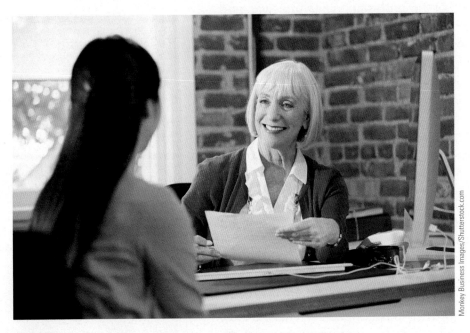

▲ **FIGURE 8-4** Your school advisor can help you find employment.

Your willingness to work hard is a key ingredient to your success. The commitment you make now in terms of time and effort will pay off later in the workplace, where your energy will be appreciated and rewarded. Having enthusiasm for getting the job done can be contagious, and when everyone works hard, everyone benefits. You can begin to develop this enthusiasm by establishing good work habits as a student.

ACTIVITY

Soft Skill Check

For one week, keep a daily record of your performance in the following areas. Use the results to gauge your areas of improvement as well as gain a better sense of your strengths when it comes time to toot your own horn in an interview. Compare your results with those of a few of your fellow students and give each other additional feedback.

- Positive attitude
- Punctuality
- Diligent practice of newly learned techniques
- Teamwork
- Professional appearance
- Regular class and clinic attendance
- Interpersonal skills
- Helping others

A SHOP SURVEY

The beauty and wellness industry is enormous, employing over a million professionals in almost as many different establishments[i]. The industry is also extremely diverse in terms of the professionals themselves and the types of shops they work in. This year, like every year, thousands of graduates will find their first position in one of the eight basic types of salon, spa, or barbershops described below. As you research places of employment, focus on the type of establishment that you believe will be the best fit for you. Note that some disciplines will emphasize some of these types over others, and other types may not be represented at all. The purpose of this list is to appreciate the variety of institutions out in the world and the different opportunities they offer.

SMALL INDEPENDENT SHOPS

Owned by an individual or two or more partners, this kind of operation makes up the majority of professional salons, spas, and barbershops. The typical independent shop has five stations, but many can have up to 40. Usually, the owners are beauty professionals who maintain their own clientele while managing the business. There are nearly as many types of independent shops as there are owners. Their image, decor, services, prices, and clientele all reflect the owner's experience and taste (**Figure 8-5**). Depending on the owner's willingness to help a newcomer learn and grow, a beginning professional can learn a great deal in an independent salon, spa, or barbershop while also earning a good living.

INDEPENDENT CHAINS

These are usually chains of five or more shops that are owned by one individual or two or more partners. Independent chains range from basic to full-service salons, barbershops, and day spas. These shops offer everything from low-priced to very high-priced services.

In large high-end shops, beauty professionals can advance to specialized positions for specific services—color, nail care, skin care, or

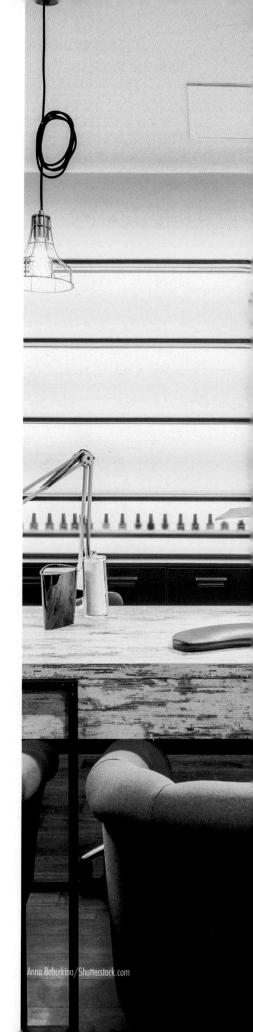

Anna Baburkina/Shutterstock.com

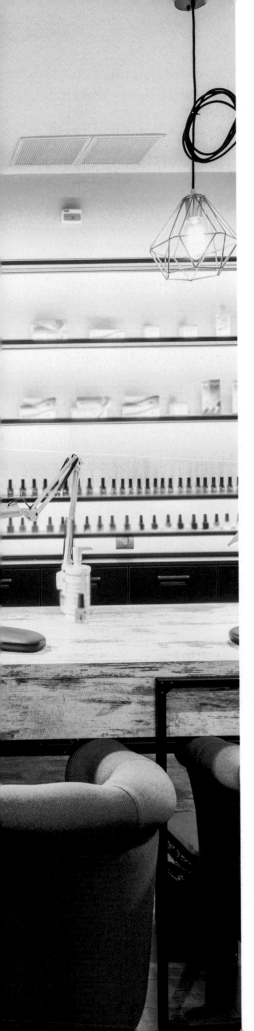

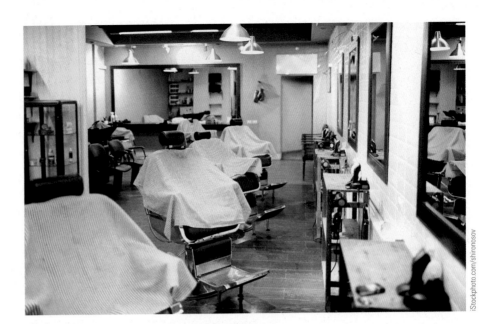

▲ **FIGURE 8-5** An independent barbershop.

other chemical services (using cosmetology as an example). Some larger shops also employ education directors and style directors and may hire beauty professionals to manage particular locations.

LARGE NATIONAL CHAINS

These companies operate salons, spas, or barbershops throughout the country, and even internationally. They can be budget or value priced, basic or full service, mid-priced or high end. Some operate within department store chains. Management and marketing professionals at the corporate headquarters make all the decisions for each salon, spa, or barbershop, such as size, decor, hours, services, prices, advertising, and profit targets. Many newly licensed professionals seek their first jobs in national chains because of the secure pay and benefits, additional paid training, management opportunities, and corporate advertising. Also, because the chains are large and widespread, employees have the added advantage of being able to transfer from one location to another.

FRANCHISES

Another chain organization, the franchise salon, spa, or barbershop has a national name and a consistent image and business formula that are used at every location. Franchises are owned by individuals who pay a fee to use the name; these individuals then receive a business plan and can take advantage of national marketing campaigns. Decisions such as size, location, decor, and prices are determined in advance by the parent company. Franchises are generally not owned by beauty professionals, but by investors who seek a return on their investment.

Franchise shops commonly offer employees the same benefits as corporate-owned chains, including on-the-job training, health-care benefits, and advancement opportunities.

BASIC VALUE-PRICED OPERATIONS

Often located in busy, low-rent shopping center strips that are anchored by a nearby supermarket or other large business, value-priced outlets depend on a high volume of walk-in traffic. They hire recent graduates and generally pay them by the hour, sometimes adding commission-style bonuses if an individual employee's sales pass a certain level. Services are usually reasonably priced and professionals are trained to work fast, with no frills.

MID-PRICED FULL-SERVICE SHOPS

These salons, spas, or barbershops offer a complete menu of services along with retail products. Successful mid-priced shops promote their most profitable services and typically offer service and retail packages to entice clients. They also run strong marketing programs to encourage client returns and referrals. These shops train their professional team to be as productive and profitable as possible. If you are inclined to give more time to each client during the consultation, you may like working in a full-service shop. Here, you will have the opportunity to build a relationship with clients that may last over time (**Figure 8-6**).

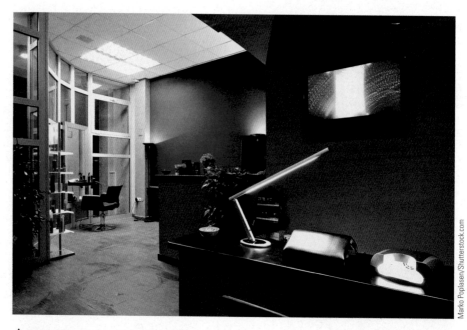

▲ FIGURE 8-6 A full-service salon.

HIGH-END SHOPS OR DAY SPAS

This type of business employs well-trained beauty professionals and assistants who offer higher-priced services to clients. They also offer luxurious extras, such as head, neck, and shoulder massages and luxurious spa manicures and pedicures. Most high-end shops are located in trendy, upscale sections of large cities; others may be located in elegant mansions, high-rent office and retail towers, or luxury hotels and resorts. Clients expect a high level of personal service; such salons, spas, and barbershops hire professionals whose technical expertise, personal appearance, and communication skills meet their high standards. Medical spas, often owned by physicians, are offshoots of day spas.

BOOTH RENTAL ESTABLISHMENTS

Booth renting, also called *chair rental*, is possibly the least expensive way of owning your own business. However, this type of business is regulated by complex laws. For a detailed discussion of booth rental see Chapter 10: "The Beauty Business."

TARGETING THE ESTABLISHMENT

It bears repeating that one of the most important steps in the process of job hunting is narrowing your search. Listed below are some points to keep in mind when targeting potential employers.

- Accept that your first job will probably not be your dream job. Few people are so fortunate.
- Do not wait until graduation to begin your search. If you do, you may be tempted to take the first offer you receive instead of carefully investigating all possibilities before making a decision.
- Locate a salon, spa, or barbershop that serves the type of clients you wish to serve. Finding a good fit with the clients and staff is critical from the outset of your career (**Figure 8-7**).
- Make a list of area salons, spas, and barbershops. The Internet will be your best source for this. If you are considering relocating to another area, a simple Google search for your area of interest and city, using key words such as *haircolor salon Portland*, can be a good place to start.

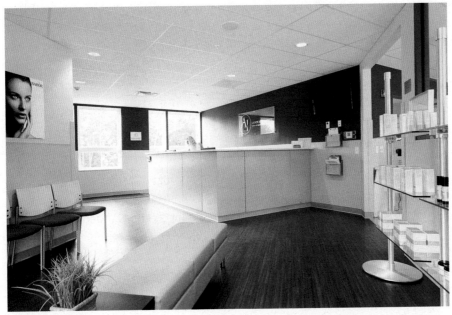

▲ FIGURE 8-7 Independent shops reflect the owner's taste, which gives you clues as to whether you'll fit in.

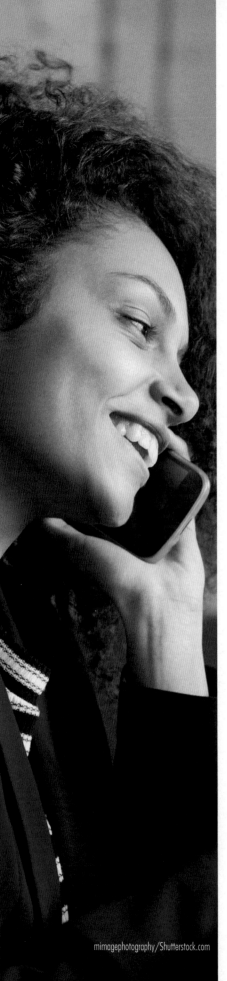

mimagephotography/Shutterstock.com

- Watch for salons, spas, or barbershops that advertise locally to get a feel for the market each one is targeting. Then check the business's website or see if it is part of a social network, such as Facebook.
- Check out websites and social networking sites for various salons, spas, and barbershops. If you contact them, don't waste their time. Get right to the point that you are a student and ask specific questions about the profession.
- Keep the salon, spa, or barbershop's culture in mind. Do the employees dress like you? Are the clients in different age groups or just one? Look for the business that will be best for you and your goals.

MAKING CONTACT

Once you've identified some establishments with potential, it's time to actually get out there, visit some salons, spas, and barbershops, and talk to owners, managers, educators, and professionals. Whether your first contact is online, in person, or on the phone, sooner or later you'll want to arrange a face-to-face meeting or an exploratory visit. To set up a shop visit, consider the following:

- If you call, use your best telephone manner; speak with confidence and self-assurance. If you e-mail, be brief, and check spelling and punctuation. Do not text message owners or managers unless they request that you do so.
- Explain that you are preparing to graduate from beauty school, that you are researching the market for potential positions, and that you have a few quick questions.
- If the person is receptive, ask whether the salon, spa, or barbershop is in need of any new professionals and how many they currently employ.
- Ask if you can make an appointment to observe during the next few weeks. If the shop representative is agreeable, be on time! When timing allows, confirm the appointment the day before, via e-mail (**Figure 8-8**).

Remember that a rejection is not a negative reflection on you. Many professionals are too busy to make time for this kind of networking. The

Dear Ms. (or Mr.) _____,

This is just a quick reminder that I'll be visiting your shop this Friday, June 12th, at 2:00 PM. I am looking forward to meeting with you, and I am eager to observe your shop and staff at work. If you should need to reach me before that time for any reason, please call or text me at _____, or e-mail me at _____.

Sincerely,
(Your name)

▲ FIGURE 8-8 Sample appointment confirmation.

good news is that you are bound to discover many genuinely kind people who remember what it was like when they started out and who are willing to devote a bit of their time to help others who are beginning their careers.

THE SHOP VISIT

When you visit a salon, spa, or barbershop, take along a checklist to ensure that you observe all the key areas that might ultimately affect your decision making. The checklist will be similar to the one used for field trips that you probably have taken to area businesses while in school. Keep the checklist on file for future reference, so that you can make informed comparisons among establishments (**Figure 8-9**).

SHOP VISIT CHECKLIST

When you visit a salon, spa, or barbershop, observe the following areas and rate them from 1 to 5, with 5 considered being the best.

_____ **SHOP IMAGE:** Is the shop's image consistent and appropriate for your interests? Is the image pleasing and inviting? What is the decor and arrangement? If you are not comfortable or if you find it unattractive, mark the shop off your list of employment possibilities.

_____ **PROFESSIONALISM:** Do the employees present the appropriate professional appearance and behavior? Do they give their clients the appropriate levels of attention and personal service, or do they act as if work is their time to socialize?

_____ **MANAGEMENT:** Does the shop show signs of being well managed? Is the phone answered promptly with professional telephone skills? Is the mood of the shop positive? Does everyone appear to work as a team?

_____ **CLIENT SERVICE:** Are clients greeted promptly and warmly when they enter the shop? Are they kept informed of the status of their appointment? Are they offered a magazine or beverage while they wait? Is there a comfortable reception area?

_____ **PRICES:** Compare price for value. Are clients getting their money's worth? Do they pay the same price in one shop but get better service and attention in another? If possible, take home shop brochures and price lists.

_____ **RETAIL:** Is there a well-stocked retail display offering clients a variety of product lines and a range of prices? Do the professionals and receptionist (if applicable) promote retail sales?

_____ **IN-SHOP MARKETING:** Are there posters or promotions throughout the shop? If so, are they professionally made, and do they reflect contemporary styles?

_____ **SERVICES:** Make a list of all services offered by each shop and the product lines they carry. This will help you decide what earning potential the professionals have in each shop.

SHOP NAME: _____

SHOP MANAGER: _____

▲ FIGURE 8-9 Shop visit checklist.

After your visit, always remember to follow up with a handwritten note or e-mail thanking the shop representative for their time (**Figure 8-10**). Do this even if you did not like the business and would never consider working there (**Figure 8-11**).

Dear Ms. (or Mr.) _____,

I appreciate having had the opportunity to observe your shop in operation last Friday. Thank you for the time you and your staff gave me. I was impressed by the efficient and courteous manner in which your professionals served their clients. The atmosphere was pleasant, and the mood was positive. Should you ever have an opening for a professional with my skills and training, I would welcome the opportunity to apply. You can contact me at the e-mail address and phone number listed below. I hope we will meet again soon.

Sincerely,

(your name, address, telephone, e-mail address)

▲ FIGURE 8-10 Sample thank-you note.

Dear Ms. (or Mr.) _____,

I appreciate having had the opportunity to observe your shop in operation last Friday. I know how busy you and all your staff are, and I want to thank you for the time that you gave me. I hope my presence didn't interfere with the flow of your operations too much. I certainly appreciate the courtesies that were extended to me by you and your staff. I wish you and your shop continued success.

Sincerely,

(your name)

▲ FIGURE 8-11 Thank-you note to a shop at which you do not expect to seek employment.

NETWORKING

Never burn your bridges. Instead, build a network of contacts who have a favorable opinion of you (**Figure 8-12**). Networking (NET-werk-ing) is a subtle approach to increasing the breadth and scope of your contacts.

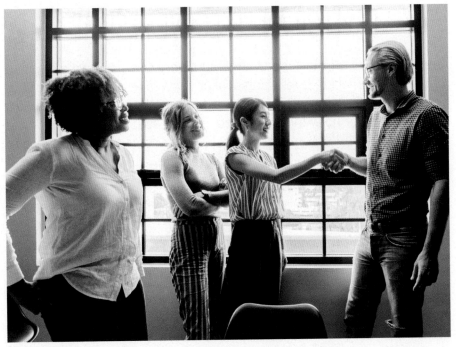

▲ FIGURE 8-12 Networking is a good way to increase contacts that can enhance your career.

It is far less intimidating than a direct request for a job interview and is a useful exercise in developing important communication skills. Students can begin to develop networking skills in many ways. The following list of suggestions will help you get started.

- Join professional organizations. Most offer student discounts and encourage membership.
- Attend industry trade shows and educational seminars. Talk to presenters and participants.
- Create a list of ideal affiliations for your discipline (for example, an esthetician may want to connect with dermatologists, massage therapists, and nutritionists). Develop a "script" for introducing yourself.
- Subscribe to trade publications and get in the habit of checking into calendars of events.
- Ask your instructors about local, regional, and national happenings.
- Investigate online communities and social media networks in which you can participate.
- Participate in field trips sponsored by your school.
- Keep a list of guest speakers who have visited your school, for future reference.
- Become involved in a charity project.
- Be open-minded and attend business functions or health seminars that will provide positive learning experiences, even if they are not completely focused on your technical expertise.

CHECK IN

List the different types of salons, spas, and barbershops that a beauty professional might work in.

DEVELOP AN EFFECTIVE RESUME

A resume (RES-uh-may) is a written summary of a person's education and work experience. It tells potential employers at a glance what your achievements and accomplishments are. If you are a new graduate, you may have little or no work experience; in this case, your resume should focus on skills and accomplishments. Here are some basic guidelines to follow when preparing your professional resume.

- Keep it simple and limit it to one page.
- Print a hard copy from your electronic version, using good-quality paper.
- Include your name, address, phone number, and e-mail address on both the resume and your cover letter.
- List recent, relevant work experience.
- List relevant education, the name of the institution from which you graduated, and relevant courses completed.
- List your professional skills and accomplishments.
- Focus on information that is relevant to the position you are seeking.

The average time that a potential employer will spend scanning your resume before deciding whether to grant you an interview is about 20 seconds. That means you must market yourself in such a manner that the reader will want to meet you. If your work experience has been in an unrelated field, show how the position helped you develop transferable skills. Restaurant work, for example, helps employees develop customer-service skills and learn to deal with a wide variety of customers.

As you list former and current positions on your resume, focus on achievements instead of detailing duties and responsibilities. Accomplishment statements enlarge your basic duties and responsibilities. The best way to show concrete accomplishment is to include numbers or percentages whenever possible. As you describe former and current positions on your resume, ask yourself the following questions:

- How many regular clients did I serve?
- How many clients did I serve weekly?
- What was my service ticket average?
- What was my client retention rate?
- What percentage of my client revenue came from retailing?
- What percentage of my client revenue came from color or texture services?

If you cannot express your accomplishment numerically, can you address which problems you solved or other results you achieved? For instance, did your office job help you develop excellent organizational skills?

This type of questioning can help you develop accomplishment statements that will interest a potential employer. There is no better time for you to achieve significant accomplishments than while you are in school. Even though your experience may be minimal, you must still present evidence of your skills and accomplishments. This may seem a difficult task at this early stage in your working career, but by closely examining your training and school clinic performance, extracurricular activities, and the full- or part-time jobs you have held, you should be able to create a good, attention-getting resume.

For example, consider the following questions:

- Did you receive any honors during your course of training?
- Were you ever selected to be student of the month?
- Did you receive special recognition for your attendance or academic progress?
- Did you win any competitions while in school?
- What was your attendance average while in school?
- Did you work with the student body to organize any fundraisers? What were the results?

Answers to these types of questions may indicate your people skills, personal work habits, and personal commitment to success (**Figure 8-13**).

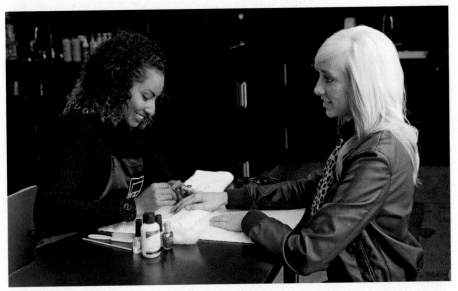

▲ **FIGURE 8-13** Excelling in school can help you build a good resume to accompany your technical skills.

Since you have not yet completed your training, you still have the opportunity to make some of the examples listed above become a reality before you graduate. Positive developments of this nature while you are still in school can do much to improve your resume.

RESUME GUIDELINES

You will save yourself from experiencing problems and disappointment right from the beginning of your job search if you keep a clear idea in your mind of what to do when it comes to creating a resume.

- **Always put your complete contact information on your resume.** If your cell phone is your primary phone, list its number first. Add a landline if you have one.
- **Make it easy to read.** Use concise, clear sentences and avoid over-writing or flowery language.

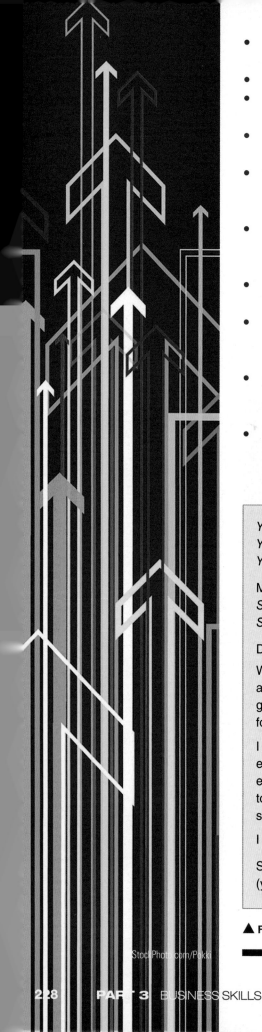

- **Know your audience.** Use vocabulary and language that will be understood by your potential employer.
- **Keep it short.** One page is preferable.
- **Stress accomplishments.** Emphasize past accomplishments and the skills you used to achieve them.
- **Focus on career goals.** Highlight information that is relevant to your career goals and the position you are seeking.
- **Emphasize transferable skills.** The skills mastered at other jobs that can be put to use in a new position are transferable skills (tranz-FUR-able SKILLZ).
- **Use action verbs.** Begin accomplishment statements with action verbs, such as *achieved*, *coordinated*, *developed*, *increased*, *maintained*, and *strengthened*.
- **Make it neat.** A poorly structured, badly typed resume does not reflect well on you.
- **Include professional references.** Use only professional references on your resume; make sure you give potential employers the person's title, place of employment, and telephone number.
- **Be realistic.** Remember that you are just starting out in a field that you hope will be a wonderful and fulfilling experience. Be realistic about what employers may offer to beginners.
- **Always include a cover letter.** See **Figure 8-14** for an example, which assumes you have targeted and visited a salon, spa, or barbershop in advance, as advised in this chapter.

Your Name
Your Address
Your Phone Number

Ms. (or Mr.) _____
Shop Name
Shop Address

Dear Ms. (or Mr.) _____,

We met in August when you invited me to observe your shop and staff while I was still in training. Since that time, I have graduated and have received my license. I have enclosed my resume for your review and consideration.

I would appreciate the opportunity to meet with you and discuss either current or future career opportunities at your shop. I was extremely impressed with your staff and business, and I would like to share with you how my skills and training might add to your shop's success.

I look forward to meeting with you again soon.

Sincerely,
(your name)

▲ **FIGURE 8-14** Sample resume cover letter.

iStockPhoto.com/Pokki

- **Note any skills with new technologies.** Include software programs, web development tools, and computerized client management systems.
- **Avoid salary references.** Don't state your salary history.
- **Avoid information about why you left former positions.**
- **Tell the truth**. Misinformation or untruthful statements usually catch up with you.

If you don't feel comfortable writing your own resume, consider seeking a professional resume writer or a job coach. There may be employment agencies that can help you as well; many online job-search websites offer easy-to-use resume templates.

DID YOU KNOW?

Use your creativity and artistic abilities as a beauty professional to create a resume that represents your style and sets you apart from the competition. Do a search for contemporary resumes on Pinterest, for instance, for ideas on color options, new styles, and formatting to create a unique resume.

Review **Figure 8-15**, which represents an achievement-oriented resume for a recent graduate of a beauty and wellness course. Remember that you are a total package, not just a resume. With determination, you will find the right position to begin your career. Use all available resources during your resume development and job search process. For example, there is an abundance of best practice information available on the Internet, or you can communicate with an individual you may already know who has gone through the hiring process and can provide recommendations. Milady also has fantastic resources at MiladyPro.com that can provide you with additional assistance when you begin your job search.

CHECK IN
What are 10 resume-writing guidelines?

PREPARE FOR A JOB INTERVIEW IN THE BEAUTY INDUSTRY

After you have graduated and completed the first two steps in the process of securing employment—targeting and observing salons, spas, and barbershops—you are ready to pursue employment in earnest. The next step is to contact the establishments that you are most interested in by sending them a resume and requesting an interview. Choosing a salon, spa, or barbershop that is the best match to your skills will increase your chances of success.

Many salons, spas, and barbershops have websites with special employment areas; others post on beauty and wellness or job-related websites. Follow the instructions exactly for filling out forms or sending resumes. (Some businesses don't want attachments sent with resumes, such as letters of recommendation or digital portfolios.) In rare instances,

SAMI STYLES

143 Fern Circle • Anytown, USA, 12345 • 123.555.1234 • SamiStyles@mye-mail.net • StyledToTheNines.blogspot.com

Objective

My objective is to obtain an apprentice position in an upscale shop and continue my education so I may become a seasoned beauty professional.

Education

ABC Academy of Beauty, Chicago, IL, May 2020
Awards: Received Award for Best Student Haircut - International Beauty Show 2016

Oak Park River Forest High School, Oak Park, IL, May 2017
Overall GPA: 3.0
Clubs: Paint/Sketch Club, Theater Club, Yearbook Committee

Qualifications

- Creative, energetic and devoted to the beauty industry
- Holds a current Illinois license and has a strong knowledge of trends
- Proven ability to retain clients and was booked solid with requests during my final four months of training
- Served as mentor to new students of the ABC Academy of Beauty

Professional Experience

Creative

- Won the student contest for best makeover
- Developed an outstanding digital portfolio of photos showing cut, color, nails, and makeovers

Sales

- Increased chemical services to 30 percent of my clinic volume by graduation
- Named Student of the Month for best attendance, best attitude, highest retail, and most services delivered

Client Retention

- Developed and retained a school clinic client base of over 75 individuals

Team Spirit

- Mentored new students and was their peer resource for the first three months of training
- Volunteered myself as the go-to person for other students to consult regarding formal styles
- Created the official ABC Academy of Beauty Facebook page, where I regularly shared new industry information

Administration

- Supervised a student "shop team" that developed a business plan for opening a 12-chair, full-service shop; earned an A and was recognized for thoroughness, accuracy, and creativity
- Reorganized a school facial room for greater efficiency and client comfort
- Led the reorganization of the school dispensary, allowing for increased inventory control and the streamlining of clinic operations
- Internet savvy with abilities in Microsoft Word, Excel, and PowerPoint

References

Please see the attached page for references.

▲ FIGURE 8-15 A resume for those with little work experience focuses on achievements.

you may need to send a resume and cover letter by traditional snail mail. Comply with the guidelines set by the salon, spa, or barbershop.

Mark your calendar to remind yourself to make a follow-up contact. A week after submitting your resume is generally sufficient. When you call or e-mail, try to schedule an interview appointment. Keep in mind that some establishments may not have openings and may not be granting interviews. When this is the case, send a resume, if you have not already, and ask the salon, spa, or barbershop to keep it on file should an opening arise in the future. Be sure to thank your contacts for their time and consideration.

INTERVIEW PREPARATION

When preparing for an interview, make sure that you have all the necessary information and materials in place (**Figure 8-16**), including the following items:

IDENTIFICATION

- Social security number
- Driver's license number
- Names, mailing addresses, e-mail addresses, and phone numbers of former employers
- Name, phone number and e-mail address of the nearest relative not living with you

INTERVIEW WARDROBE

Your appearance is crucial, especially since you are applying for a position in the image and beauty industry (**Figure 8-17**). It is recommended that you obtain one or two interview outfits. You may be requested to return for a second interview, hence the need for the second outfit. Consider the following points:

- Is the outfit appropriate for the position?
- Is it fashionable, flattering, and similar to what the employees of the salon, spa, or barbershop wear? (If you haven't visited the location, walk by or check out its website to gauge its style culture so that you can dress accordingly.)
- Are your accessories both fashionable and functional (for example, not noisy or so large that they would interfere with performing services)?
- Are your nails well groomed?
- Is your hairstyle current? Does it flatter your face and your overall style?
- Is your makeup current? Does it flatter your face and your overall style?
- Are you clean shaven? If not, is your beard properly trimmed?
- Is your perfume or cologne subtle (or nonexistent)?

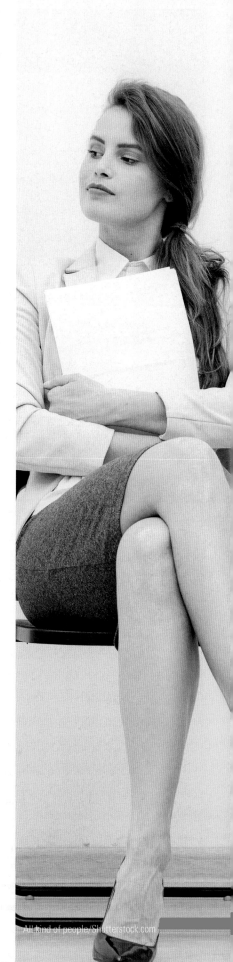

All kind of people/Shutterstock.com

PREPARING FOR THE INTERVIEW CHECKLIST

RESUME COMPOSITION

☐ Does it present your abilities and what you have accomplished in your jobs and training?

☐ Does it make the reader want to ask, "How did you accomplish that?"

☐ Does it highlight accomplishments rather than detailing duties and responsibilities?

☐ Is it easy to read, short, and does it stress past accomplishments and skills?

☐ Does it focus on information that's relevant to your own career goals?

☐ Is it complete and professionally prepared?

PORTFOLIO CHECKLIST

☐ Diploma, secondary, and post-secondary

☐ Awards and achievements while in school

☐ Current resume focusing on accomplishments

☐ Letters of reference from former employers

☐ List of, or certificates from, trade shows attended while in training

☐ Statement of professional affiliations

☐ Statement of civic affiliations and/or activities

☐ Before and after photographs of technical services you have performed

☐ Any other relevant information

Ask yourself: Does my portfolio portray me and my career skills in the manner that I wish to be perceived? If not, what needs to be changed?

GENERAL INFORMATION

- Describe specific methods or procedures you will employ in the shop to build your clientele.

- Describe how you feel about retail sales in the shop and give specific methods you would use in the shop to generate sales.

- State why you feel consumer protection and safety is so important in the beauty industry.

- After careful thought, explain what you love about your new career. Describe your passion for your discipline.

▲ FIGURE 8-16 Preparing for the interview checklist.

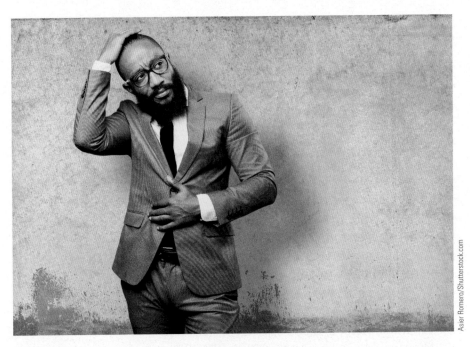

▲ FIGURE 8-17 Dressed for an interview.

Asier Romero/Shutterstock.com

HERE'S A TIP

When you contact a salon, spa, or barbershop to make an appointment for an interview, you may be told that they are not currently hiring but would be happy to conduct an interview for future reference. Never think that this would be a waste of time. Take advantage of the opportunity. Not only will it give you valuable interview experience, but it may also provide opportunities that you would otherwise miss.

SUPPORTING MATERIALS

- **Resume.** Even if you have already sent a resume, take a paper copy with you.
- **Facts and figures.** Have ready a list of names and dates of former employment, education, and references.
- **Employment portfolio.** Even if you have just two photos in your portfolio and they are pictures of haircolor, makeup, skin care, or nails you did for friends, bring them along. And if you have created a digital portfolio to share, be sure to bring a printed copy as well in case of technical issues.

REVIEW AND PREPARE FOR ANTICIPATED INTERVIEW QUESTIONS

Certain questions are typically asked during an interview. Being familiar with these questions will allow you to reflect on your answers ahead

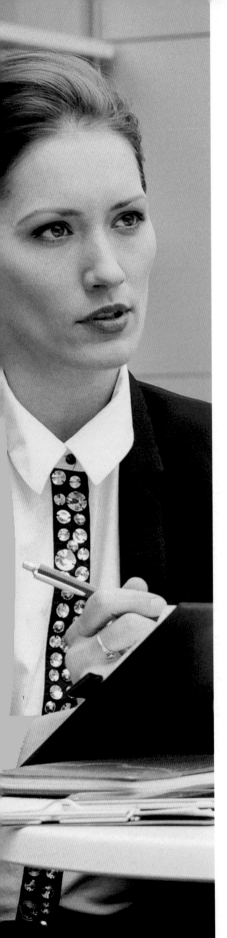

Anton Gvozdikov/Shutterstock.com

of time. You might even consider role-playing an interview situation with friends, family, or fellow students. Typical questions include the following:

- Why do you want to work here?
- What did you like best about your training?
- Are you punctual and regular in attendance?
- Will your school director or instructor confirm this?
- What skills do you feel are your strongest?
- In which areas do you consider yourself to be less strong?
- Are you a team player? Please explain.
- Do you consider yourself flexible? Please explain.
- What are your career goals?
- What days and hours are you available for work?
- Are there any obstacles that would prevent you from keeping your commitment to full-time employment? Please explain.
- What assets do you believe that you would bring to this business and this position?
- What computer skills do you have?
- How would you handle a problem client?
- How do you feel about retailing?
- Would you be willing to attend our company's training program?
- Describe ways that you provide excellent customer service.
- What consultation questions might you ask a client?
- Are you prepared to train for a year before you have your own clients?

DID YOU KNOW?

It can be difficult for new graduates to afford the two or three outfits necessary to project a confident and professional image when going out into the workplace. Fortunately, several nonprofit organizations have been formed to address this need. These organizations receive donations of clean, great-looking clothes in good repair from individuals and manufacturers. These are then passed along to individuals who need them. For more information, visit Wardrobe for Opportunity at wardrobe.org and Dress for Success at dressforsuccess.org.

BE PREPARED TO PERFORM A SERVICE

Some salons, spas, or barbershops require applicants to perform a service in their chosen discipline as part of the interview; many ask that you bring your own model. Be sure to confirm whether this is a requirement. If it is, make sure that your model is appropriately dressed and properly prepared for the experience and that you bring the necessary supplies, products, and tools to demonstrate your skills.

HERE'S A TIP

Any time that you are applying for any position, you will be required to complete an application, even if your resume already contains much of the requested information. Your resume and the list you have prepared prior to the interview will assist you in completing the application quickly and accurately.

THE INTERVIEW

On the day of the interview, try to make sure that nothing occurs that will keep you from completing the interview successfully. You should practice the following behaviors in connection with the interview itself:

- Always be on time or, better yet, early. If you are unsure of the location, find it the day before, so there will be no reason for delays.
- Turn off your cell phone! Do not arrive with ear buds or a hands-free cell phone device in your ear.
- Project a warm, friendly smile. Smiling is the universal language.
- Walk, sit, and stand with good posture.
- Be polite and courteous.
- Do not sit until you are asked to do so or until it is obvious that you are expected to do so.
- Never smoke or chew gum, even if one or the other is offered to you.
- Do not come to an interview with a cup of coffee, a soft drink, snacks, or anything else to eat or drink.
- Never lean on or touch the interviewer's desk. Some people do not like their personal space broached without an invitation.
- Try to project a positive first impression by appearing as confident and relaxed as you can be (**Figure 8-18**).

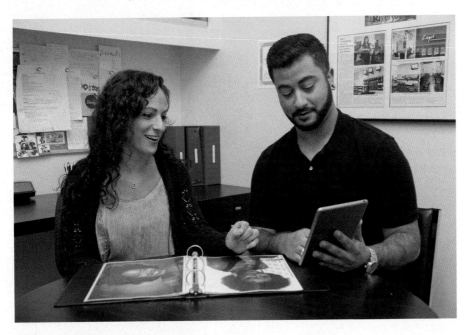

▲ FIGURE 8-18 Interview in progress.

- Speak clearly. The interviewer must be able to hear and understand you.
- Answer questions honestly. Think about the question and answer carefully. Do not speak before you are ready and do not speak for more than two minutes at a time.
- Never criticize former employers.
- Always remember to thank the interviewer at the end of the interview.

ACTIVITY

Mock Interviews

Find a partner among your fellow students and role-play the employment interview. Each of you can take turns as the applicant and the employer. After each session, conduct a brief discussion regarding how it went; that is, what did and did not work. Discuss how your performance could be improved. Bear in mind that a role-playing activity will never predict exactly what will occur in a real interview. However, the process will help prepare you for the interview and boost your confidence.

Another critical part of the interview comes when you are invited to ask the interviewer questions of your own. You should think about those questions ahead of time and bring a list, if necessary. Doing so will show that you are organized and prepared. Some questions that you might consider include the following:

- What are you looking for in a beauty professional?
- Is there a job description? May I review it?
- Is there a salon, spa, or barbershop manual? May I review it?
- How does the salon, spa, or barbershop promote itself?
- How long do beauty professionals typically work here?
- Are employees encouraged to grow in skills and responsibility? How so?
- Does the salon, spa, or barbershop offer continuing education opportunities?
- What does your training program involve?
- Is there room for advancement? If so, what are the requirements for promotion?
- What key benefits does the salon, spa, or barbershop offer, such as advanced training and medical insurance?
- What outside and community activities is the salon, spa, or barbershop involved in?
- What is the form of compensation?
- When will the position be filled?
- May I contact you in a week regarding your decision?
- May I have a tour of the salon, spa, or barbershop?

Do not feel that you have to ask all of your questions. The point is to create as much of a dialogue as possible. Be aware of the interviewer's reactions and make note of when you have asked enough questions. By obtaining the answers to at least some of your questions, you can compare the information you have gathered about other salon, spa, or barbershops and choose the one that offers the best package of income and career development.

Remember to follow up the interview with a thank-you note or e-mail. It should simply thank the interviewer for the time he or she spent with you. Close with a positive statement that you want the job (if you do). If the interviewer's decision comes down to two or three possibilities, the one expressing the most desire may be offered the position. Also, if the interviewer suggests that you call to learn about the employment decision, by all means do so.

Daxiao Productions/Shutterstock.com

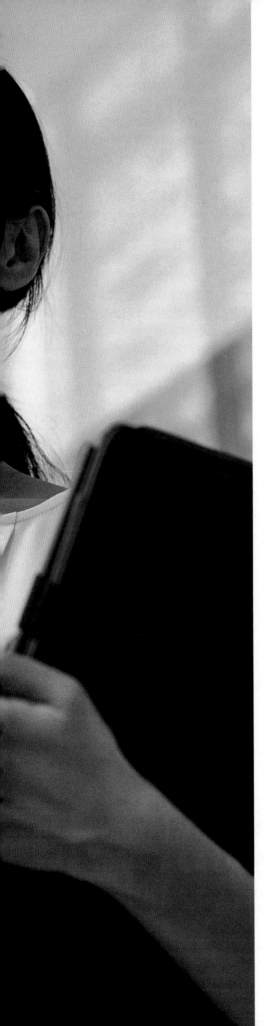

LEGAL ASPECTS OF THE EMPLOYMENT INTERVIEW

Over the years, a number of legal issues have arisen about questions that may or may not be included in an employment application or interview, including ones that involve race/ethnicity, religion, national origin, marital status, sexual orientation, and whether you have children. Generally, there should be no questions in any of these categories. Additional categories of appropriate and inappropriate questions are listed below:

- **Age or date of birth.** It is permissible to ask the age of applicants if they are younger than 18. Otherwise, age should not be relevant in most hiring decisions; therefore, date-of-birth questions prior to employment are improper.
- **Disabilities or physical traits.** The Americans with Disabilities Act prohibits general inquiries about health problems, disabilities, and medical conditions.
- **Drug use or smoking.** Questions regarding drug or tobacco use are permitted. In fact, the employer may obtain the applicant's agreement to be bound by the employer's drug and smoking policies and to submit to drug testing.
- **Citizenship.** Employers are not allowed to discriminate because an applicant is not a U.S. citizen. However, employers can request to see a green card or work permit.

It is important to recognize that not all potential employers will understand that they may be asking improper or illegal questions. If you are asked such questions, you might politely respond that you believe the question is irrelevant to the position you are seeking, and that you would like to focus on your qualities and skills that are suited to the job and the mission of the establishment.

DID YOU KNOW?

These are examples of illegal questions as compared to legal questions:

Illegal Questions
How old are you?
Please describe your medical history.
Are you a U.S. citizen?
What is your native language?

Legal Questions
Are you over the age of 18?
Are you physically able to perform this job?
Are you authorized to work in the United States?
In which languages are you fluent?

EMPLOYEE CONTRACTS

Employers can legally require you to sign contracts as a condition of employment. In the salon, spa, and barbershop business, the most common are non-compete and confidentiality agreements. Owners often invest a great deal in training and don't want you taking all that education to a competing business across the street once your apprenticeship or initial training is complete. Non-compete agreements address this issue, prohibiting you from seeking employment within a given time period and geographic area after you leave employment with them. Often, non-compete agreements also forbid employees from gathering and keeping client records, including client phone numbers. A contract cannot interfere with your right to work; as a result, these contracts must be very specific and are sometimes controversial. If you are presented with any contract, take it home, read it, and make certain you completely understand it. If you do not completely understand any part of it, consult with a labor-law attorney before signing it.

DOING IT RIGHT

You are ready to set out on your exciting new career as a beauty professional. The right way to proceed is by learning important study and test-taking skills early and applying them consistently.

Think ahead to your employment opportunities and use your time in school to develop a record of interesting, noteworthy activities that will make your resume more exciting. When you compile a history that shows how you have achieved your goals, your confidence will grow.

Always take one step at a time. Be sure to take the helpful preliminary steps that we have discussed when preparing for employment.

Develop a dynamic portfolio. Keep your materials, information, and questions organized in order to ensure a high-impact interview.

Once you are employed, take the necessary steps to learn all that you can about your new position and the establishment you will be serving. Read all you can about the industry. Attend trade shows and take advantage of as much continuing education as you can manage. Become an active participant in efforts to make the beauty and wellness industry even better.

As you transition into your new career as a beauty professional, let Milady continue the journey with you. Be sure to visit the MiladyPro.com website. In addition to helping you prepare for your state board exam, MiladyPro.com offers access to materials designed to help you hit the ground running and grow your skill set, assuring long-term success no matter where you may take your career.

CHECK IN
What questions are illegal to be asked when interviewing for a job?

APPLY CAREER PLANNING

Congratulations on completing this chapter! Before you move on, take a moment to think about how these Career Planning topics apply to your particular discipline. Discuss with a classmate or study group what procedures you will need to practice for your practical exam; what types of salons, spas, or barbershops can be found locally and which you prefer; what you expect interviews in your discipline will require; and so on.

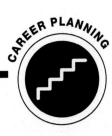

COMPETENCY PROGRESS

How are you doing with Career Planning? **Check off the Chapter 8 Learning Objectives below that you feel you have mastered; leave unchecked those objectives you will need to return to:**

☐ EXPLAIN CAREER PLANNING.

☐ REVIEW THE STATE LICENSING EXAMINATION PROCESS.

☐ DISCOVER POTENTIAL EMPLOYERS.

☐ DEVELOP AN EFFECTIVE RESUME.

☐ PREPARE FOR A JOB INTERVIEW IN THE BEAUTY INDUSTRY.

GLOSSARY

deductive reasoning dee-DUCK-tiv REE-son-ing	p. 214	the process of reaching logical conclusions by employing logical reasoning
networking NET-werk-ing	p. 224	a method of increasing contacts and building relationships to further one's career
practical exams PRAC-ti-cal ex-AMZ	p. 215	hands-on testing on a live model
resume RES-uh-may	p. 226	a written summary of a person's education and work experience
stem STEM	p. 214	the basic question or problem
test-wise TEST-whys	p. 211	understanding the strategies for successful test taking
transferable skills tranz-FUR-able SKILLZ	p. 228	skills mastered at other jobs that can be put to use in a new position

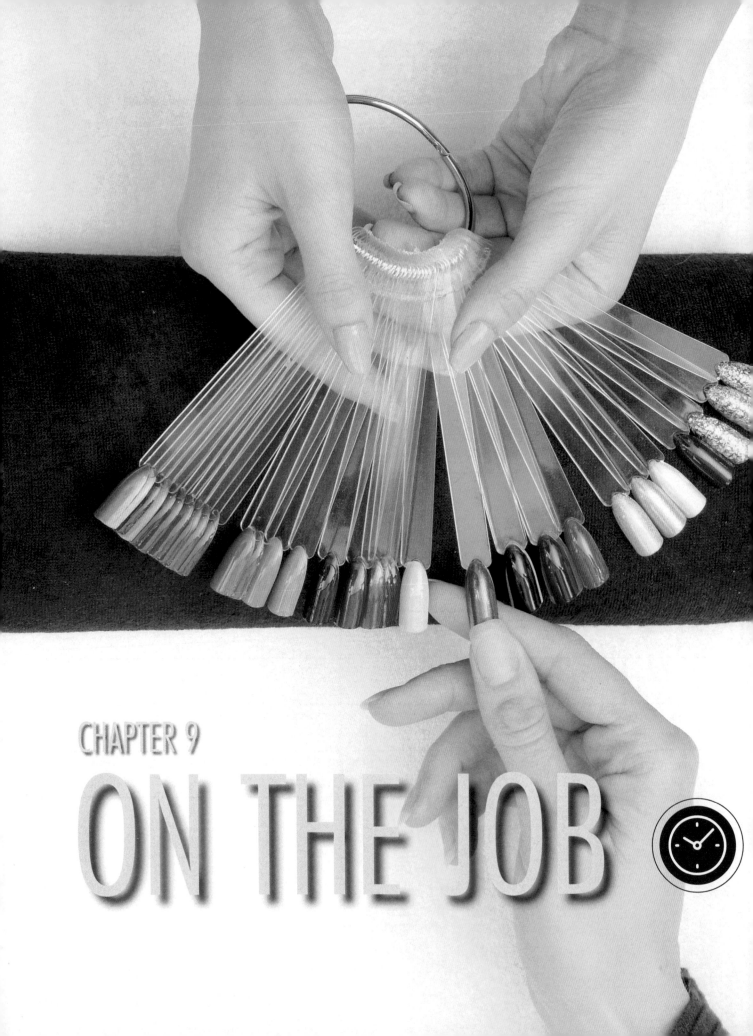

CHAPTER 9
ON THE JOB

"Do what you have to do until you can do what you want to do."
-Oprah Winfrey

AFTER COMPLETING THIS CHAPTER, YOU WILL BE ABLE TO:

1. EXPLAIN WHAT IT'S LIKE ON THE JOB.

2. DESCRIBE THE EXPECTATIONS OF MOVING FROM SCHOOL TO WORK.

3. SUMMARIZE EMPLOYMENT OPTIONS IN THE REAL WORLD.

4. PRACTICE MONEY MANAGEMENT.

5. MASTER SELLING IN THE SALON, SPA, AND BARBERSHOP.

6. USE MARKETING TO EXPAND YOUR CLIENT BASE.

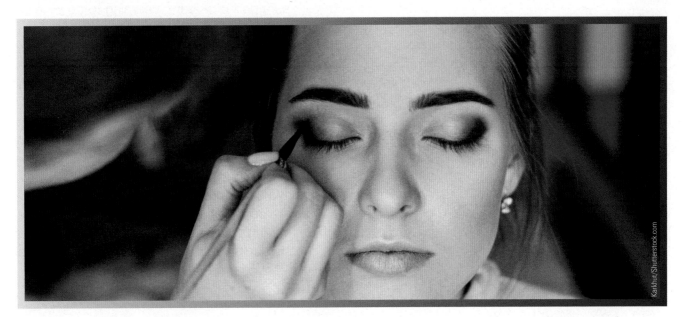

Karkhut/Shutterstock.com

EXPLAIN WHAT IT'S LIKE ON THE JOB

Congratulations! You've worked hard in school, passed your state's licensing exam, and been offered your first job in the field. Now, more than ever, you need to prioritize your goals and commit to personal rules of conduct and behavior. Your goals and rules should guide you throughout your career. If you let them do so, you can expect to always have work and to enjoy all the freedom that your chosen profession can offer (**Figure 9-1**).

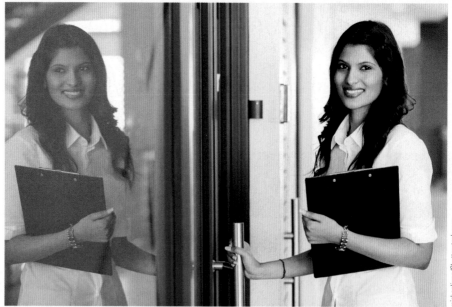

▲ FIGURE 9-1 On to the next step in your career.

Beauty professionals should study and have a thorough understanding of what it is like on the job because:

- Working in a salon, spa, or barbershop requires each staff member to belong to and work as a part of a team. Learning to do so is an important aspect of being successful in the work environment.
- There are a variety of ways that an employer may compensate their employees. Being familiar with each one and knowing how it works will help you determine if the compensation system at a particular business can work for you and what to expect from it.
- Once you are working as a beauty professional, you will also have financial obligations and responsibilities to attend to, so learning the basics of financial management while you are building your clientele and business is invaluable.
- As you gather clientele and settle into your professional life, there will be opportunities for you to use a variety of techniques for increasing your income, such as retailing and upselling services. Knowing and using these techniques will help you promote yourself, build a loyal client base, and create a sound financial future for yourself.

DESCRIBE THE EXPECTATIONS OF MOVING FROM SCHOOL TO WORK

Making the transition from school to work can be difficult. While you may be thrilled to have a job, working for a paycheck includes a number of duties and responsibilities that you may not have considered.

Beauty and wellness school is a forgiving environment. You are given the chance to do a certain procedure over and over again until you get it right. Making and fixing mistakes is an accepted part of the process, and your instructors and mentors are there to help you. Schedules can be adjusted if necessary, and you are given some leeway in juggling your personal life with the demands of your schooling (**Figure 9-2**).

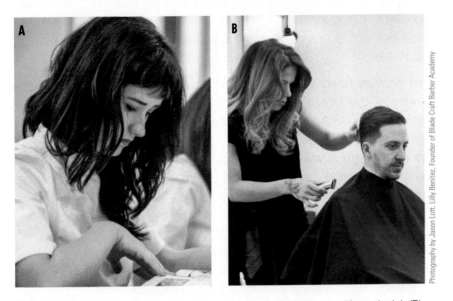

▲ FIGURE 9-2 Time to transition from your school life (A) to your life on the job (B).

When you become an employee, however, you will be expected to put the needs of the business and its clients ahead of your own. You will need to be on time for every scheduled shift and be prepared to perform whatever services or functions are required of you, regardless of what is happening in your personal life. For example, if a friend offers you tickets for a concert on a day when you are scheduled to work, you cannot just take the day off. If you did, you would definitely inconvenience your clients; they might even decide not to return to the salon, spa, or barbershop. It could also burden your coworkers, who might feel resentful if they are asked to take on your appointments.

Many graduates believe they should be rewarded with a high-paying job, performing only the kinds of services they want to do, as soon as they graduate from school. It does not work out that way for most people. In a job, you may be asked to do work or perform services that are not your first choice. The good news is that when you are really working in the trenches, you are also learning every moment, and there is no substitute for that kind of experience.

DID YOU KNOW?

Network with mentors, professionals, educators, and classmates and ask questions, take advice, listen, and consider all your options! By doing this, you will open yourself to knowledge, resources, and terrific beauty and wellness industry information.

THRIVING IN A SERVICE PROFESSION

The first reality of a service position is that your career revolves around serving your clients. There will always be people who do not treat others with respect; however, the majority of the people you encounter will truly appreciate the work you perform for them. They will look forward to seeing you and will show their appreciation for your hard work with their loyalty.

Here are some points that will help guide you as you meet your clients' needs:

- **Put others first.** You will have to quickly get used to putting the needs of the business and the client ahead of your feelings or desires. This means performing what is expected of you (unless you are physically unable to do so).
- **Be true to your word.** Choose your words carefully and honestly. Be someone who can be counted on to tell the truth and to do what you say you will do.
- **Be punctual.** Scheduling is central to the beauty business. Getting to work on time shows respect not only for your clients but also for your coworkers (who will have to handle your clients if you are late).
- **Be a problem solver.** No job or situation comes without its share of problems. Be someone who recognizes problems promptly and finds ways to resolve them constructively.
- **Be a lifelong learner.** Valued employees continue to learn throughout their careers. Thinking that you are done learning once you are out of school is immature and limiting. Your career might go in all kinds of interesting directions, depending on what new things you learn. This applies to every aspect of your life. Besides learning new technical skills, you should continue gaining more insight into your own behavior and better ways to deal with people, problems, and issues.

PART OF THE TEAM

Working in a salon, spa, or barbershop requires that you practice and perfect your people skills. These kinds of workplaces are very much team environments. To become a good team player, you should do your best to practice the following workplace principles:

- **Strive to help.** Be concerned not only with your own success, but also with the success of others. Be willing to help a teammate by staying a little later or coming in a little earlier.
- **Pitch in.** Be willing to help with whatever needs to be done in the shop—from folding towels to making appointments—when you are not busy servicing clients (**Figure 9-3**).
- **Share your knowledge.** Be willing to share what you know. This will make you a respected member of any team. At the same time, be willing to learn from your coworkers by listening to their perspectives and techniques.

pikselstock/Shutterstock.com

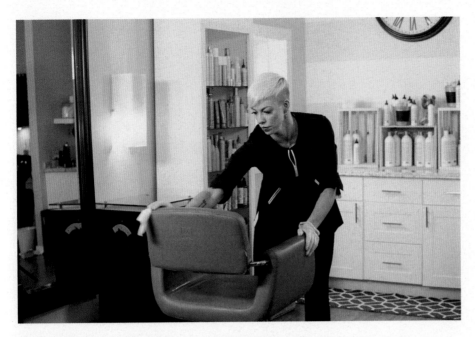

▲ **FIGURE 9-3** Pitch in whenever you're needed.

- **Remain positive.** Resist the temptation to give in to maliciousness and gossip.
- **Become a relationship builder.** Just as there are different kinds of people in the world, there are different types of relationships within the beauty and wellness world. You do not have to be someone's best friend to build a good working relationship with that person.
- **Be willing to resolve conflicts.** The most difficult part of being in a relationship is conflict. Conflict and tension are bad for the people who are in it, those who are around it, and the business as a whole. Nevertheless, conflict is a natural part of life. If you can work constructively toward resolving conflict, you will always be a valued member of the team. If you have a conflict, discuss it privately with the individual, not with others who are not involved.
- **Be willing to be subordinate.** No one starts at the top. Keep in mind that beginners almost always start out lower down in the pecking order.
- **Be sincerely loyal.** Loyalty is vital to the workings of a salon, spa, or barbershop. Beauty professionals need to be loyal to the business and its management. Management needs to be loyal to the staff and clients. Ideally, clients will be loyal to the employee and the business. As you work on team-building characteristics, you will start to feel a strong sense of loyalty to your workplace (**Figure 9-4**).

While each individual may be concerned with getting ahead and being successful, a good teammate knows that no one can be successful alone. You will be truly successful if your entire business is successful!

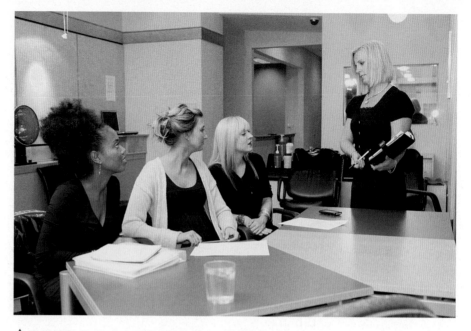

▲ FIGURE 9-4 Communication is the key to teamwork.

CHECK IN

What workplace principles should you practice to become a good team player?

SUMMARIZE EMPLOYMENT OPTIONS IN THE REAL WORLD

It is important to determine which type of position is right for you by being honest with yourself as you evaluate your skills. Ask your instructor for advice if you need help and direction with sorting out the specifics of the various workplaces you are considering during your job hunt. You will be off to a great start if you choose your first salon, spa, or barbershop carefully, based on its culture and the type of shop and benefits you prefer.

THE JOB DESCRIPTION

When you take a job, you will be expected to behave appropriately, perform services asked of you, and conduct your business professionally. To do this to the best of your abilities, you should be given a job description (JOHB des-CRIP-shun), a document that outlines the duties and responsibilities of a particular position. Many businesses have preprinted job descriptions available. If you find yourself at a shop that does not use job descriptions, you may want to write one for yourself. You can then present it to your manager for review, ensuring that you both have a good understanding of what is expected of you.

Once you have your job description, be sure you understand it. While reading it over, make notes and jot down questions you want to ask your manager. When you assume your new position, you are agreeing to do everything as it is written down in the job description. If you are unclear about something or need more information, it is your responsibility to ask.

Remember, you will be expected to fulfill all the functions listed in the job description. How well you fulfill these duties will influence your future at the business, as well as your financial rewards.

The best businesses cover all the bases when crafting a job description. They outline not only the employee's duties and responsibilities, but also the attitudes that they expect their employees to have and the opportunities that are available to them. Like the salons, spas, and barbershops that generate them, job descriptions come in all sizes and shapes and feature a variety of requirements, benefits, and incentives.

EMPLOYMENT CLASSIFICATIONS

When you assess a job offer, your first concern will probably be the compensation for your work. The way you will be paid for services performed on the job will depend primarily on your status as an employee, independent contractor, or booth renter. Many beauty professionals work as independent contractors or booth renters, although plenty of employee positions are also available in salons, spas, and barbershops. The U.S. Internal Revenue Service (IRS) categorizes independent contractors and booth renters as self-employed workers; these professionals have certain required criteria and restrictions that separate them from being designated as an employee for tax liability purposes.

HERE'S A TIP

Most employers require you to take a certain amount of continuing education, even after you have been on the job for years. That's a good thing! The more you learn, the more you will earn, and industry compensation studies prove it.

Online continuing education is not only travel-free and affordable; it also opens up a universe of global ideas and can be taken on your own time. Head to Milady.com and MiladyPro.com for online resources that include personal and professional development, webinars, infection control, articles, videos, networking opportunities, marketing tools, and more.

EMPLOYEE STATUS

As an employee (em-PLOY-ee), you might work on a salary, commission, or salary-plus-commission basis. You can expect to be told when and where to work, how to perform the job, and whether a uniform is required. Your clients will more than likely be booked for you, and you probably will not handle any money for services other than your tips. Training may be offered or required, depending on the needs of the business, and some establishments may provide insurance or vacation benefits.

As an employee, your employer is responsible for withholding income and Medicare taxes; paying a portion of your Social Security tax; paying unemployment taxes; and providing you with a Form W-2, Wage and Tax Statement. Your responsibilities as an employee include reporting all

Dmytro Zinkevych/Shutterstock.com

wages, reporting tips of $20.00 or more per month and commissions for product sales, and filing your personal income tax statement.

INDEPENDENT CONTRACTOR STATUS

As an independent contractor (in-deh-PEN-dant CON-tract-uhr), you may rent a chair or work for a percentage of the proceeds of services you perform; however, you must apply for a tax identification number and provide your own business insurance coverage. You are also responsible for your own income and self-employment taxes and should receive a Form 1099-MISC from the shop's owner when you earn over $600.00 a year. Although your business expenses may be tax deductible, all income and tips are to be reported and estimated quarterly tax payments may be required. To prove that you are working as an independent contractor for tax purposes, there must be a written agreement or contract between you and the owner. This agreement must include how you will be compensated, your responsibilities, what is included in the chair rental, an end date for your work, and additional stipulations as required. When set up properly, independent contractor agreements may be renewable. It is recommended that you seek the guidance of an accountant to ensure the agreement conforms to current federal tax laws.

BOOTH RENTER STATUS

In a booth rental (BOOTH ren-tal) arrangement, you are actually setting up a small business. This requires a contract with the shop owner, appropriate business licenses, insurance, a tax ID number, and tax designation as a booth renter or independent businessperson. As a booth renter, you lease space from the business owner and are solely responsible for your own clientele, supplies, record keeping, workstation maintenance, and accounting. You handle all money transactions and are responsible for booking your own appointments. Usually, the only obligation to the owner is the weekly or monthly rent. You should be given a key to the establishment and be able to set your own hours and schedule.

One of the main advantages of booth rental is that you can become self-employed for a relatively small investment. The initial expenses are fairly low and usually limited to the costs incurred for rent, supplies, products, and personal promotion or advertising. For some booth renters, a very low overhead may balance equitably with the income generated as a beginning beauty professional with a small clientele. However, a good rule to follow is to make sure your clientele is large enough to cover all overhead costs and still pay you a salary.

Chair or booth rental may also be ideal for individuals who are interested in part-time employment, want to supplement another income, or prefer to take a stepping-stone approach to business ownership. Regardless of the motivation, a booth rental arrangement provides the means for an individual to retain most of the control and decision making as it applies to work schedules and professional goals.

Position availability, personal choice, convenience, and the level of responsibility you care to assume will influence the capacity in which you work. Be sure to familiarize yourself with applicable state and federal tax laws. Working as an independent contractor and working as a booth renter are forms of self-employment, meaning that paid holidays or vacation benefits are nonexistent. Instead, you will have to plan ahead and set aside savings for times when you are not working or an emergency arises.

Table 9-1 provides a summary of the differences between working as an employee, independent contractor, or booth renter.

TABLE 9-1: EMPLOYMENT CLASSIFICATION OVERVIEW

EMPLOYEE	INDEPENDENT CONTRACTOR	BOOTH RENTER
Work instructions are provided; job performance is evaluated	No instruction, training, or evaluation is provided	No instruction, training, or evaluation is provided
Training may be provided or required	May require personal investment in advanced training	Requires personal investment in advanced training
Operating hours are set or scheduled	Sets own hours and schedule with agreement	Sets own hours and work schedule
Appointments are scheduled by business	May schedule own appointments	Schedules own appointments
Services revenue most often collected at front desk	Services revenue may be collected at front desk	Services revenue is collected by booth renter
Equipment and facilities are provided	May pay for certain equipment or arrange an agreement; opportunity for profit and loss exists	Certain equipment included in lease; opportunity for profit and loss
Benefits may be provided	No benefits are provided	No benefits are provided
No rental agreement exists	Independent contractor agreement required. Requires agreement with an end date, wage payment information, responsibilities, etc.	Booth rental agreement is required. Requires lease with dates, fee, booth renter responsibilities, etc.
Expenses may be reimbursed	Expenses are not usually reimbursed	Expenses are not reimbursed
May be paid on hourly, salaried, commission, or salary-plus-commission basis	May work on percentage, commission, or flat fee; and agreements may be renewed. May work in more than one location	Responsible for collecting all service revenues
Uniforms may be required	Attire may be discussed in agreement	Generally the renter's decision
Income tax, portion of social security tax, Medicare tax, and unemployment tax are paid by employer	Is responsible for all taxes, licenses, and insurance	Is responsible for all taxes, licenses, insurance, and advertising
Amount of tips are recorded by employer	Responsible for own tips and taxes	Responsible for own tips and taxes
Employer is required to provide Form W-2, Wage and Tax Statement	May work within confines of shop hours. Owner is required to provide 1099 form	Requires submitting 1099 form to owner for rent paid

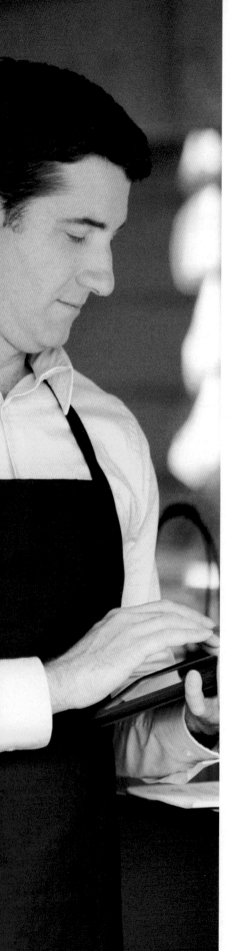

Monkey Business Images/Shutterstock.com

WAGE STRUCTURES

As discussed previously, booth rental involves paying the shop owner a fixed amount of rent for the space. All the profits brought in from the performance of services are basically yours after you pay for the rent and supplies. For the employee or independent contractor, however, compensation may be structured in one of several different ways.

SALARY

Being paid an hourly rate is usually the best way for a new beauty professional to start out, because new professionals rarely have an established clientele. An introductory hourly rate is usually based on the minimum wage, or may be slightly higher to encourage new beauty pros to take the job and stick with it. In this situation, if you earn $10 per hour and you work 40 hours, you will be paid $400 that week. If you work more hours, you will get more pay. If you work fewer hours, you will get less pay. Regular taxes will be taken out of your earnings.

Remember, if you are offered a set salary in lieu of an hourly rate, that salary must be at least equal to the minimum wage for the number of hours you work. You are entitled to overtime pay if you work more than 40 hours per week. The only exception would be if you were in an official management position.

COMMISSION

A **commission** (kahm-ISH-un) is a percentage of the revenue generated from services performed by a professional. Commission is usually offered once an employee has built up a loyal clientele. A commission payment structure is very different from an hourly wage: Any money you are paid is a direct result of the total amount of service dollars you generate for the salon, spa, or barbershop. Commissions are paid based on a percentage of your total service dollars and can range anywhere from 25 to 70 percent, depending on your length of time with the business, your performance level, and the benefits that are part of your employment package.

Suppose, for example, that at the end of the week, when you add up all the services you have performed, your total is $1,000. If you are at the 50 percent commission level, then you would be paid $500 (before taxes). Keep in mind that until you have at least two years of servicing clients under your belt, you may not be able to make a living on straight commission compensation. Additionally, many states do not allow straight commission payments unless they average out to be at least minimum wage.

SALARY PLUS COMMISSION

A salary-plus-commission structure is another common way to be compensated in the beauty business. Here, you receive both a salary and a commission. This arrangement is sometimes called a *guarantee,* as it guarantees a minimum base salary. This kind of structure is often used to motivate employees to perform more services, thereby increasing their productivity. For example, imagine that you earn an hourly wage of $300 per week and perform about $600 worth of services every week. Your manager may offer you an additional 25 percent commission on any services you perform over your usual $600 per week. Or, perhaps you receive a straight hourly wage but can receive as much as a 15 percent commission on all the retail products you sell. This variant is sometimes called *salary plus bonus*. With this structure, your salary is based on an average of what you would have made if you were paid commission, but you also get a bonus on anything over and above. You can see how this kind of structure quickly leads to significantly increased compensation (**Figure 9-5**).

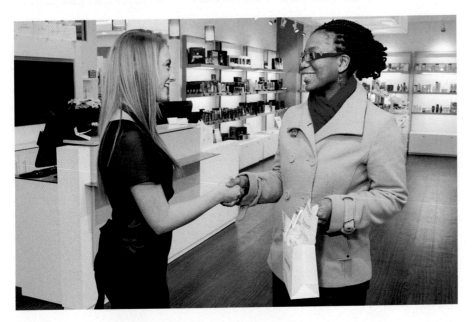

▲ FIGURE 9-5   Commissions on retail sales boost income.

TIPS

When you receive satisfactory service at a hotel or restaurant, you are likely to leave your server a tip. It has become customary for clients to acknowledge their beauty professionals in this way, too. Some salons, spas, and barbershops have a tipping policy; others have a no-tipping policy. This is determined by what the business feels is appropriate for its clientele.

Tips are income in addition to your regular compensation and must be tracked and reported on your income tax return. Reporting tips will be beneficial to you if you wish to take out a mortgage or another type of loan and want your income to appear as strong as it really is.

As you can see, there are a number of ways to structure compensation for a beauty professional. You will probably have the opportunity to try each of these methods at different points in your career. When deciding whether a certain compensation method is right for you, it is important to be aware of what your monthly expenses are and to have a personal financial budget in place. Budget issues are addressed later in this chapter.

Your
SMILE
is your
LOGO,
Your
PERSONALITY
is your
BUSINESS
CARD,

HOW YOU LEAVE OTHERS
FEELING AFTER AN
EXPERIENCE WITH YOU
BECOMES YOUR
TRADEMARK.

– JAY DANZIE

HERE'S A TIP

Accepting a commission-paying position can have positive and negative aspects for new professionals. If you think you have enough clients to work on commission and can earn a large enough paycheck to pay your expenses, then go ahead and give it a try—it could be a great way to work toward better commission percentages or even booth renting. (Note that some states do not recognize booth rental as an acceptable method of doing business. Check with your state to be aware of all the latest news and regulations.)

If you don't think you can make enough money being paid on a commission basis alone, then take a job in a salon, spa, or barbershop that is willing to pay you an hourly wage until you build your client base. After you have honed your technical skills and built a solid client base, you can consider working on commission.

EMPLOYEE EVALUATION

The best way to keep tabs on your progress is to ask for feedback from your manager and coworkers. Most likely, your employer will have a structure in place for evaluation purposes. Commonly, evaluations are scheduled 90 days after hiring and once a year after that. But you should feel free to ask for help and feedback any time you need it. This feedback can help you improve your technical abilities as well as your customer service skills.

Ask a senior professional to sit in on one of your client consultations and to make note of areas where you can improve. Ask your manager to observe your technical skills and to point out ways in which you can perform your work more quickly and efficiently. Have a trusted coworker watch and evaluate your skills when it comes to selling retail products. All of these evaluations will benefit your learning process enormously.

FIND A ROLE MODEL

One of the best ways to improve your performance is to model your behavior after someone who is having the kind of success that you wish to have (**Figure 9-6**).

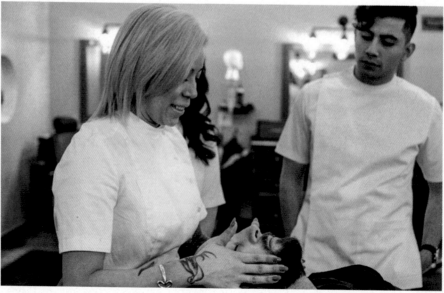

▲ FIGURE 9-6 A good role model can provide guidance as you start out.

Photography by Jason Lott; Lilly Benitez, Founder of Blade Craft Barber Academy

Watch other professionals in your shop. You will easily be able to identify who is really good and who is just coasting along. Focus on the skills of those who are really good. How do they treat their clients? How do they treat the staff and manager? How do they book their appointments? How do they handle their continuing education? What process do they use when formulating color or selecting a product? What is their attitude toward their work? How do they handle a crisis or conflict?

DID YOU KNOW?

These beauty professionals can increase their chances of building a solid and loyal clientele more quickly:

- They live in a large city or choose areas within their cities that have a large number of potential clients.
- They select a location where the competition for clients is less saturated.
- They have advanced training, skills, and certifications.
- They have and use their artistic abilities.
- They employ marketing and publicity strategies.
- They concentrate on an unusual niche within the beauty business (e.g., teens).

Go to these standout professionals for advice. Ask for a few minutes of their time, but be willing to wait for it, as it may not be easy to find time to talk during a busy workday. If you are having a problem, explain your situation and ask if the mentor can help you see things differently. Be prepared to listen and not argue your points. Remember that you asked for help, even when what your coworker is saying is not what you want to hear. Thank your coworker for their help and reflect on the advice you have been given.

A little help and direction from skilled, experienced coworkers will go a long way toward helping you achieve your goals.

CHECK IN
What are three common employment statuses for beauty professionals?

PRACTICE MONEY MANAGEMENT

Although a career in the beauty and wellness industry is very artistic and creative, it also requires financial understanding and planning. Too many beauty professionals live for the moment and do not plan for the future. They may end up feeling cheated out of the benefits that their friends and family in other careers are enjoying.

In a corporate structure, the human resources department of the corporation handles a great deal of the employees' financial planning for them. For example, health and dental insurance, retirement accounts, savings accounts, and many other items may be automatically deducted and paid out of the employees' salary. Most beauty professionals, however, must research and plan for all of those expenses on their own. This may seem difficult, but in fact it is a small price to pay for the kind of freedom, financial reward, and job satisfaction that a career in beauty and wellness can offer. And the good news is that managing money is something everyone can learn to do.

REPAYMENT OF YOUR DEBTS

In addition to making money, responsible adults are concerned with paying off their debts. Throughout your life and your career, you will undoubtedly incur debt in the form of car loans, home mortgages, or student loans. While it is easy for some people to merely ignore their responsibility in repaying these loans, it is extremely irresponsible and immature to accept a loan and then shrug off the debt. Not paying back your loans is called *defaulting*, and it can have serious consequences for your personal and professional credit. Legal action can be taken against you if you fail to repay your loans. The best way to meet all your financial responsibilities is to know precisely what you owe and what you earn so that you can make informed decisions regarding your finances. Before committing to a loan, make sure you understand the payment terms, the interest rate, and what you realistically can afford.

REPORTING YOUR INCOME

As you enter your new career and strive to become established, you most likely will be in a commissioned or salaried structure. When you receive your paycheck, taxes and other deductions will already be taken out according to your state's laws. You may earn all other income outside of your salon, spa, or barbershop, such as performing services on location for weddings or parties or at a private residence. When you file your annual state taxes, it is critical that you report cash tips and all other income that is not shown on your paycheck. There are serious legal consequences for not reporting such income:

- fines and even potential jail time
- decreasing your borrowing power as it is based on your reported income
- reducing the amount of Social Security benefits for retirement
- lowering the Bureau of Labor's endorsement as a sustainable industry, leading to decreased availability of federal loans and grants

The best way to record your tips and additional income is to keep a daily log. At the end of each week, add the total amount of your additional income. Next, add the total for the month. Keep your monthly totals on a single page in the front of your log book or spreadsheet. At the end of the year, you will be able to easily report your total cash income for your taxes. Ethical beauty professionals take the responsibility to comply with tax laws seriously and report their income accurately at the end of each year.

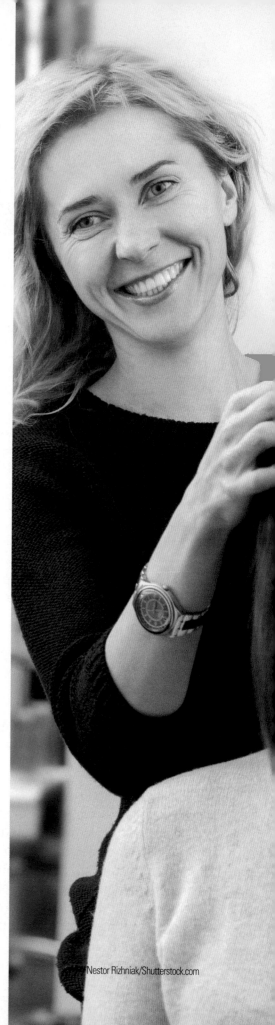
Nestor Rizhniak/Shutterstock.com

Business Technology

Today, it is common for most salons, spas, and barbershops to use computer technology to support their business, a trend that can be advantageous for technology-savvy students. You may be able to master business software more easily than other professionals. These programs now handle cash flow management, inventory tracking, payroll automation, client appointment books, performance evaluation tracking, and more. Just remember, these client records are usually considered the property of the business and are protected by confidentiality guarantees.

If you are accustomed to working with technology, you may be able to help your business set up e-mail access, a website, social networking pages, and more. With many clients enjoying the freedom of online booking and text-message appointment reminders, and with shops benefiting from e-mail or even electronic marketing programs, it is important for you to have a basic grasp of technology. Many resources—including your fellow students and future coworkers—are available if you feel you need help with specific applications.

PERSONAL BUDGET

It is amazing how many people work hard and earn very good salaries but never take the time to create a personal budget. Many people are afraid of the word *budget* because they think that it will be too restrictive on their spending or that they will have to be mathematical geniuses to work with one. Thankfully, neither fear is rooted in reality.

Personal budgets range from extremely simple to extremely complex. The right one for you depends on your needs. At the beginning of your career, a simple budget should be sufficient. To get started, take a look at the Personal Monthly Budget Worksheet (**Figure 9-7**). It lists the standard monthly expenses that most people budget. It also includes school loan repayments, savings, and payments into an individual retirement account (IRA).

Keeping track of where your money goes is one step toward making sure that you always have enough. It also helps you to plan ahead and save for bigger expenses, such as a vacation, your own home, or even your own business. All in all, sticking to a budget is a good practice to follow faithfully for the rest of your life.

THE B-WORD

Go through the Personal Monthly Budget Worksheet and fill in the amounts that apply to your current living and financial situation. If you are unsure of the amount of an expense, put in the amount you have averaged over the past three months (or give it your best guess). You may need to have three or four months of employment history to complete the income item, but fill in what you can. If the balance is a minus number, start listing ways you can decrease expenses or increase income.

Personal Monthly Budget Worksheet

A. Expenses

1. Monthly rent (or share of the rent) $_____
2. Car payment   _____
3. Car insurance   _____
4. Auto fuel/upkeep and maintenance   _____
5. Electricity   _____
6. Gas   _____
7. Health insurance   _____
8. Entertainment (movies, dining, etc.)   _____
9. Groceries   _____
10. Dry cleaning   _____
11. Personal grooming   _____
12. Prescriptions/medical   _____
13. Cell phone   _____
14. Internet/television/home phone   _____
15. Student loan   _____
16. IRA   _____
17. Savings deposit   _____
18. Other expenses   _____

TOTAL EXPENSES $_____

B. Income

1. Monthly take-home pay   _____
2. Tips   _____
3. Other income   _____

TOTAL INCOME $_____

C. Balance

Total Income (B)   _____
Minus Total Expenses (A)   _____

BALANCE $_____

▲ FIGURE 9-7   Use this budget worksheet, or one like it, to get a picture of how your monthly expenses compare to your income.

GIVING YOURSELF A RAISE

Once you have taken some time to create, use, and work with your personal budget, you may want to look at ways in which you can have more money left over after paying bills. You might automatically jump to the most obvious sources, such as asking your employer for a raise or asking for a higher percentage of commission. While these tactics are certainly valid, you will also want to think about other ways to increase your income. Here are a few tips:

- **Spend less money.** Although it may be difficult to reduce your spending, it is certainly one way to increase the amount of money that is left over at the end of the month. These dollars can be used to invest, save, or pay down debt.

- **Work more hours.** If possible, choose times when the shop is busiest, which are the most convenient for clients. Come early and stay late to accommodate clients' booking needs. Saturday is a peak workday in most salons, spas, and barbershops.
- **Increase service prices.** It will probably take some time before you are in a position to increase your service prices. For one thing, to do so you need a loyal **client base** (KLY-ent bays), customers who are loyal to a particular professional, which in this case is you! You must also have fully mastered all the services that you are performing. When you do have a loyal client base and service mastery, there is nothing wrong with increasing your prices every year or two, as long as you do so by a reasonable amount. Do a little research to determine what your competitors are charging for similar services, and increase your fees accordingly.
- **Retail more.** Most employers pay a commission on every product you recommend and sell to your clients. If you sell more products, you make more money!

SEEK PROFESSIONAL ADVICE

Just as you will want your clients to seek out your advice and services for their beauty and wellness needs, sometimes it is important for you to seek out the advice of experts, especially when it comes to your finances. You can research and interview financial planners who will be able to give you advice on reducing your credit card debt, investing your money, and funding for retirement. Speak to the officers at your local bank; they may be able to suggest bank accounts that offer you greater returns or flexibility with your money, depending on what you need.

When seeking out advice from other beauty professionals, be sure not to take anyone's advice without carefully considering whether it makes sense for your particular situation and needs. Before you buy into anything, be an informed consumer about available goods and services. Ask yourself these questions as you begin to think about keeping to a budget:

- How do your expenses compare to your income?
- What is your balance after all your expenses are paid?
- Were there any surprises for you in this exercise?
- Do you think that keeping a budget is a good way to manage money?
- Do you know of any other methods people use to manage money?

CHECK IN
What are four tips for increasing your income?

MASTER SELLING IN THE SALON, SPA, AND BARBERSHOP

Another area that touches on the issue of you and money is selling. As a beauty professional, you will have plentiful opportunities to sell retail products and upgrade service tickets. **Ticket upgrading** (TIK-it UP-grayd-ing), also known as *upselling services*, is the practice of recommending and selling additional services to your clients. These services may be performed by you or other professionals licensed in a different field. Retailing (REE-tail-ing) is the act of recommending and selling products to your clients for at-home use (**Figure 9-8**). These two activities can make all the difference in your economic picture.

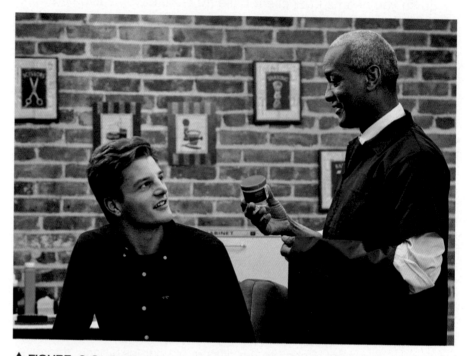

▲ FIGURE 9-8 Retailing is vitally important to increasing revenue.

PRINCIPLES OF SELLING

Some beauty professionals shy away from sales. They think that selling is being pushy. A close look at how selling works can set your mind at ease. Not only can you become very good at selling once you understand the principles behind it, but you can also feel good about providing your clients with a valuable service.

To be successful in sales, you need ambition, determination, and a pleasing personality. The first step in selling is to sell yourself. Clients must like and trust you before they will purchase services, skin care items, shampoos and conditioners, or other merchandise.

Remember, every client who enters the salon, spa, or barbershop is a potential purchaser of additional services or merchandise. Recognizing the client's needs and preferences lays the foundation for successful selling (**Figure 9-9**).

To become a proficient salesperson, you must be able to apply the following principles of selling products and services:

- Be familiar with the features and benefits of the various services and products that you are trying to sell and recommend only those that the client really needs. You should try to test all the products available yourself.

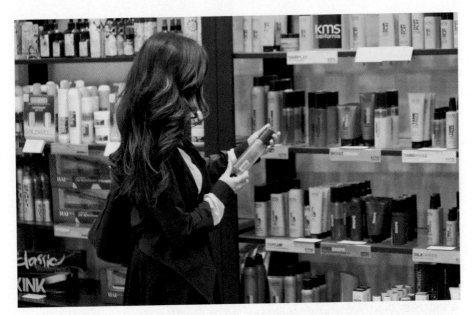

▲ FIGURE 9-9 Every client is a potential purchaser of additional services and products.

- Adapt your approach and technique to meet the needs and personality of each client. Some clients may prefer a soft sell that involves informing them about the product, without stressing that they purchase it. Others are comfortable with a hard-sell approach that focuses emphatically on why a client should buy the product.
- Be self-confident when recommending products for sale. You become confident by knowing about the products you are selling and by believing that they are as good as you say.
- Generate interest and desire in the customer by asking questions that determine a need.
- Never misrepresent your services or products. Making unrealistic claims will lead only to your client's disappointment, making it unlikely that you will ever again make a sale to that client.
- Do not underestimate the client's intelligence or their knowledge of their own home care regimen or particular needs.
- To sell a product or service, deliver your sales talk in a relaxed, friendly manner. If possible, demonstrate the use of the product (**Figure 9-10**).
- Recognize the right psychological moment to close any sale. Once the client has offered to buy, quit selling. Do not oversell; simply praise the client for making the purchase and assure the client that they will be happy with it.

HERE'S A TIP

For quick reference, keep these five points in mind when selling:

1. Establish rapport with the client.
2. Determine the client's needs.
3. Recommend products/services based on these needs.
4. Emphasize benefits.
5. Close the sale.

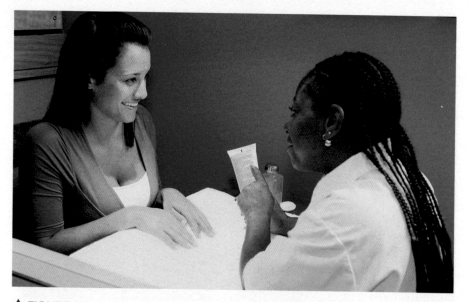

▲ FIGURE 9-10 Demonstrate products whenever possible.

FOCUS ON

Overcoming Objections

Making sales won't always be easy. Sometimes a client is stuck on a color that isn't flattering. Other times, the client may not feel convinced a product is any better than a drugstore brand or may have a genuine price objection.

To overcome an objection, reword the objection in a way that addresses the client's need. For instance, let's say you recommend a shampoo based on the fact that your client has dry hair and has just had it colored. In response, they say they already have a shampoo for color-treated hair.

First, acknowledge what they said. Then reword their objection that they already had the right shampoo in a different way, which gets them thinking. For example:

"I know, but not all shampoos for color-treated hair are alike. This shampoo not only protects your color from fading, it will moisturize it as well, which is what adds the shine you told me you wanted. I can leave it at the front desk, so you can think about it."

If the objection is a price objection, base your reaction on the client's. For strong objections, acknowledge the price and offer a free sample, if you can. If the objection is moderate, acknowledge it and reiterate the product's benefits.

"It is a little more expensive, but if you really want your color to last and your hair to feel good and look shiny, this is the best product I've found. We used it on you today. See what you think, and let me know."

Always state things in terms of the client's benefit, based on the information you gathered during the consultation.

THE PSYCHOLOGY OF SELLING

Most people have reasons for doing what they do, and when you are selling something, it is your job to figure out the reasons that will motivate a person to buy. You will find that your clients' motives for buying beauty and wellness products vary widely. Some may be concerned with issues of vanity—they want to look better. Some are seeking personal satisfaction—they want to feel better about themselves. Others need to solve a problem that is bothersome—they want to spend less time maintaining their look.

Sometimes a client may inquire about a product or service but still be undecided or doubtful. In this type of situation, you can help the client by offering honest and sincere advice. When you explain a service to a client, address the results and benefits of that service. Always keep in mind that the best interests of the client should be your first consideration. You will need to know exactly what your client's needs are, and you need to have a clear idea as to how those needs can be fulfilled.

Here are a few tips on how to get the conversation started on retailing products:

- Ask all your clients what products they are using for home maintenance of their hair, skin, and nails.
- Discuss the products you are using as you use them. For instance, tell the client why you are using this particular mousse or scrub and what it will do for them. Also explain how the client should use the product at home.
- Place the product in the client's hands whenever possible or have the product in view.
- Advise the client about how the recommended service will provide personal benefit (a closer shave or stronger nails, for instance).
- Keep retail areas clean, well lit, and appealing.
- Inform clients of any promotions and sales that are going on in the salon, spa, or barbershop.
- Be informed about the merits of using a professional product, as opposed to generic store brands.
- If you have time, offer a quick styling lesson. If your client has difficulty home styling, they will appreciate your guidance. After demonstrating, watch as the client mimics the recommended styling technique, so you can guide them.

ACTIVITY

Discover the Selling You
While you realize that retailing products is a service to your clients, you may not be sure how to go about it. Pick a partner from class and role-play the dynamics of a sales situation. Take turns being the customer and the beauty professional. Evaluate each other on how you did, with suggestions about where you can improve. Then try this exercise with someone else because no two customers are the same. Explore different topics, such as retailing or upselling, with different types of objections, such as cost or brand.

 CHECK IN
What are the principles of selling products and services in the salon, spa, or barbershop?

USE MARKETING TO EXPAND YOUR CLIENT BASE

Once you have mastered the basics of good service, including retailing and upselling, take a look at some marketing techniques that will expand your client base—the customers who keep coming back to you for services.

The following are only a few suggestions; there are many others that may work for you. The best way to decide which techniques are most effective is to try several!

- **Provide consistently good service.** It seems basic enough, but it is amazing how many professionals work hard to get clients only to lose them because they rush through a service, leaving clients feeling dissatisfied. Providing good-quality service must always be your first concern.
- **Be reliable.** Always be courteous, thoughtful, and professional. Be at the salon, spa, or barbershop when you say you will be there, and do not keep clients waiting. Give your clients the style they ask for, not something else. Recommend a retail product only when you have tried it yourself and know what it can and cannot do.
- **Be respectful.** When you treat others with respect, you become worthy of respect yourself. Being respectful means that you do not gossip or make fun of anyone or anything related to your workplace. Negative energy brings everyone down, especially you.
- **Be positive.** Be one of those people who always sees the glass as half full. Look for the positive in every situation. No one enjoys being around a person who is always unhappy.
- **Be professional.** Sometimes a client may try to make your relationship more personal than it ought to be. It is in your best interest, and your client's best interest, not to cross that line.
- **Send birthday cards.** Ask clients for their birthday information (just the month and day, not the year) on the client consultation card and then use it as a tool to get them into the shop again. About one month prior to the client's birthday, send a card with a special offer. Make it valid only for the month of their birthday. This form of advertisement is not expensive, and it is always greatly appreciated.
- **Ask for your clients' e-mail addresses.** E-mail is now the preferred mode of communication for many people. In fact, many clients prefer to book appointments using e-mail.
- **Utilize social media.** The Internet is a powerful medium to build your reputation and attract new clients. Use social media tools such as Facebook and Yelp to establish your credibility, showcase your work, and provide a space for satisfied clients to recommend you. Create a Facebook page dedicated to your business, and make it a place to share beauty and wellness tips, trends, and shop information and promotions. Post before and after photos to illustrate your skills (but always get approval from your clients before sharing their photos). Yelp is a powerful tool to build your brand. If the salon, spa, or barbershop has a Yelp listing, be sure

to use it as a way to strengthen your business. Satisfied clients are able to post a review of your services and provide a rating of their overall experience. It is always a good practice to casually invite your clients to provide a review; however, it is not ethical to pressure anyone to do so.

- **Business card referrals.** Make up a special business card with your information on it, but leave room for a client to put their name on it as well. If your client is clearly pleased with your work, give them several cards. Ask them to put their name on the cards and to refer their friends and associates to you. For every card you receive from a new customer with the client's name on it, give them 10 percent off their next service or a complimentary added service to their next appointment. This gives the client lots of motivation to recommend you to others, which in turn helps build up your clientele (**Figure 9-11**).

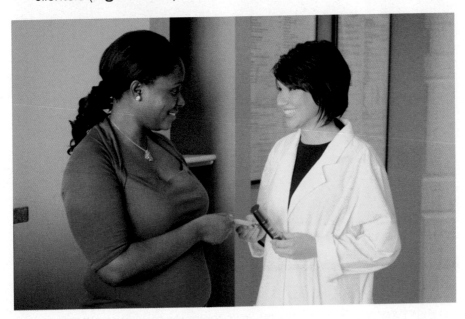

▲ FIGURE 9-11 Referral cards help build a client base.

- **Local business referrals.** Another terrific way to build business is to work with local businesses to get referrals. Look for gyms, diners, boutiques, tattoo parlors, and other small businesses near your salon, spa, or barbershop. Offer to have a card swap and commit to referring your clients to them when they are in the market for goods or services that your neighbors can provide, if they will do the same for you. This is a great way to build a feeling of community among local vendors and to reach new clients you may not be able to otherwise.

- **Public speaking.** Make yourself available for public speaking at local groups, the PTA, organizations for young people, and anywhere else that will put you in front of people in your community who are all potential clients. Put together a short program (20 to 30 minutes) in which, for example, you might discuss professional appearance with emphasis in your chosen field and other grooming tips for people looking for jobs or who are already employed.

REBOOKING CLIENTS

The best time to think about getting your clients back into your salon, spa, or barbershop is while they are still there. It may seem a little difficult to assure your clients that you are concerned with their satisfaction on this visit while you are talking about their next visit, but the two go together. The best way to encourage your clients to book another appointment before they leave is to simply talk with them, ask questions, and listen carefully to their answers (**Figure 9-12**).

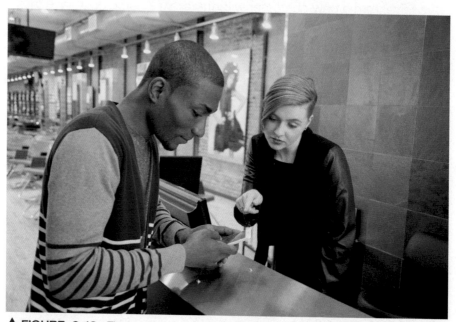

▲ FIGURE 9-12 The best time to rebook a client is before they leave the salon, spa, or barbershop.

If you are working on a client's hair, for instance, talk about the condition of their hair, their hairstyling habits at home, and the benefits of regular or special shop maintenance. Listen carefully to what your clients tell you during their visit because they will often give the careful listener many good clues as to what is happening in their lives. Those clues will open the door to a discussion about their next appointment.

FOCUS ON

Building Your Efficiency

Some professionals believe that the more time they spend with their clients performing services, the better the service will be. Not so! Unless your salon, spa, or barbershop has a lounge, your client should be in the shop only as long as is necessary for you to adequately complete a service.

Be aware of how much time it takes you to perform your various services, and then schedule accordingly. As you become more and more experienced, you should see a reduction in the amount of time it takes you to perform these services. That means clients wait less, and you can increase the number of services you perform each day. The increase in services naturally increases your income.

ON YOUR WAY

Your first job in this industry will most likely be the most difficult. Getting started in this business means spending some time on a steep learning curve. Be patient with yourself as you transition from the "school you" to the "professional you." Always remember that in your work life, as in everything else you do, practice makes perfect. You will not know everything you need to know right at the start, but be confident in the fact that you are graduating from school with a solid knowledge base. Make use of the many generous and experienced professionals you will encounter and let them teach you the tricks of the trade. Make the commitment to perfecting your technical and customer service skills.

HERE'S A TIP

There are plenty of books and Web articles that give great strategies for building a client base and keeping those clients coming back to you. Look into these and make a list of the suggestions that seem like a good fit for you; your client base; and your salon, spa, or barbershop. Then choose one strategy to try every two to three months, and see how well it works. If it helped you accomplish your goal of getting and keeping new clients, then put a star next to it and save the idea to use again when the time is right!

Above all, always be willing to learn. If you let the concepts that you have learned in this book be your guide, you will be well on the way toward enjoying your life and reaping the amazing benefits of a career in the beauty and wellness industry (**Figure 9-13**).

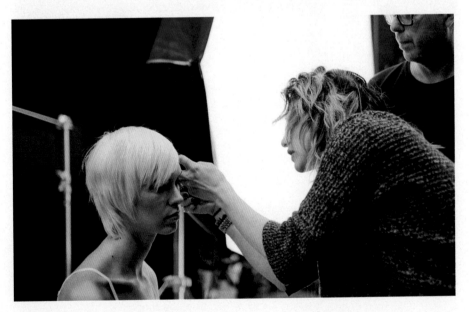

▲ FIGURE 9-13 Welcome to your new career in the beauty business!

CHECK IN

What are three possible marketing techniques for maintaining and expanding your client base?

APPLY ON THE JOB

Congratulations on completing this chapter! Before you move on, take a moment to think about how these On the Job topics apply to your particular discipline. Discuss with a classmate or study group what employment status you would prefer to have; any concerns you have about retailing or upselling; how you plan to handle repaying your student loans; and so on.

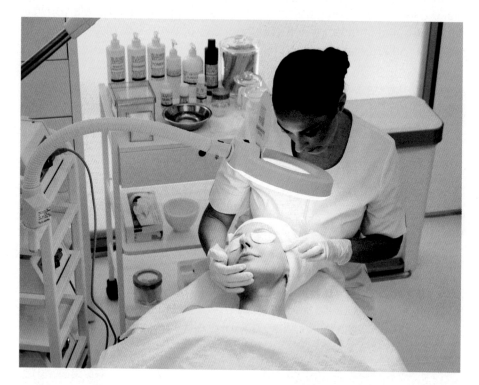

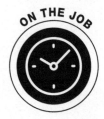
COMPETENCY PROGRESS

How are you doing with Electricity and Electrical Safety? **Check off the Chapter 9 Learning Objectives below that you feel you have mastered; leave unchecked those objectives you will need to return to:**

☐ EXPLAIN WHAT IT'S LIKE ON THE JOB.

☐ DISCUSS THE EXPECTATIONS OF MOVING FROM SCHOOL TO WORK.

☐ SUMMARIZE EMPLOYMENT OPTIONS IN THE REAL WORLD.

☐ PRACTICE MONEY MANAGEMENT.

☐ DEMONSTRATE SELLING IN THE SALON, SPA, AND BARBERSHOP.

☐ USE MARKETING TO EXPAND YOUR CLIENT BASE.

GLOSSARY

booth rental (BOO-th ren-tal)	p. 248	also known as *chair rental*; a form of self-employment, business ownership, and tax designation, distinguished by renting a booth or station in a salon, spa, or barbershop
client base (KLY-ent bays)	p. 257	customers who are loyal to a particular beauty professional
commission (kahm-ISH-un)	p. 250	percentage of the revenue generated from services performed by a professional
employee (em-PLOY-ee)	p. 247	employment classification in which the employer withholds certain taxes and has a high level of control
independent contractor (in-dee-PEN-dant CON-tract-uhr)	p. 248	form of self-employment and tax designation with specific responsibilities for bookkeeping, taxes, insurances, and so on
job description (JOHB des-CRIP-shun)	p. 246	document that outlines all the duties and responsibilities of a particular position
retailing (REE-tail-ing)	p. 258	act of recommending and selling products to your clients for at-home use
ticket upgrading (TIK-it UP-grayd-ing)	p. 257	also known as *upselling services*; the practice of recommending and selling additional services to your clients

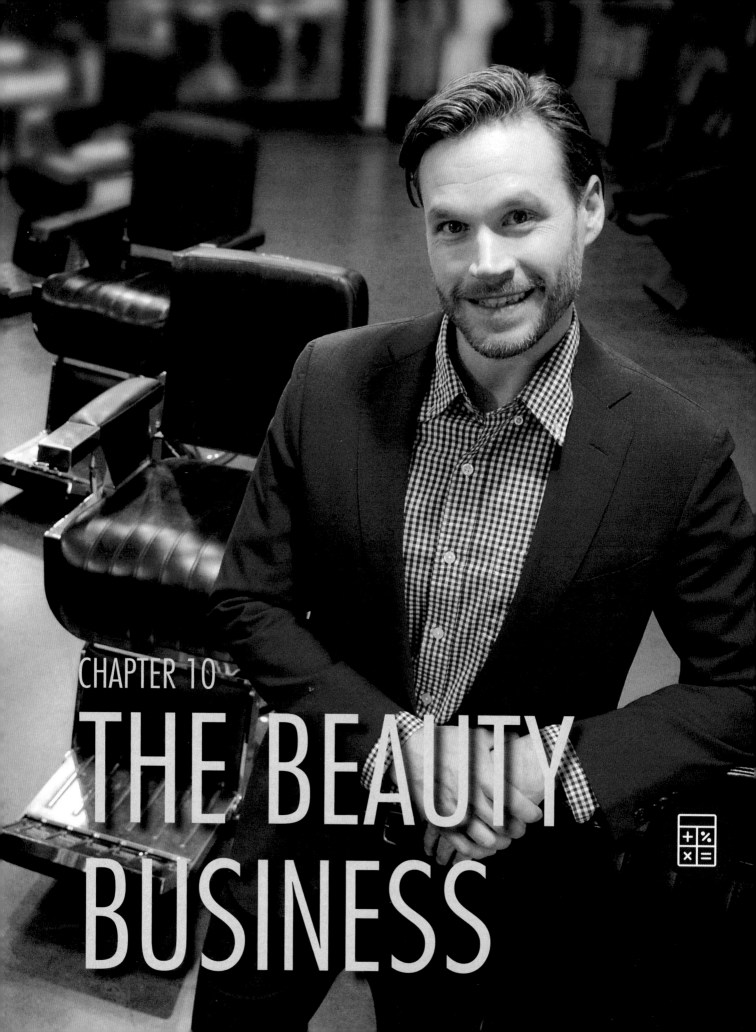

CHAPTER 10

THE BEAUTY BUSINESS

"Your future is created by what you do today, not tomorrow"

-Robert Kiyosaki

AFTER COMPLETING THIS CHAPTER, YOU WILL BE ABLE TO:

1. EXPLAIN THE BEAUTY BUSINESS.

2. OUTLINE THE REQUIREMENTS OF OWNING A BUSINESS.

3. DESCRIBE BOOTH RENTAL.

4. IDENTIFY THE ELEMENTS OF A SUCCESSFUL SALON, SPA, OR BARBERSHOP.

5. LIST MARKETING STRATEGIES FOR BUILDING YOUR BUSINESS.

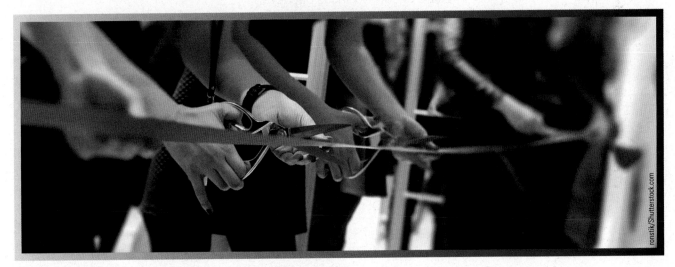

ronstik/Shutterstock.com

EXPLAIN THE BEAUTY BUSINESS

If you reach a point in your life when you feel that you are ready to become your own boss, you will have two main options to consider: (1) owning your own business, or (2) renting a booth in an existing salon, spa, or barbershop. Both options are extremely serious undertakings that require significant financial investment and a strong line of credit.

Entire books have been written on each of the topics touched on in this chapter, so be prepared to research your business ideas extensively before making any final decisions about opening a business. The following information is only meant to be a general overview; however, the better prepared you are to be both a great artist and a consummate businessperson, the greater your chances of success (**Figure 10-1**).

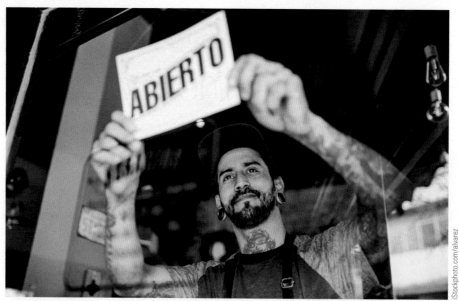

▲ **FIGURE 10-1** The successful beauty business brings together artistic talent and business acumen.

Beauty professionals should study and have a thorough understanding of the beauty business because:

- As they become more proficient in their craft and their ability to manage themselves and others, beauty pros may decide to become an independent booth renter or even a business owner. In fact, most owners once worked as professionals.
- Even if they spend their entire career as an employee of someone else's establishment, beauty pros should be familiar with the rules of business that affect the salon, spa, or barbershop of which they are a part. It is also important they look at their career as their own business.
- To become a successful entrepreneur, they will need to attract employees and clients to their business and maintain their loyalty over long periods of time.
- Even if they think they will be involved in the artistic aspect of the industry forever, business knowledge will serve beauty pros well in managing their career and professional finances as well as their business practices.

OUTLINE THE REQUIREMENTS OF OWNING A BUSINESS

Business owners have a very different job than beauty professionals. Typically, owners continue to service clients while they manage the business. This is extremely time-consuming, and there is no guarantee of profits, which is why the adventure of owning your own salon, spa, or barbershop is definitely not for everyone.

THE BUSINESS PLAN

Regardless of the type of business you plan to own, it is imperative to have a thorough and well-researched business plan in place. A business plan (BIZ-ness plahn) is a written description of your business as you see it today and as you foresee it in the next five years (detailed by year). A business plan is more of an agreement with yourself and not legally binding. However, if you wish to obtain financing, it is essential that you have a business plan in place first. Many books, classes, DVDs, and websites offer much more detailed information than can be provided here, but below is a sampling of the kinds of information and materials that a business plan should include.

- **Executive Summary.** A summary of your plan and list of your objectives
- **Vision Statement.** A long-term picture of what the business is to become and what it will look like when it gets there
- **Mission Statement.** A description of the key strategic influences of the business, such as the market it will serve, the kinds of services it will offer, and the quality of those services
- **Organizational Plan.** An outline of employee and management levels and a description of how the business will run administratively
- **Marketing Plan.** An outline of all of the research obtained regarding the clients your business will target and their needs, wants, and habits
- **Financial Documents.** Projected financial statements, actual (historical) statements, and financial statement analysis
- **Supporting Documents.** The owner's resume, personal financial information, legal contracts, and any other agreements
- **Business Policies.** Policies that even small shops and booth renters should adhere to and that ensure that all clients and employees are treated fairly and consistently

OPENING YOUR OWN BUSINESS

Opening your own salon, spa, or barbershop is a huge undertaking—financially, physically, creatively, and mentally—because you will face challenges that are complex and unfamiliar to you. In addition to the business plan, before you can open your doors you'll need to decide what products to use and carry, what types of marketing and promotions you will employ, the best method and philosophy for running the business and creating a culture, and whom to hire if you need additional staff.

Whether you're opening a small destination spa, large franchise nail salon, or modest independent barbershop, you must carefully consider some basic issues and perform fundamental tasks as outlined in the following section.

CREATE A VISION AND MISSION STATEMENT FOR THE BUSINESS

A vision statement (VIZ-uhn state-ment) is a sweeping picture of the long-term goals for the business: what it is to become and what it will look like when it gets there. A mission statement is a guide to the actions of the organization: it spells out the overall goals, provides a path, and contains the core values to help guide decision making. The mission statement lays the foundation for how your company's strategies are created. Goals (GOHLZ) are an essential set of benchmarks that, once achieved, help you to realize your mission and your vision. It is important to set realistic goals for both the short term and long term.

CREATE YOUR BRAND IDENTITY

Creating your brand identity at the start is essential to building a unique, successful business. To create your brand, start by identifying a few simple concepts to use as building blocks for your brand identity.

- What is your point of difference? What is going to make a client want to visit your business versus the one across the street?
- What are you selling? Every salon, spa, or barbershop sells beauty services; think beyond the obvious. Are you selling a luxury experience, a family-friendly environment, or a cost-conscious express service?
- What is your aesthetic? Will there be a consistent color, theme, or uniform for your staff?

Identifying the answers to the three main questions above will solidify your concepts and serve as reference. Refer to them frequently for inspiration, guidance, and a reminder of what your business is built upon.

CREATE A BUSINESS TIMELINE

While initially you will be concerned with the first two aspects of the timeline, once your business is successful, you will need to think about the others as well.

- **Year 1:** It could take a year or more to determine and complete all of the aspects of starting the business.
- **Years 2 to 5:** This time period is for tending to the business, its clientele, and its employees and for growing and expanding the business so that it is profitable.
- **Years 5 to 10:** This time period, if successfully achieved, can be for adding more locations, expanding the scope of the business, constructing a larger space, or including anything else you or your clients need and want.
- **Years 11 to 20:** In this time period, you may want to move from being a working beauty professional into a full-time manager of the overall business and begin planning for your eventual retirement.

THE REAL SECRET OF SUCESS IS ENTHUSIASM.

– Walter Chrysler

- **Year 20 and onward:** This may be the perfect time to consider selling your successful business or changing it in some way, such as taking on a junior partner and training them to take over the day-to-day operations of the business so you can have time away to explore interests or hobbies.

DETERMINE BUSINESS FEASIBILITY

Determining whether the business you envision is feasible means addressing certain practical issues. For example, do you have a special skill or talent that can help you set your business apart from other salons, spas, or barbershops in your area? Does the town or area in which you are planning to locate the business offer you the appropriate type of clientele for the products and services you want to offer? Based on what you envision for the business, how much money will you need to open the business? Is this funding available to you?

CHOOSE A BUSINESS NAME

The name you select for your business explains what it is and can also identify characteristics that set your business apart from competitors in the marketplace. The name you select for your business will also influence how clients and potential clients perceive the business. The name will create a picture of your business in clients' minds. Note that once that picture exists, it can be very difficult to change it if you are not satisfied. In addition, once your business is named, it is complicated to make all of the legal, banking, and tax updates if you later want to change the name.

CHOOSE A LOCATION

You will want to base your business location on your primary clientele and their needs. Select a location that has good visibility, high traffic, easy access, sufficient parking, and handicap access (**Figure 10-2**).

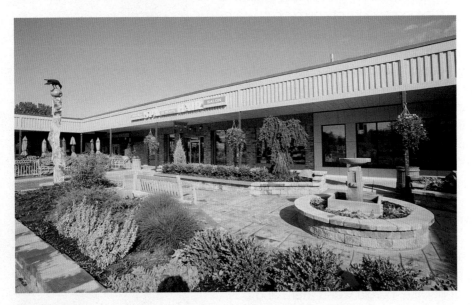

▲ **FIGURE 10-2** Scout the best location for your business.

WRITTEN AGREEMENTS

Many written agreements (RIT-en uh-GREE-mentz) and documents govern the opening of a business, including leases, vendor contracts, employee contracts, and more. These agreements detail, usually for legal purposes, who does what and what is given in return. You must be able to read and understand them. Your business plan, although not legally binding, falls under this category; it will follow your business throughout the entire process from start-up through many years in the future.

The plan should include a general description of the business and the services that it will provide; area demographics (dem-oh-GRAF-iks), which consist of information about a specific population, including data on race, age, income, and educational attainment; expected salaries and cost of related benefits; an operations plan that includes pricing structure and expenses, such as equipment, supplies, repairs, advertising, taxes, and insurance; and projected income and overhead expenses for up to five years. A certified public accountant (CPA) can be invaluable in helping you gather accurate financial information. The chamber of commerce in your proposed area typically has information on area demographics.

BUSINESS REGULATIONS AND LAWS

Business regulations and laws (BIZ-ness reg-u-LAY-shuns AND LAWZ), are any and all local, state, and federal regulations and laws that you must comply with when you decide to open your business or rent a booth. Since the laws change from year to year and vary from state to state and from city to city, it is important that you contact your local authorities regarding business licenses, permits, and other regulations, such as zoning and inspections. Additionally, you must know and comply with all federal Occupational Safety and Health Administration (OSHA) guidelines, including those requiring that information about the ingredients of cosmetic preparations be available to employees. OSHA requires Safety Data Sheets (SDSs) for this purpose. There are also many federal laws that apply to hiring and firing, payment of benefits, contributions to employee entitlements (for example, social security and unemployment), and workplace behavior.

Understanding the laws and rules of owning a business is imperative to running a successful salon, spa, or barbershop. The laws and rules not only lay the foundation of acceptable guidelines regarding hiring and firing, they also build a framework for day-to-day policies and procedures and safety. Not following the laws and rules can result in costly fines and heavy penalties. It is important to become very familiar with the local, state, and federal laws and rules before you open your business.

When you do open your business, you will need to purchase insurance (in-SHUR-ance) that guarantees protection against financial loss from malpractice, property liability, fire, burglary and theft, and business interruption. You will need to have disability policies as well. Make sure that your policies cover you for all the monetary demands you will have to meet on your lease.

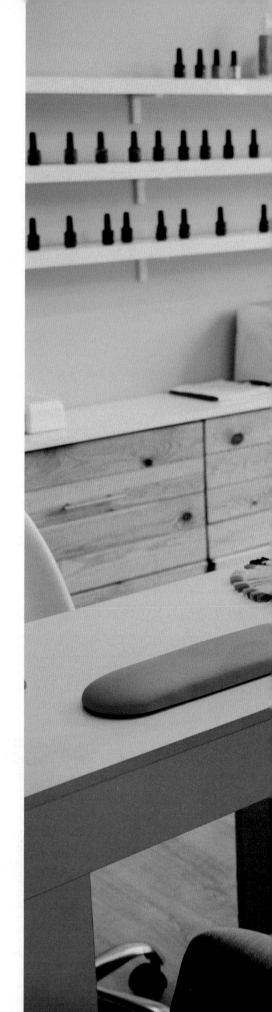

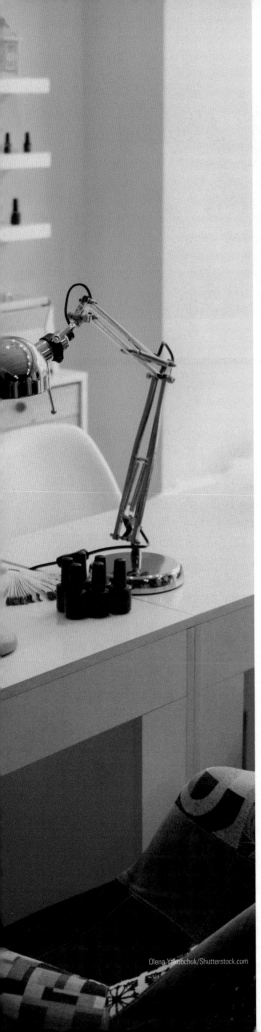

Olena Yakobchuk/Shutterstock.com

DAILY OPERATION

As you can see, a new business has numerous requirements, documents, and considerations that must be sorted out before opening. Many of these will extend through the life of the business and inform how your salon, spa, or barbershop is run day to day. **Business operation** (BIZ-ness op-er-AYE-shun) refers to these recurring processes or activities involved in the running of a business for the purpose of producing income and value.

Business policies (BIZ-ness POL-ih-sees) is the term for the rules and regulations adopted by a business to ensure that all clients and associates are being treated fairly and consistently. Even small shops and booth renters should have such policies in place. A final, foundational part of daily business is **record keeping** (REK-urd keeping), the act of maintaining accurate and complete records of all financial activities in your business. A strong accounting and record-keeping system will serve you well in a number of ways, especially around tax time.

TYPES OF BUSINESS OWNERSHIP

A salon, spa, or barbershop can be owned and operated by an individual, a partnership, or a corporation or franchise. Before deciding which type of ownership is most desirable for your situation, research each option thoroughly. There are excellent reference tools available. You can also consult a small business attorney for advice.

INDIVIDUAL OWNERSHIP

If you like to make your own rules and are responsible enough to meet all the duties and obligations of running a business, individual ownership may be the best arrangement for you.

The **sole proprietor** (SOHL pro-PRY-eh-tor) is the individual owner and, most often, the manager of the business, who determines policies and has the last say in decision making, as well as assumes expenses, receives profits, and bears all losses.

PARTNERSHIP

In a **partnership** (PART-nur-ship) business structure, two or more people share ownership—although not necessarily equally. One reason for going into a partnership arrangement is to have more **capital** (KAP-uh-tal), or money to invest in a business; another is to have help running your operation. Partners can pool their skills and talents, making it easier to share work, responsibilities, and decision making. Keep in mind that partners must assume one another's liability for debts.

Partnerships may mean more opportunity for increased investment and growth. They can be fantastic if the right chemistry exists; they can be disastrous if you find yourself legally linked to the wrong person. Your partner can incur losses or debts that you may not even be aware of unless you use a third-party accountant. Trust is just one of the requirements for this arrangement (**Figure 10-3**).

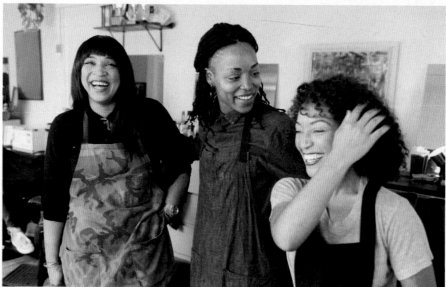

▲ FIGURE 10-3 Business partners share the responsibilities and the rewards.

CORPORATION

A corporation (kor-pour-AYE-shun) is an ownership structure controlled by one or more stockholders. Incorporating is one of the best ways that a business owner can protect their personal assets. Most people choose to incorporate solely for this reason, but there are other advantages as well. For example, the corporate business structure saves you money in taxes, provides greater business flexibility, and makes raising capital easier. It also limits your personal financial liability if your business accrues unmanageable debts or otherwise runs into financial trouble.

Characteristics of corporations are generally as follows:

- Corporations raise capital by issuing stock certificates or shares.
- Stockholders (people or companies that purchase shares) have an ownership interest in the company. The more stock they own, the bigger that interest becomes.
- You can be the sole stockholder (or shareholder), or you can have many stockholders.
- Corporate formalities, such as director and stockholder meetings, are required to maintain a corporate status.
- Income tax is limited to the salary that you draw and not the total profits of the business.
- Corporations cost more to set up and run than a sole proprietorship or partnership. For example, there are the initial formation fees, filing fees, and annual state fees.
- A stockholder of a corporation is required to pay unemployment insurance taxes on their salary, whereas a sole proprietor or partner is not.

Your accountant may suggest that your business become an S corporation (small business corporation), which is a business elected for S corporation status through the Internal Revenue Service (IRS).

This status allows the taxation of the company to be similar to a partnership or sole proprietor, as opposed to paying taxes based on a corporate tax structure. Or your accountant may suggest that your business become registered as a limited liability company (LLC), which is a type of business ownership combining several features of corporation and partnership structures. Owners of an LLC also have the liability protection of a corporation. An LLC exists as a separate entity, much like a corporation. Members cannot be held personally liable for debts unless they have signed a personal guarantee.

DID YOU KNOW?

When you open your own business, you should consult an attorney and an accountant before filing any documents to legalize your business. Your attorney will advise you of the legal documents and obligations that you will take on as a business owner, and your accountant can inform you of the ways in which your business may be registered for tax purposes. It is helpful to find professionals who have previous experience in the beauty business.

FRANCHISE OWNERSHIP

A franchise is a form of business organization in which a firm that is already successful (the franchisor) enters into a continuing contractual relationship with other businesses (franchisees) operating under the franchisor's trade name in exchange for a fee. When you operate a franchise salon, spa, or barbershop, you usually operate under the franchisor's guidance and must adhere to a contract with many stipulations. These stipulations ensure that all locations in the franchise are run in a similar manner, look the same way, use the same logos, and, sometimes, even train in the same way or carry the same retail products (**Figure 10-4**).

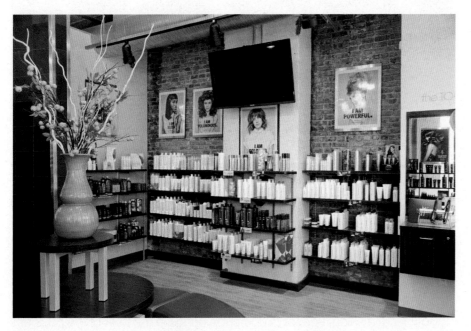

▲ FIGURE 10-4 Franchise ownership can have many benefits.

Franchises offer the advantage of a known name and brand recognition, and the franchisor does most of the marketing for you. Also, many have protected territories, meaning another franchise with the same name cannot open up within your fixed geographic area. However, franchise agreements vary widely in what you can and cannot do on your own. Owning a franchise is no guarantee of making a profit, and you should always research the franchise; talk to other owners of the franchise's shops; and have an attorney read the contract and explain anything you do not understand, including your precise obligations and arrangements for paying the franchise fee. In most cases, whether or not you are profitable, you must pay the fee.

PURCHASING AN ESTABLISHED BUSINESS

Purchasing an existing salon, spa, or barbershop could be an excellent opportunity, but, as with anything else, you have to look at all sides of the picture (**Figure 10-5**). If you choose to buy an established business, seek professional assistance from an accountant and a business lawyer. You may have the option of purchasing all the assets of a shop or some or all of

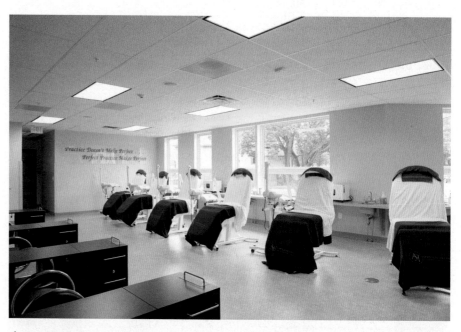

▲ FIGURE 10-5 Purchasing an established business can be an excellent opportunity that requires careful handling.

its stock. It is important to know, however, that you are not purchasing the staff or clientele. There is no guarantee that with new ownership the staff will be retained or that the clients will continue to return. In general, any agreement to buy an established business should include the following items:

*   Financial audit to determine the actual value of the business once the current owner's bookings are taken out of the equation—often, the owner of a salon, spa, or barbershop brings in the bulk of the business income, and it is unlikely you will retain all the former owner's clients without a lot of support and encouragement from that former owner

- Written purchase and sale agreement to avoid any misunderstandings between the contracting parties
- Complete and signed statement of inventory (goods, fixtures, and the like) indicating the value of each article
- If applicable, a transfer of a note, mortgage, lease, or bill of sale, including an investigation by the buyer to determine whether there are defaults in the payment of debts
- Confirmed identity of owner
- Use of the business's name and reputation for a definite period of time
- Disclosure of any and all information regarding the shop's clientele and its purchasing and service habits
- Disclosure of the conditions of the facility—if you are buying the actual building, a full inspection is in order; many other legalities also apply, as noted by your realtor and attorney
- Non-compete agreement stating that the seller will not work in or establish a new salon, spa, or barbershop within a specified distance from the present location
- Employee agreement, either formal or informal, that lets you know if the employees will stay with the business under its new ownership—existing employee contracts should be transferable

ACTIVITY

Practically in Business

Form student teams to plan the practical side of your own salons, spas, or barbershops. Designate certain tasks to specific team members or decide if everyone will work on every task as a group. Each team should perform the following tasks:

- Decide on a name for their business.
- Determine what services will be offered.
- Create fun signage for the shop's exterior.
- Write a vision statement.
- Write a mission statement.
- Create an organizational plan and a marketing plan.

Most students will not be able to develop complex budgets, but if you feel up to it, decide on a specific budget and allocate it to key areas, such as decorating, equipment, supplies, and personnel. Ask your instructors to provide feedback about whether your budget is realistic.

DRAWING UP A LEASE

In most cases, owning your own business does not mean that you own the building that houses your business. When renting or leasing space, you must have an agreement with the building's owner that has been well thought out and well written. The lease should specify clearly who owns what and who is responsible for which repairs and expenses. You should also secure the following:

- Exemption of fixtures or appliances that might be attached to the salon, spa, or barbershop so that they can be removed without violating the lease

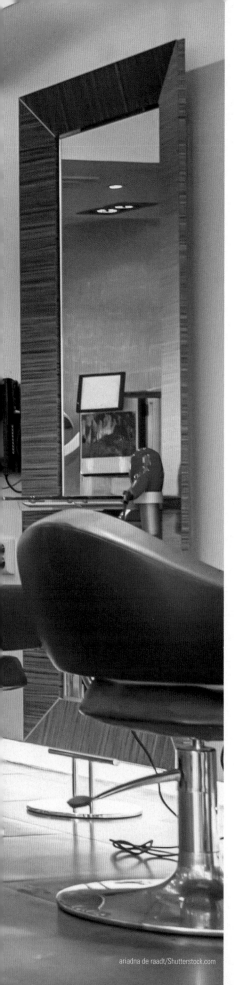

- Agreement about necessary renovations and repairs, such as painting, plumbing, fixtures, and electrical installation
- Option from the landlord that allows you to assign the lease to another person – obligations for the payment of rent are thus kept separate from the responsibilities of operating the business should you decide to bring in another person or owner

PROTECTION AGAINST FIRE, THEFT, AND LAWSUITS

As a business owner, you must protect the business, clients, and staff on several levels. Here are some of the ways you can reduce risk and ensure this protection:

- Ensure that your business has adequate locks as well as a fire alarm system, a burglar alarm system, and a surveillance system.
- Purchase liability, fire, malpractice, and burglary insurance and do not allow these policies to lapse while you are in business.
- Become thoroughly familiar with all laws governing your discipline and with the safety and infection control codes of your city and state.
- Keep accurate records of the number of employees, their salaries, lengths of employment, and Social Security numbers as required by various state and federal laws that monitor the social welfare of workers.
- Always check with your regulatory agency if you have any questions about a law or regulation. Ignorance of the law is no excuse for violating it.

BUSINESS OPERATIONS

Whether you are an owner or a manager, there are certain skills that you must develop in order to successfully run a salon, spa, or barbershop. To run a people-oriented business, you need:

- excellent business aptitude, good judgment, and solid diplomatic skills
- knowledge of sound business principles.

Because it takes time to develop these skills, you would be wise to establish a circle of contacts—business owners, both within your industry and without—who can give you advice along the way. Consider joining a local entrepreneurs' group or your city's chamber of commerce in order to extend the reach of your networking. The chamber of commerce is a local organization of businesses and business owners whose goal is to promote, protect, and further the interests of businesses in a community. Smooth business management depends on the following factors:

- Sufficient investment capital
- Efficient management
- Good business procedures
- Strong computer skills
- Cooperation between management and employees
- Trained and experienced personnel
- Excellent customer service
- Proper pricing of services (**Figure 10-6**)

ariadna de raadt/Shutterstock.com

MENU

Hair Removal

Eyebrow Waxing	$7.00
Full Leg Wax	$75.00
Bikini Wax (American)	$40.00
Hands/Feet Wax	$15.00
Upper Lip or Chin Wax	$15.00
Underarm Waxing	$30.00
Chest Wax	$25.00

Facials

Express Facial	$25.00
Basic Facial	$45.00
Back Facial	$80.00
Microdermabrasion	$80.00 and up
Body Mask	$100.00

Makeup

Basic Makeup	$30.00
Tinting ashes	$15.00

Salon Services

Child's Haircut (under 12)	$25.00 and up
Shampoo & Blowdry	$35.00 and up
Permanent Haircolor (cut not included)	$65.00 and up
Haircolor Refresher	$30.00 and up
Hair Extensions	Free consultation required
Thermal Hair Straightening	$85.00 and up

Barbering Services

Shampoo & Cut	$40.00
Beard & Mustache Trim	$15.00 and up
Hot Shave	$35.00
Gentleman's Manicure	$20.00
Gentleman's Pedicure	$50.00
Neck Shave	$15.00

Nails

Manicure	$25.00
Pedicure	$35.00
Gel Manicure	$30.00
Nail Designs	$5.00 and up
Pink/White	$30.00
Nail Repair	$4.00

▲ FIGURE 10-6   Example of a service menu.

ALLOCATION OF MONEY

As a business operator, you must always know where your money is being spent. A good accountant and an accounting system are indispensable. The figures in **Table 10-1** provide a guideline for money allocation in a beauty business, but will vary depending on locality and discipline.

THE IMPORTANCE OF RECORD KEEPING

Good business operations require a simple and efficient record-keeping system. Proper business records are necessary to meet the requirements of local, state, and federal laws regarding taxes and employees. Records are of value only if they are correct, concise, and complete. Proper bookkeeping methods include keeping an accurate record of all income and expenses. Income is usually classified as receipts from services and retail sales. Expenses include rent, utilities, insurance, salaries, advertising, equipment, and repairs. Retain all check stubs, cancelled checks, receipts, and invoices. A professional accountant or a full-charge bookkeeper is recommended to help keep records accurate.

TABLE 10-1 FINANCIAL BENCHMARKS FOR SALONS, SPAS, AND BARBERSHOPS IN THE UNITED STATES

EXPENSES	PERCENT OF TOTAL GROSS INCOME
Salaries and Commissions (Including Payroll Taxes)	53.5
Rent	13.0
Supplies	5.0
Advertising	3.0
Depreciation	3.0
Laundry	1.0
Cleaning	1.0
Light and Power	1.0
Repairs	1.5
Insurance	0.75
Telephone	0.75
Miscellaneous	1.5
Total Expenses	85.0
Net Profit	15.0
Total	100.0

Courtesy Kopsa Otte CPAs & Advisors in York, NE, nationally known as the only accounting firm that specializes in salons and spas.

Table 10-1 is a generalization, and percentages can vary from city to city. For example, rent in New York City may be a different percentage of sales than in Duluth, Minnesota.

The term *full-charge bookkeeper* refers to someone who is trained to do everything from recording sales and payroll to generating a profit-and-loss statement. The most important part of record keeping is having the ability to defend your business in the case of an audit by the federal or state government and to have accurate proof of all sales made and taxes paid.

PURCHASE AND INVENTORY RECORDS

The purchase of inventory and supplies should be closely monitored. Purchase records help you maintain a perpetual inventory, which prevents overstocking or a shortage of needed supplies, and alert you to any incidents of theft. Purchase records also help establish the net worth of the business at the end of the year.

Keep a running inventory of all supplies and classify them according to their use and retail value. Those to be used in the daily business operation are consumption supplies (kon-SUMP-shun sup-LYZ). Those to be sold to clients are retail supplies (REE-tail sup-LYZ). Both categories have different tax responsibilities, so be sure to check with your accountant that you are charging the proper taxes.

SERVICE RECORDS

Always keep service records or client cards that describe the treatments given and merchandise sold to each client. Using a salon-, spa-, or barbershop-specific software program for this purpose is highly recommended. All service records should include the name and address of the client, the date of each purchase or service, the amount charged, the products used, and the results obtained. Clients' preferences and tastes should also be noted.

CHECK IN
What are the components of a basic business plan?

DESCRIBE BOOTH RENTAL

Booth rental, also known as *chair rental*, involves renting a booth or station in a salon, spa, or barbershop. This practice is popular in shops all over the United States. Many people see booth rental or renting a station as a more desirable alternative to owning a business.

DID YOU KNOW?

Currently, booth rental is legal in every state except Pennsylvania, where there is a law prohibiting it. In New Jersey, the state board does not recognize booth rental as an acceptable method of doing business. Check with your state to be aware of all the latest laws and regulations.

In a booth rental arrangement, a professional generally rents a station or work space in a salon, spa, or barbershop for a weekly fee paid to the owner. Booth renters are solely responsible for their own clientele, supplies, record keeping, and accounting, and have the ability to be their own boss with very little capital investment.

Booth rental is a desirable situation for many beauty professionals who have a large, steady clientele and who do not have to rely on a business's general clientele to keep busy. Unless you are at least 70 percent booked all the time, however, it may not be advantageous to rent a booth.

Although it may sound like a good option, booth renting has its share of obligations, such as the following:

- Keeping records for income tax purposes and other legal reasons
- Paying all taxes, including higher Social Security (double that of an employee)
- Carrying adequate malpractice insurance and health insurance
- Complying with all IRS obligations for independent contractors—go to irs.gov and search for independent contractors to learn more
- Using your own telephone and booking systems
- Collecting all service fees, whether they are paid in cash or via a credit card
- Creating all professional materials, including business cards and a service menu
- Purchasing all supplies, including back bar and retail supplies and products
- Tracking and maintaining inventory

- Managing the purchase of products and supplies
- Budgeting for advertising or offering incentives to ensure a steady flow of new clients
- Paying for all continuing education
- Working in an independent atmosphere where teamwork usually does not exist and where shop standards are interpreted on an individual basis
- Adhering to state laws and regulations—to date, two states (Pennsylvania and New Jersey) do not allow booth rental at all; others may require that each renter in an establishment hold their own establishment license and carry individual liability insurance; always check with your state regulatory agency

As a booth renter, you will not enjoy the same benefits as an employee of a salon, spa, or barbershop would, such as paid days off or vacation time. Remember, as a booth renter, when you do not work, you do not get paid. Perhaps most importantly, you must continually attract new clients and maintain the ones you have, which means working the hours your clients need you to be available. For more information on booth rental as a business option, reference Milady's *Booth Renting 101: A Guide for the Independent Stylist*.

CHECK IN
What responsibilities does a booth renter assume?

IDENTIFY THE ELEMENTS OF A SUCCESSFUL SALON, SPA, OR BARBERSHOP

The only way to guarantee that you will stay in business and have a prosperous business is to take excellent care of your clients. Clients visiting your shop should feel that they are being well taken care of, and they should always have reason to look forward to their next visit. To accomplish this, your salon, spa, or barbershop must be physically attractive, well organized, smoothly run, and, above all, sparkling clean.

PLANNING THE LAYOUT

One of the most exciting opportunities ahead of you is planning and constructing the best physical layout for the type of business you envision. Maximum efficiency should be the primary concern. For example, if you are opening a low-budget establishment offering quick service, you will need several stations and a small- to medium-sized reception area because clients will be moving in and out fairly quickly. Retail sales are essential to a profitable beauty business. Make sure the products you carry and the space you design reflect the importance of high retail sales (**Figure 10-7**).

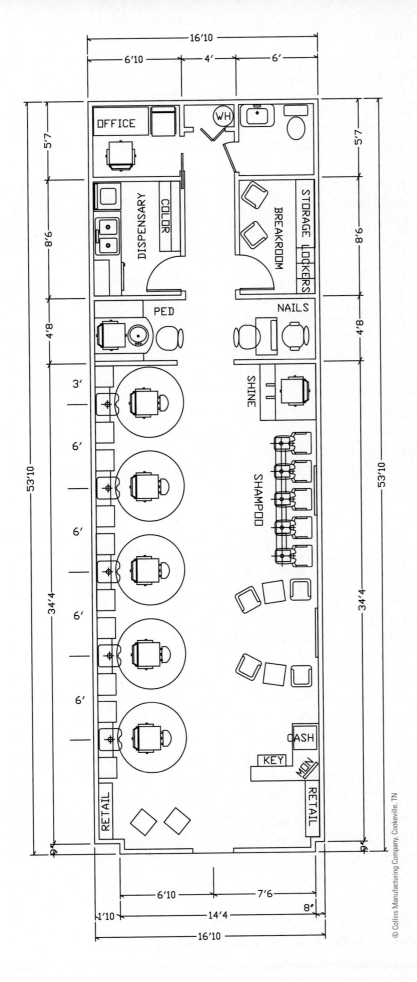

© Collins Manufacturing Company, Cookeville, TN

However, if you are opening a high-end business, where clients expect the quality of the service to be matched by the environment, you may want to plan for more room in the waiting area. In fact, you might choose to have several areas in which clients can lounge and enjoy light snacks or beverages—from soda and coffee to alcoholic beverages. Most salons, spas, and barbershops also provide complimentary Wi-Fi access to their guests.

CAUTION

If you plan to serve alcoholic beverages at your business, check with your local and state laws to make sure you obtain all proper licenses and insurance.

Layout is crucial to the smooth operation of a salon, spa, or barbershop. Once you have decided on the type of business that you wish to run, seek the advice of an architect with plenty of experience in designing for the beauty industry. For renovations, a professional equipment and furniture supplier will be able to help you (**Figure 10-8**).

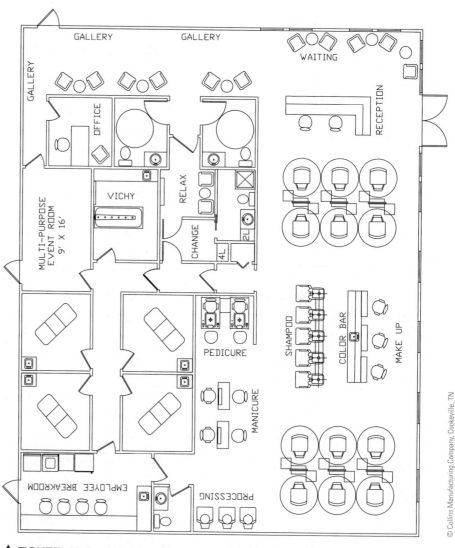

▲ **FIGURE 10-8** Typical layout for a larger salon or spa.

© Collins Manufacturing Company, Cookeville, TN

Ideally, the design you develop should include the following:

- Ample aisle space
- Space for each piece of equipment
- Quality mirrors
- Fixtures, furniture, and equipment chosen on the basis of cost, durability, utility and appearance
- Decoration and paint that is thematic and pleasing to the eye
- Restrooms for clients and employees
- Handicap-accessible facilities and doors
- Good plumbing and lighting for services
- Heating, ventilation, and air-conditioning
- Sufficient electrical outlets and current adequate to service all equipment
- Storage areas
- Display areas
- Attractive, furnished and comfortable reception or waiting area

Costs to create even a small salon, spa, or barbershop in an existing space can range from $75 to $125 per square foot, if not more. Renovating existing space requires familiarity with building codes and the landlord's restrictions before you do anything. All the plumbing should be in the same area, and electrical wiring must be up to code. If they are not, you'll pay thousands of dollars extra. Before you begin, get everything in writing from contractors, design firms, equipment manufacturers, and architects. It is a good idea to get three quotes on everything from contractors and cleaning services to work stations and equipment. Don't be afraid to negotiate whenever you can.

Try to estimate how much each area in the business will earn, so you can use space efficiently. An inviting retail display in your reception area is a good investment; on the other hand, an employee break area produces no income. In addition to start-up costs for creating your business, you'll need financing for operational expenses. Realistically, you should plan to have at least several months and up to one year of expenses available to help get you up and running. It takes most new shops about six months to begin operating at full capacity.

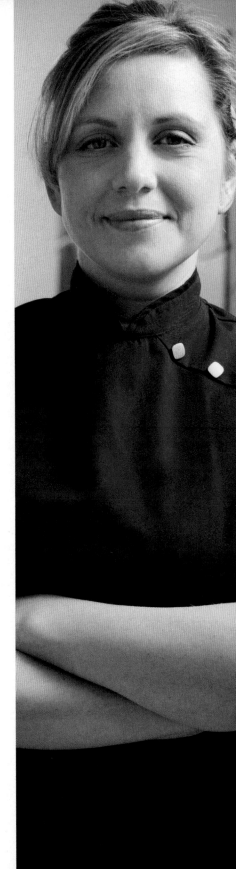

SpeedKingz/Shutterstock.com

ACTIVITY

Legendary Layout

What would your dream salon, spa, or barbershop look like? Try your hand at designing a business that would attract the kinds of clients you want; offer the services you would like to specialize in; and provide an efficient, comfortable working environment for beauty professionals.

Draw pictures, use words, or try a combination of both. Pay attention to practical requirements, but feel free to dream a little, too. Skylights? Waterfalls? A mechanical bull? You name it, it's your dream! Consider how you might target all five of the senses.

PERSONNEL

Your personnel (per-son-EL) is your staff or employees. The size of your business will determine the size of your staff. Large salons, spas, or barbershops may require receptionists, assistants, and housekeepers in addition to beauty professionals with a variety of specializations. Smaller establishments often employ personnel who are expected to perform more than one type of service. For example, a barber might also be the shop's colorist. Ultimately, whether your business is large or small, high end or economical, its success depends on the attitude and quality of work done by the staff.

When interviewing potential employees, consider the following:

- **Level of skill.** What is their educational background? When was the last time they attended an educational event? How long have they been in the industry? What can they bring to the organization beyond their technical skills?
- **Personal grooming.** Do they look like professionals you would consult for personal grooming advice?
- **Image as it relates to the business.** Are they too progressive or too conservative for your environment? Does their image reflect the image of your business?
- **Overall attitude.** Are they mostly positive or mostly negative in their responses to your questions? Do they seem self-motivated and self-directed?
- **Communication skills.** Are they able to understand your questions? Can you understand their responses?
- **Work history.** Have they been at a previous business for many years, or do they hop from shop to shop? Are they bringing a clientele, or do they expect you to build one for them?

Making good hiring decisions is crucial. Undoing bad hiring decisions is costly and painful for all involved and can be more complicated than one might expect.

PAYROLL AND EMPLOYEE BENEFITS

In order to have a successful business, one in which everyone feels appreciated and is happy to work hard to service clients well, you must be willing to share your success with your staff whenever it is financially feasible to do so. You can do this in a number of ways:

- Make it your top priority to meet your payroll obligations. In the allotment of funds, this comes first. It will also be your largest expense.
- Whenever possible, offer hardworking and loyal employees as many benefits as possible. Either cover the cost of these benefits, or simply make them available to employees, who can decide if they can cover the cost themselves.
- Provide staff members with a schedule of employee evaluations. Make it clear what is expected of them if they are to receive pay increases.
- Create and stay with a tipping policy. It is a good idea both for your employees and your clients to know exactly what is expected. It is also important to be familiar with the tax laws around tipping.
- Put your entire pay plan in writing.
- Create incentives by giving your staff opportunities to earn more money, prizes, or tickets to educational events and trade shows; rewards can inspire employees to achieve more.
- Create business policies and stick to them. Everyone should be governed by the same rules, including you!

MANAGING PERSONNEL

As a new business owner, one of your most challenging tasks will be managing your staff. At the same time, leading your team can also be very rewarding. If you are good at managing others, you can make a positive impact on their lives and their ability to earn a living. If managing people does not come naturally, don't despair. People can learn how to manage other people, just as they learn how to drive a car or perform hair services. Keep in mind that managing others is a serious job. Whether or not it comes naturally to you, it takes time to become comfortable with the role.

Human resources (HR) is an entire specialty in its own right. It not only covers how you manage employees, but also what you can and cannot say when hiring, managing, or firing. All employers must be familiar with various civil rights laws, including Equal Employment Opportunity Commission (EEOC) regulations and the Americans with Disabilities Act (ADA), which pertains to hiring and firing as well as business design for accessibility. Every business should have a written personnel policies and procedures manual, and every employee must read and sign it. If you choose to use a payroll company, they can provide HR services and employee manuals for a nominal fee. The more documented systems you have for managing human resources, the better.

There are many excellent books, both within and outside the beauty industry, that you can use as resources for learning about managing employees and staff. Spend an afternoon online or at your local bookstore researching the topic and purchasing materials or registering for classes that will educate and inform you. Once you have a broad base of information, you will be able to select a technique or style that best suits your personality and that of your salon, spa, or barbershop.

THE FRONT DESK

Most owners believe that the quality and pricing of services are the most important elements of running a successful salon, spa, or barbershop. Certainly these are crucial, but too often the front desk—the operations center of the business—is overlooked. The best businesses employ professional receptionists to handle the job of answering phones, scheduling appointments, greeting clients, and attending to client needs.

THE RECEPTION AREA

First impressions count, and since the reception area is the first thing clients see, it needs to be attractive, appealing, and comfortable. This is your business's nerve center, where retail merchandise will be on display, where the phone system is centered, where financial transactions will be carried out, and where your receptionist will stand (should you employ one).

Make sure that the reception area is stocked with business cards and a prominently displayed price list that shows at a glance what your clients should expect to pay for various services.

iStockPhoto.com/Antonio_Diaz

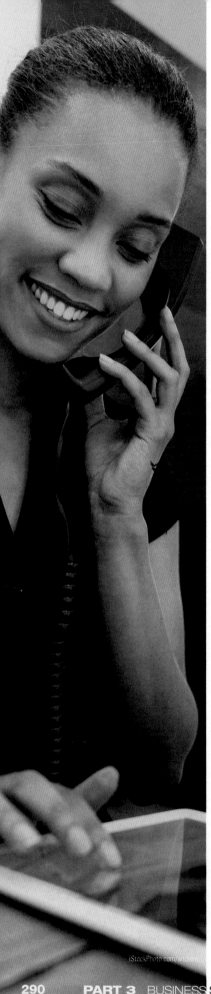

THE RECEPTIONIST

A well-trained receptionist is crucial to the life of the business, as the receptionist is the first and last person the client contacts. The receptionist should have an image that reflects your brand, be pleasant and patient, greet each client with a smile, and address each client by name. Efficient, friendly, and consistent service fosters goodwill, confidence, and satisfaction.

In addition to filling the crucial role of greeter, the receptionist handles other important functions, including answering the phone, booking appointments, informing beauty professionals that a client has arrived, preparing daily appointment information for the staff, and recommending additional services and products to clients. The receptionist should have a thorough knowledge of all retail products carried by the shop so that they can also serve as a salesperson and information source for clients.

During slow periods, it is customary for the receptionist to perform certain other duties and activities, such as straightening up the reception area and maintaining inventory and daily reports. Personal calls or personal projects are done on personal time, not at work.

BOOKING APPOINTMENTS

The key duty of the receptionist is booking appointments. This must be done with care because services are sold in terms of time on the appointment page. Appointments must be scheduled to make the most efficient use of everyone's time—both the client and the beauty pro. Under ideal circumstances, a client should not have to wait for a service, and a professional should not have to wait for the next client.

Booking appointments is primarily the receptionist's job, but when they are not available, the owner or manager, or one of the other professionals in small businesses, can help with scheduling. It is important for each person involved in working the reception area to understand how to book an appointment and how much time is needed for each service. Regardless of who actually makes the appointment, anyone who answers the phone or deals with clients must have a pleasing voice and personality.

THE APPOINTMENT BOOK

The appointment book helps professionals arrange time to suit their clients' needs. It should accurately reflect what is taking place in the salon, spa, or barbershop at any given time. In larger establishments, the receptionist prepares the appointment schedule for staff members; in smaller shops, each person may prepare their own schedule (**Figure 10-9**).

Increasingly, the appointment book is computerized and easily accessed through the business's computer system. Or, it may be an actual hardcopy book located on the reception desk. Some shops have websites with online booking systems, which tie into scheduling software.

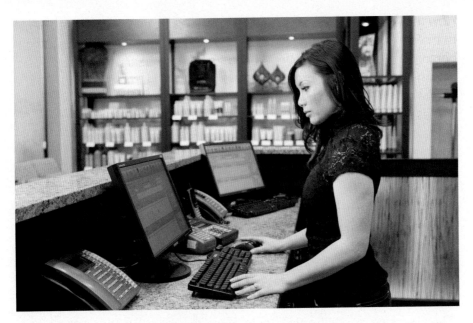

▲ FIGURE 10-9 Computerized appointment book.

THE TELEPHONE

The majority of beauty business is handled over the telephone. Good telephone habits and techniques make it possible for the owner and employees to increase business and improve relationships with clients and suppliers. With each call, a gracious, appropriate response will help build the shop's reputation. For example, "Thank you for calling Spa Milady, Shannon speaking. How may I help you?"

GOOD PLANNING

Because it can be noisy, business calls to clients and suppliers should be made at a quiet time of the day or from a quiet area of the shop. Telephone etiquette is as follows:

- Use a pleasant telephone voice, speak clearly, and use correct grammar. A smile on your face will be reflected in your voice and counts for a lot.
- Show interest and concern when talking with a client or a supplier.
- Be polite, respectful, and courteous to all (even when people may test the limits of your patience).
- Be tactful. Do not say anything to irritate the person on the other end of the line.

INCOMING TELEPHONE CALLS

An incoming call is often your client's first impression of your business. Clients usually call ahead for appointments with a preferred beauty pro but may call to cancel or reschedule. The person answering the phone should have the necessary telephone skills to handle these calls.

When you answer the phone, say, "Good morning (afternoon or evening), thank you for calling The Milady Salon. How may I help you?" or "Thank you for calling Milady Barbers. This is Jonathan speaking.

How may I help you?" Some businesses require that you give your name to the caller. The first words you say tell the caller something about your personality. Let callers know that you are glad to hear from them.

Answer the phone promptly. A good rule of thumb is to pick up the phone by the fourth ring. On a system with more than one line, if a call comes in while you are talking on another line, ask to put the first person on hold, answer the second call, and ask that person to hold while you complete the first call. Take calls in the order in which they are received.

If you do not have the information requested by a caller, either put the caller on hold and get the information, or offer to call the person back with the information as soon as you have it.

Do not talk with a client standing nearby while you are speaking with someone on the phone. Have one conversation at a time to avoid doing a disservice to both clients.

BOOKING APPOINTMENTS BY PHONE

When booking appointments, write down the client's first and last name, their phone number, their e-mail address, and the service booked. Many businesses call the client to confirm the appointment one or two days before it is scheduled. Automated systems can send an e-mail or even a text message confirmation.

All employees should be familiar with all the services and products available in the salon, spa, or barbershop and their costs as well as which professionals perform specific services, such as color correction or microdermabrasion. Be fair when making assignments. Don't schedule six appointments for one professional and only two for another (unless it's necessary because you are working with specialists).

However, if someone calls to ask for an appointment with a particular professional on a particular day and time, make every effort to accommodate the client's request. If that beauty pro is not available, handle the situation in one of the following ways:

- Suggest other times that the professional is available.
- If the client cannot come in at any of those times, suggest another professional.
- If the client is unwilling to try another professional, offer to call the client if there is a cancellation at the desired time.

HANDLING COMPLAINTS OVER THE PHONE

Handling complaints, particularly over the phone, is a difficult task. The caller is probably upset and possibly short-tempered. Respond with self-control, tact, and courtesy, no matter how trying the circumstances. Only then will the caller feel that they have been treated fairly.

The tone of your voice must be sympathetic and reassuring. Your manner of speaking should convince the caller that you are really con-cerned about the complaint. Do not interrupt the caller. After hearing the complaint in full, try to resolve the situation quickly and effectively.

CHECK IN
List the four elements of a successful salon, spa, or barbershop.

LIST MARKETING STRATEGIES FOR BUILDING YOUR BUSINESS

A new salon, spa, or barbershop owner will want to get the business up and running as soon as possible to start earning some revenue and to begin paying off debts. This is where marketing (MAR-ket-ing)—a strategy for how goods and services are bought, sold, and exchanged—comes in. Think of marketing as the methods you'll use to attract and retain satisfied clients. It is the means for selling and promoting your business.

According to a survey conducted by the Professional Beauty Association (PBA), the top three ways that clients find a service provider are

1. recommendations or referrals,
2. a convenient location, and
3. advertisements.

With this is mind, the focus of many of your marketing strategies will likely be aimed at answering one question: What are your clients telling their friends about your business?

VIRAL MARKETING

The modern version of word of mouth is *viral marketing*, which, despite the different media, often still takes the form of referrals and recommendations. It is the personal communication about a service or product between target clients and their friends, relatives, and associates. The viral marketing technique can further pass your message along to hundreds and thousands of potential clients through social media sites and e-mail campaigns.

Viral marketing is a phenomenon of the digital age that you can use, and may already have used, to spread your brand, by way of clients who are so motivated about your services that they tell their friends and family, along interpersonal networks that can reach into the thousands.

SOCIAL MEDIA FOR THE BUSINESS OWNER

Social media as a business tool has been covered in other chapters, but it is worth repeating the strength of this platform to engage and communicate with a community of people and as an ideal vehicle for viral marketing. Social media allows you to bridge geographical and cultural distances to reach a variety of people with the same interests and desires. It is a means to attract a following and have other people promote you and your business via viral marketing.

This is accomplished by consistently providing content that is seen as valuable and relevant to your audience and by providing your online community with avenues to interact with your brand outside of the salon, spa, or barbershop itself. The following are a few ways you might use social media to provide consistent content oriented around your business:

- Write a blog reflecting your knowledge, talent, and skills with beauty and wellness tips and resources.
- Post beauty and wellness tips of the day.

- Network with cosmetic and beauty brands and give your personal review of new products.
- Start a beauty and wellness advice column.

Don't forget to follow your social media best practices from Chapter 2: "Professional Image"!

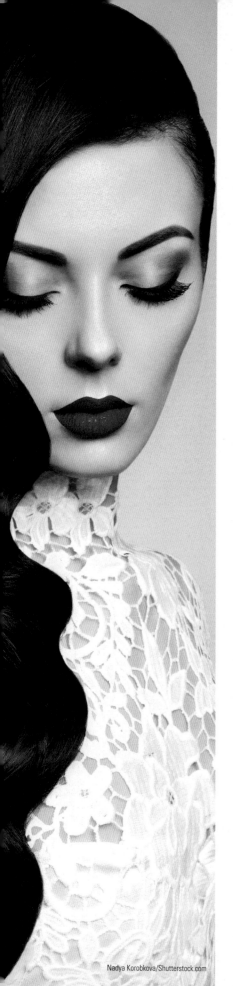

HERE'S A TIP

This chapter provides a general overview of the complex issues involved in salon, spa, and barbershop ownership. There are many resources on the Internet for further study. These can get you started:

Design

- http://www.beautydesign.com
  Click on the Design Center tab (at the top) to see various salon layouts and photos of salons from all over the world.
- http://www.collinsmfgco.com
  Check out the gallery and design options at this manufacturer of salon, spa, and barbershop equipment.

Human Resources

- http://www.dol.gov/compliance/guide
  This is the U.S. Department of Labor's online employment law guide.
- http://www.eeoc.gov
  Research relevant equal employment opportunity regulations at the U.S. Equal Employment Opportunity Commission website; check out the compliance manual.
- http://www.hr.blr.com
  This site offers human resources-related business and legal reports. Find a forum, dozens of topics, and regulations by state.

Small Business Ownership and Operation

- http://www.business.com
  Find advice on business topics from A to Z and business resources for accounting, sales, marketing, technology, and more.
- http://www.isquare.com
  The Small Business Advisor.
- http://www.salonbuilder.com
  Find information on starting a beauty business.
- http://www.strategies.com
  This site offers salon and spa business growth seminars, training, and coaching.

Salon, Spa, and Barbershop Software

- http://www.harms-software.com
- http://www.shortcuts.net
- http://www.salonbizsoftware.com
- http://www.saloniris.com
- http://www.salon-software.com

ADVERTISING

The term *advertising* encompasses promotional efforts that are paid for and are directly intended to increase business.

Advertising includes all activities that promote your salon, spa, or barbershop favorably, from newspaper ads to radio spots to charity events that the business participates in, such as fashion shows or community outreach. In order to create a desire for a service or product, advertising must attract and hold the attention of readers, listeners, or viewers.

Nadya Korobkova/Shutterstock.com

Once again, satisfied clients are the very best form of advertising, so make your clients happy (**Figure 10-10**)! Then, have your clients work for you. Develop a referral program and a loyalty program in which the referring client reaps a reward.

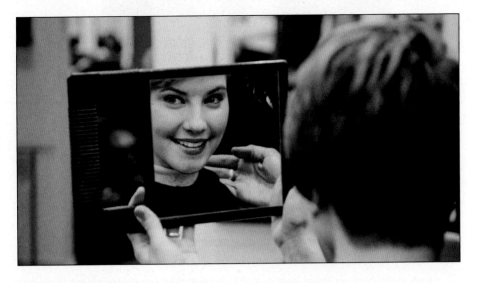

▲ **FIGURE 10–10**   Customer satisfaction is your best advertising.

If you have some experience developing ads, you may decide to do your own advertising. Or you can hire an agency or ask a local newspaper or radio station to help you produce an ad. As a general rule, an advertising budget should not exceed 3 percent of your gross income. Make sure you plan well in advance for holidays and special yearly events, such as proms, New Year's Eve, or the wedding season.

Make certain you know what you are paying for. Get everything in writing. No form of advertising can promise that you'll get business. Sometimes, local circulars can work well. You must know your clientele, which types of media they use, and what kinds of messages attract them.

Here are some tools you may choose to use to attract customers to your salon, spa, or barbershop:

* Newspaper ads and coupons
* A website
  If you don't have a large budget now, buy your domain name and keep that ownership current. You can set up a site very inexpensively and as your business grows, you can build it to have many pages and features. A website is an easy way for new clients to find you through Internet searches or friends sharing links.
* E-mail newsletters and discount offers to all clients who agree to receive such mailings (**Figure 10-11**)
  Always include an *Unsubscribe* link. You can also purchase e-mail lists targeted to your demographic to help you build your subscriber list.
* Website offerings, including those on your own website, social networking websites, and blogs
* Direct mail to mailing lists and your current client list
* Classified advertising

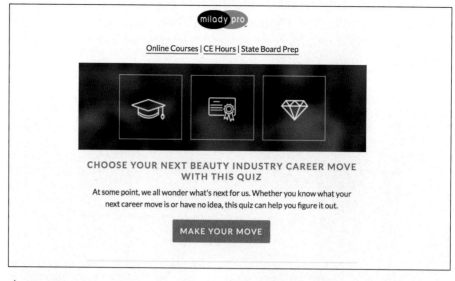

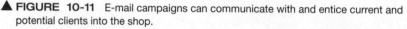

▲ FIGURE 10-11 E-mail campaigns can communicate with and entice current and potential clients into the shop.

- Giveaway promotional items, such as branded combs, or retail packages, like shampoos and colognes
- Window displays that attract attention and feature the shop and your retail products
- Radio advertising
- Television advertising
- Community outreach: Volunteer at men's and women's clubs, church functions, political gatherings, charitable affairs, and on TV and radio talk shows
- Donations of your services for local organizations like school fundraisers
- Client referrals
- In-shop videos promoting your services and products
- An on-hold message featuring your business's best attributes

Many of these vehicles can help you attract new clients, but the first goal of every business should be to maintain current clients. It takes at least three visits for a new client to become a loyal current client. Encourage your staff to have their guests pre-book their appointments: Just because a client has visited the shop 100 times doesn't mean they will come again. By having a pre-booking system in place, you are guaranteeing future business. Once you have a loyal client base, it is far less expensive to market to that base. That is why you should follow up every visit to determine the client's satisfaction and personally contact any client who has not been in for more than eight weeks.

SELLING IN THE SALON, SPA, AND BARBERSHOP

An important aspect of a beauty business's financial success revolves around *upselling* (adding on additional services), *cross promoting* (encouraging a client who is booked for one service to add another), and *retailing* (selling take-home or maintenance products). No matter the size or style of your business, adding services and retail sales to your service ticket means additional revenue. Remember: Your client will spend money during their visit. It is your job to encourage your client to invest in retail and services that will keep them coming back for more, while also helping to maintain the look you just gave them!

It is important that we as professionals feel confident in selling services and retail. Remove any negative feelings or stereotypes you have toward sales or sales people and start fresh. Helpful and knowledgeable professionals make customer care their top priority. These people play a major role in the lives of their customers and are very valuable to clients because they offer good advice. In fact, the successful owner, like the successful professional, makes their living by giving complete beauty and wellness advice every day (**Figure 10-12**).

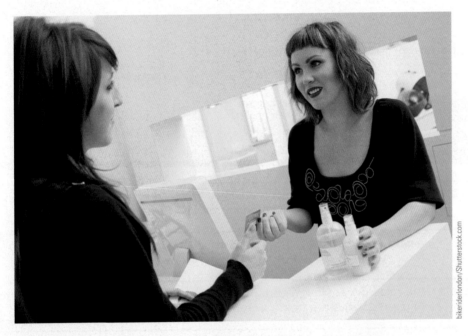

▲ FIGURE 10-12 Selling retail products benefits everyone.

CHECK IN
Name five advertising tools you might use to attract customers to your salon, spa, or barbershop.

APPLY THE BEAUTY BUSINESS

Congratulations on completing this chapter! Before you move on, take a moment to think about how these Beauty Business topics apply to your particular discipline. Discuss with a classmate or study group what ownership type you would be most interested in (or if you would rather rent a booth, or neither own nor rent!); any design elements or features you would have to have for your own salon, spa, or barbershop; where you would locate your business, who your clientele would be; what you would specialize in; and so on.

COMPETENCY PROGRESS

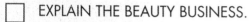

How are you doing with The Beauty Business? **Check off the Chapter 10 Learning Objectives** below that you feel you have mastered; leave unchecked those objectives you will need to return to:

☐ EXPLAIN THE BEAUTY BUSINESS.

☐ OUTLINE THE REQUIREMENTS OF OWNING A BUSINESS.

☐ DESCRIBE BOOTH RENTAL.

☐ IDENTIFY THE ELEMENTS OF A SUCCESSFUL SALON, SPA, OR BARBERSHOP.

☐ LIST MARKETING STRATEGIES FOR BUILDING YOUR BUSINESS.

GLOSSARY

business operation (BIZ-ness op-er-AYE-shun)	p. 275	the recurring processes or activities involved in the running of a business for the purpose of producing income and value
business plan (BIZ-ness plahn)	p. 271	a written description of your business as you see it today and as you foresee it in the next five years (detailed by year)
business policies (BIZ-ness POL-ih-sees)	p. 275	the rules or regulations adopted by a business to ensure that all clients and associates are being treated fairly and consistently
business regulations and laws (BIZ-ness reg-u-LAY-shuns AND LAWZ)	p. 274	any and all local, state, and federal regulations and laws that you must comply with when you decide to open your business or rent a booth
capital (KAP-uh-tal)	p. 275	money needed to invest in a business
consumption supplies (kon-SUMP-shun sup-LYZ)	p. 282	supplies used in the daily business operation
corporation (kor-pour-AYE-shun)	p. 276	an ownership structure controlled by one or more stockholders
demographics (dem-oh-GRAF-iks)	p. 274	information about a specific population, including data on race, age, income, and educational attainment
goals (GOHLZ)	p. 272	a set of benchmarks that, once achieved, help you to realize your mission and your vision

insurance (in-SHUR-ance)	p. 274	guarantees protection against financial loss from malpractice, property liability, fire, burglary and theft, and business interruption
marketing (MAR-ket-ing)	p. 293	a strategy for how goods and services are bought, sold, and exchanged
partnership (PART-nur-ship)	p. 275	business structure in which two or more people share ownership, although not necessarily equally
personnel (per-son-EL)	p. 287	your staff or employees
record keeping (REK-urd keep-ing)	p. 275	maintaining accurate and complete records of all financial activities in your business
retail supplies (REE-tail sup-LYZ)	p. 282	supplies sold to clients
sole proprietor (SOHL pro-PRY-eh-tor)	p. 275	individual owner and, most often, the manager of a business
vision statement (VIZ-uhn state-ment)	p. 272	a long-term picture of what the business is to become and what it will look like when it gets there
written agreements (RIT-en uh-GREE-mentz)	p. 274	documents that govern the opening of a business, including leases, vendor contracts, employee contracts, and more; all of which detail, usually for legal purposes, who does what and what is given in return

Chapter 2

1. Mann, Charles Riborg. *A Study of Engineering Education*. New York, NY: Carnegie Foundation, 1918. 106–107.

2. Mehrabian, Albert. *Silent Messages*. Belmont, CA: Wadsworth Publishing Company, Inc., 1971.

Chapter 6

1. United States Department of Labor's Occupational Safety & Health Administration. "OSHA QuickCard – Hazard Communication Safety Data Sheets," 2015. https://www.osha.gov/Publications/HazComm_QuickCard_SafetyData.html

Chapter 8

1. Professional Beauty Association. *Economic Snapshot of the Salon and Spa Industry – May 2014*, 2014. https://www.finance.senate.gov/imo/media/doc/Professional%20Beauty%20Association-%20 2014%20Economic%20Snapshot%20of%20the%20Salon%20Industry.pdf

C

Capital, money needed to invest in a business, 275

Carbohydrates, nutrients needed for energy to run every function within the body, 74

Carcinogen, a substance that causes or is believed to cause cancer, 176

Career planning, 209–210
discovering potential employers, 216–225
state licensing examination process, 210–216

Catalysts, substances that speed up chemical reactions, 200

Cataphoresis, process of fusing an acidic (positive) product into deeper tissues using galvanic current from the positive pole toward the negative pole, 193

Cathode, negative electrode of an electrotherapy device; the cathode is usually black and is marked with an *N* or a minus (–) sign, 192

Cation, an ion with a positive electrical charge, 165

Chelating soaps, break down stubborn films and remove the residue of products such as scrubs, salts, and masks; also known as *chelating detergents,* 125

Chemical
disposal, 173
labels, 170–171
mixing, 173
storage, 172
transportation, 171

Chemical change, a change in the chemical composition or make-up of a substance, 157–158

Chemical properties, characteristics that can only be determined by a chemical reaction and a chemical change in the substance, 158

Chemical safety, 153–154, 170–173

Chemical structure
basics of, 154–159

Circuit breaker, switch that automatically interrupts or shuts off an electric circuit at the first indication of overload, 187–188

Cleaning, a mechanical process (scrubbing) using soap and water or detergent and water to remove all visible dirt, debris, and many disease-causing germs. Cleaning also removes invisible debris that interfere with disinfection. Cleaningis what cosmetologists are required to do before disinfecting, 101, 115–116

Client base, customers who are loyal to a particular cosmetologist, 257
keeping and expanding, 262–265

Client consultation, communication with a client that determines what the client's needs are and how to achieve the desired results, 54–61

Client-cosmetologist relationship, 48

Client injury, 128, 141–143

Client intake form, also known as a *client questionnaire, consultation card,* or *health history form;* used in beauty and wellness services as a questionnaire that discloses the client's contact information, products they use, hair/nail/skin care needs, preferences and lifestyle. The form also includes all medications, both topical (applied to skin) and oral (taken by mouth), along with any known medical issues, skin or scalp disorders or allergies that might affect services, 50–53

Clients' needs, meeting, 244

Combustible, material that is capable of igniting and burning, 176

Combustion, rapid oxidation of a substance accompanied by the production of heat and light, 170

Commission, percentage of the revenue generated from services performed by a professional, 250

Communicable, able to be communicated; transferable by contact from one person to another as in a communicable disease, 104

Communication
client consultation, 54–61
client intake form, 50–53
golden rules of, 49–50
handling barriers of, 62–65
steps for effective, 48–49
for success, 68
10-step method, 56–60
workplace, 66–68

Complete electric circuit, the path of negative and positive electric currents moving from the generating source through the conductors and back to the generating source, 184

Compound molecules, also known as compounds, a chemical combination of two or more atoms of different elements in definite (fixed) proportions, 156–157

Conductor, any material that conducts electricity, 184

Consumption supplies, supplies used in the daily business operation, 282

Contagious disease, also known as *communicable disease;* disease that is capable of being spread from one person to another, 104

Contamination, the presence, or the reasonably anticipated presence, of blood or other potentially infectious materials on an item's surface, or visible debris or residues such as dust, hair, and skin, 105

Contraindication, a condition that requires avoiding certain treatments, procedures, or products to prevent undesirable side effects, 195

Corporation, an ownership structure controlled by one or more stockholders, 276–277

Creativity
enhancing, 9
success and, 8

D

Deductive reasoning, the process of reaching logical conclusions by employing logical reasoning, 214–215

Demographics, information about a specific population including data on race, age, income, and educational attainment, 274

Desincrustation, a form of anaphoresis; process used to soften and emulsify grease deposits (oil) and blackheads in the hair follicles, 194

Diagnosis, determination of the nature of a disease from its symptoms and/or diagnostic tests; federal regulations prohibit salon professionals from performing a diagnosis, 105

Direct current, abbreviated DC; constant, even-flowing current that travels in one direction only and is produced by chemical means, 185

Direct transmission, transmission of pathogens through touching (including shaking hands), kissing, coughing, sneezing, and talking, 99–100

Disease, an abnormal condition of all or part of the body, or its systems or organs, that makes the body incapable of carrying on normal function, 99
preventing spread of, 115–124
terms related to, 105

Disinfectants, chemical products approved by the EPA designed to destroy most bacteria (excluding spores), fungi, and viruses on surfaces, 96, 97, 118–125